KU-509-594

Anxiety Management in Adult Day Surgery
A Nursing Perspective

LIVERPOOL JMU LIBRARY

3 1111 01102 7396

Anxiety Management in Adult Day Surgery

A Nursing Perspective

Mark Mitchell BA, MSc, PhD, RGN, NDNCert, RCNT, RNT
University of Salford, Greater Manchester, UK

LIVERPOOL
JOHN MOORES UNIVERSITY
AVRIL ROBARTS LRC
TEL. 0151 231 4022

W

WHURR PUBLISHERS
LONDON AND PHILADELPHIA

© 2005 Whurr Publishers Ltd
First published 2005
by Whurr Publishers Ltd
19b Compton Terrace
London N1 2UN England and
325 Chestnut Street, Philadelphia PA 19106 USA

All rights reserved. No part of this publication may be
reproduced, stored in a retrieval system, or transmitted in any form
or by any means, electronic, mechanical, photocopying, recording or
otherwise, without the prior permission of Whurr Publishers Limited.

This publication is sold subject to the conditions that it shall not, by
way of trade or otherwise, be lent, resold, hired out, or otherwise
circulated without the publisher's prior consent in any form of
binding or cover other than that in which it is published and
without a similar condition including this condition being imposed
upon any subsequent purchaser.

British Library Cataloguing in Publication Data

A catalogue record for this book
is available from the British Library.

ISBN 1 86156 463 5

Typeset by Adrian McLaughlin, a@microguides.net
Printed and bound in the UK by Athenæum Press Limited, Gateshead, Tyne & Wear

Contents

Preface

This book is centrally concerned with the formal management of preoperative anxiety. The vast majority of patients experience varying degrees of anxiety when entering hospital for surgery and yet little formal intervention is commonly provided. This is the first book of its kind to be written for nurses exclusively concerning the complete formal pre- and postoperative management of anxiety in relation to modern, elective, adult day surgery. During the early 1970s classic nursing studies suggested information provision to be crucial for effective inpatient preoperative anxiety management. However, following such early recommendations no other formal aspects of psychoeducational care have impacted on mainstream surgical nursing intervention. Physical aspects of care have dominated proceedings for the last three decades or more, whereas psychoeducational aspects have largely remained informal, marginal issues. Both surgery and anaesthesia have changed dramatically during this period and nursing intervention must now do likewise.

The domination of physical nursing intervention is, however, slowly changing as the continuous global rise in elective ambulatory surgery has highlighted the need for more structured psychoeducational approaches to patient care. The psychological theories to aid preoperative anxiety management have been available for many years. However, they have not succeeded in making an impact within the clinical surgical setting, because they have not previously been constructed into a coherent, clinically realistic plan of care. The purpose of this book is therefore (1) to consider the relevant psychological concepts that can inform and guide modern surgical nursing practices, (2) to provide a comprehensive map of the wider evidence available and (3) to introduce clinically realistic nursing interventions necessary for the complete psychoeducational management of adult patients undergoing elective, ambulatory surgery.

On a philosophical level, I hope to communicate with a wide audience of nurses working in the field of adult ambulatory surgery or studying modern surgical nursing practices. We need to re-evaluate nursing knowledge for this new surgical era so that compelling nursing evidence can help to guide practice and not remain in the shadows of medical advances. This book is intended to provoke debate within the profession, present the case for change and, above all, demonstrate the ability of nursing knowledge to make a significant contribution to the care required by patients experiencing modern ambulatory surgery. Much evidence, within the nursing domain, is widely available to help guide important global nursing issues in ambulatory surgery.

The political reforms currently running through the National Health Service in the UK have resulted in nursing knowledge largely becoming marginalized. The utilization of nurses and their skills features widely in these reforms, but not the utilization of nursing skills based on nursing knowledge. Surgical self-preparation and self-recovery are now implicit aspects of the modern surgical patients' experience. Patients and their relatives did not request this new, essential role although most now welcome the social convenience and swift treatment that day surgery affords. Such advances have, however, guaranteed that many of yesterday's professional nursing interventions have become today's layperson interventions. Much physical surgical nursing is increasingly becoming obsolete because it can now be undertaken by laypeople. I am hopeful that this book will add to the debate about the future of modern surgical nursing intervention, because the trend of surrendering much pre- and postoperative care to relatives and replacing it with interventions that once were the domain of junior doctors must not remain unchallenged. 'New' nursing knowledge has much to offer the ambulatory surgery patient and we must robustly demonstrate how our professional knowledge can make this contribution. Professional knowledge and its application are powerful, liberating and motivating forces. I hope that this book empowers, liberates and motivates all who read it and that you find it as stimulating to read as I have found it to write.

Mark Mitchell

Chapter 1

Twenty-first century: a time for change

Growth of day surgery

The Department of Health (DoH 2000) has a clear vision for the future level of day surgery activity. *The NHS Plan* states 'Around three-quarters of operations will be carried out on a day case basis with no overnight stay required' (DoH 2000, p. 19). In 1985 less than 15% of all elective surgery was undertaken on a day-case basis (NHS Management Executive Value for Money Unit 1991). A day surgery candidate is defined in the UK as 'a patient who is admitted for investigation or operation on a planned non-resident basis and who nonetheless requires facilities for recovery' (Royal College of Surgeons of England 1992, p. 3). More recently, a day surgery candidate has been defined as 'A patient admitted electively during the course of a day with the intention of receiving care who does not require the use of a hospital bed overnight and who returns home as scheduled. If this original intention is not fulfilled and the patient stays overnight, such a patient should be counted as an ordinary admission' (Cook et al. 2004, p. 11).

Such a rapid change in surgical health-care delivery over the past 30 years has ensured a major shift in medical and nursing surgical intervention. Intermediate elective surgical episodes once requiring lengthy hospital admission are disappearing from the inpatient ward, never to return, e.g. inguinal hernia repair, varicose vein stripping, cataract extraction and many more (Cahill 1999) (intermediate elective surgery is defined here as planned uncomplicated surgery under general anaesthesia, which can be undertaken in an operating theatre in less than an hour.) Therefore, the extensive physical care and treatment once required by patients undergoing cholecystectomy, for example, is now becoming obsolete, as the British Association of Day Surgery has recommended that at least 50% of all such surgery should now be possible in day-case facilities (Cahill 1999). Patients undergoing cholecystectomy once remained in hospital for approximately 3 weeks and required a considerable amount of physical care, e.g. pain management, wound care, assistance with activities of living. Most adult elective surgery patients do not now require the level of physical nursing intervention once demanded by more traditional

1

surgical techniques (Bringman et al. 2001, Amarnath et al. 2002). The average length of stay in a day surgery facility within Europe is currently 6.5 hours (Pfisterer et al. 2001). In addition, inpatients increasingly spend considerably less time in hospital and one study reported the average length of stay to be 2.7 days (Tierney et al. 1999)

This change in surgical health care has had, and is increasingly having, a major impact on the delivery of the psychoeducational elements of care because the length of time patients spend in hospital has been dramatically cut (psychoeducational intervention is defined here as the purposeful attempt to provide tangible aspects of care aimed at enhancing an individual's psychological status, together with the planned provision of educational material), e.g. patients are commonly admitted 1–2 hours before day surgery with minimal time for nurse–patient interaction (Bondy et al. 1999). After surgery, patients are normally dressed and ready to go home, again within 1–2 hours. In a recent study, 13.2% of day-case patients had a postoperative stay of 3 hours or less, 55.3% of 3–6 hours and 26.2% of 6 hours or more (Junger et al. 2001). Such persistent time restrictions habitually ensure that medical aspects of care must take preference over many other nursing interventions, e.g. psychoeducational elements of care.

Day-surgery growth has developed as a result of medical advances and economic expansion. Growth in this country, although slow in the early 1980s, continues to rise, i.e. 46.4% (1994–1995) to 60% (1997–1998) of all elective surgery (De Lathouwer and Poullier 1998). In Europe and the USA different definitions and health-care practices have led to different rates of growth. In the USA, for example, day surgery or ambulatory surgery is defined as a stay of less than 23 hours whereas currently in the UK this would been considered an overnight stay. However, the government has a target of 75% of all elective surgery to be undertaken in day-surgery facilities (Department of Health 2000). This may be achieved by day-surgery units remaining open a little longer, e.g. having an 'extended day', adopting a more American-style definition of day surgery, increasing capacity (Cook et al. 2004) or by the building of new treatment centres (Fuller 2003). In addition, the complexity of surgical procedures that can be performed within day-surgery facilities continues to expand (Jarrett 1997, Cahill 1998, Garcia-Urena et al. 2000, Huang et al. 2000, Perez et al. 2000, Larner et al. 2003).

The majority of patients treated in day-case facilities have welcomed this new form of surgical health care because, crucially, it involves minimal disruption to their lifestyle (Greenwood 1993, Myles et al. 2000). In a survey by Black and Sanderson (1993) of 373 day-surgery patients, 80% preferred day surgery rather than inpatient surgery. However, a minority of patients experienced some dissatisfaction and required an overnight stay. 'The main reasons dissatisfied patients gave for wanting to stay in hospital overnight were the desire to have recovered fully from the anaesthetic and the operation before going home; anxiety about being at home if something went wrong; difficulty of getting sufficient rest once back at home and difficulties early discharge had caused family and friends' (Black and Sanderson 1993, p. 159). As can be seen in Figure 1.1 such advances in surgical health care have enabled day surgery to be advertised as a commodity or economic product advertised on the back of a buses. You could be excused for thinking that this 'all-inclusive' offer refers to a holiday and not surgical treatment. The term 'keyhole surgery', once alien to the public, is now a phrase growing in usage and synonymous in society with quick, effective surgical treatment combined with minimal hospital stay.

Figure 1.1 Modern surgery advertised on the back of a bus: Llandudno, north Wales, Spring 2002.

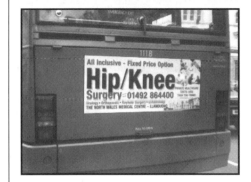
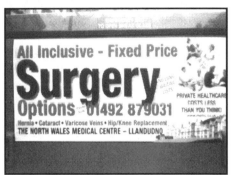

Medical advances and cost-effectiveness

This rapid growth in day surgery has arisen mainly as a result of medical advances and the desire for greater cost-effectiveness (Audit Commission for Local Authorities and the NHS in England and Wales 1990, 1992, Jarrett 1995). First, medical advances or, more accurately, surgical and pharmacological advances, have helped to achieve the expansion of day surgery in different ways. The operating time or length of time required to perform certain surgical procedures has been greatly reduced. So-called 'keyhole surgery', or more accurately 'minimal access surgery', is the reason for the considerable reduction in time. As a result of these new surgical techniques the operating theatre time once required to undertake operations necessitating large surgical incisions and the corresponding length of hospitalization needed for recovery from such surgical assaults have been dramatically reduced (Hodge 1994, Jarrett 1995, Keulemans et al. 1998, Thomas et al. 2001, Erdem et al. 2003, Lemos et al. 2003). Indeed, Montori (1998, p. 244) states: 'It is no exaggeration to say that minimally invasive surgery has opened up a new form of modern surgery.'

Laparoscopic surgery has been further enhanced by the use of more rapid acting anaesthetic agents, e.g. Diprivan (propofol) (Ratcliffe et al. 1994, Ong et al. 2000, Ture et al. 2003). Not only can larger surgical procedures now be undertaken in less time but also improved anaesthetic agents allow the patient to become fully conscious in a much shorter period. As a direct result of these advances the Royal College of Surgeons (1992, p. 2) stated that 'day surgery is now considered to be the best option for 50% of all patients undergoing elective surgical procedures, though the proportion will vary between specialities'. In a later study, it was revealed that all day-surgery units surveyed expected a steady increase in their workload (Royal College of Surgeons of England and East Anglia Regional Health Authority 1995). This is indeed proving to be the case because the original list of 'basket procedures' (list of 20 intermediate surgical procedures deemed suitable for transfer from inpatient surgery to day-case surgery) put forward by the Audit Commission (1990) has grown and is now referred to as the 'trolley of procedures' (Cahill 1999) (list of approximately 25 intermediate surgical procedures deemed suitable for transfer from inpatient surgery to day-case surgery).

Second, day surgery has the potential to be more cost-effective than inpatient surgery, i.e. more patients treated for the same amount of money. With the growth of consumerism supported by more formal mechanisms (DoH 1991), a central government initiative was launched to encourage all NHS trusts to expand their day-surgery facilities (NHS Management Executive Value for Money Unit 1991). The aim was to help decrease the time people spent waiting for operations, improve NHS efficiency and reduce overall running costs (Jarrett 1995). Many NHS trusts responded and the level of day-surgery activity increased overall by 30% (NHS Management Executive 1993). This report goes on to state that 50% of all elective surgery should be undertaken on a day-case basis by 1997–1998 with some surgical specialities being able to achieve 80% by 2000. Indeed, in a more recent report regarding day surgery (Audit Commission for Local Authorities and the NHS in England and Wales 2001) it is stated that if all hospital trusts could achieve the level of surgery undertaken by the best performing day-surgery units, a further 120 000 inpatients per year could be treated on a day-case basis. Furthermore, a recent European study (Lemos et al. 2003) established that a saving of £7.5 million each year could be achieved when a gynaecological procedure (laparoscopic tubal ligation) was undertaken on a day-case basis.

Psychoeducational management

The steady rise in day surgery has, however, presented a considerable challenge to its future effectiveness. Day-case patient preparation is dominated by medical fitness for surgery (Dunn 1998, Fellowes et al. 1999, Rose et al. 1999, Hilditch et al. 2003a, 2003b). One needs to look no further than the preassessment package released by the NHS Modernisation Agency (2002) for evidence of the domination of 'medical fitness'. Indeed, nurse-led preassessment clinics have demonstrated considerable ability to reduce the DNA (did not attend) rate and the cancellation rate on the day of surgery (Clinch 1997, Casey and Ormrod 2003, Healy and McWhinne 2003, Rai and Pandit 2003). However, in the pursuit of safe, efficient, day-case surgery to ensure a constant throughput of patients, psychoeducational aspects of care may have become marginalized (Spitzer 1998, Kleinbeck 2000, Leinonen et al. 2001). Although ensuring medical fitness for surgery is a vitally important activity, preassessment skills could be widely viewed as medically oriented tasks to ensure surgical safety and the progressive throughput of patients in the limited time available (Reid 1997, Cahill 1998). Although such work practices may have embraced challenges geared to maximize day-surgery efficiency they may have inadvertently relegated other crucial patient-centred issues, e.g. psychoeducational care. Moreover, if such an emphasis is reflective of 'normal' day-surgery practice, e.g. ensuring medical fitness for, and medical recovery from, surgery, it becomes all too apparent why information provision and its dissemination have been identified as considerable challenges for day surgery (Mitchell 1999a, 1999b).

The delivery of effective psychoeducational care is further compounded in the UK by the lack of formal anxiety management plans, e.g. the documented attempts to provide tangible aspects of care aimed at enhancing an individual's psychological status together with the planned provision of educational material. Current preoperative psychological preparation for surgery consists almost exclusively of the provision of procedural, behavioural and sensory information, and to a lesser extent cognitive coping strategies, relaxation and modelling information (Chapter 5 – see Tables 5.2 and 5.3). In addition, such information provision is rarely delivered in a systematic, structured manner. Classic studies regarding the need for information provision are frequently cited (Volicer 1973, Hayward 1975, Boore 1978, Wilson-Barnett 1984) and their recommendations pursued. Although excellent studies, their recommendations belong to a different era when (1) the amount of information provided to patients was negligible and (2) patients were admitted to hospital for a far greater length of time. However, classic work by researchers such as Volicer, Hayward, Boore and Wilson-Barnett must not be forgotten.

Indeed, such work should be built upon, expanded and adapted to meet the psychoeducational requirements of the day-surgery patient in the twenty-first century.

Historical perspective

The cause of such suboptimal psychoeducational interventions spans many decades. For many years it has been known that admission to hospital, especially for surgical intervention, can cause considerable apprehension (Shipley et al. 1978, Pickett and Clum 1982, Ridgeway and Mathews 1982). Studies spanning four decades have identified the causes of such anxiety, e.g. the anaesthetic, pain and discomfort, unconsciousness and the operation itself (Egbert et al. 1964, Ramsay 1972, Male 1981, McCleane and Cooper 1990). Several more recent studies have further highlighted the increase in anxiety experienced by patients admitted for day surgery (Mackenzie 1989, Swindale 1989, Caldwell 1991a, Markland and Hardy 1993, Mitchell 1997, 2000) (Figure 1.2). Despite such evidence, preoperative psychoeducational management is an aspect of nursing intervention, which, as yet, has no formalized strategy, i.e. no identified plan adhered to and replicated by all members of staff (Rudolfsson et al. 2003b). Individual nurses may practise informal aspects of anxiety management although no nursing plan is followed, as none exists.

It has been reported that psychological nursing care is seldom undertaken by nurses until the 'real work' is completed and then not in a systematic and documented manner (Salvage 1990, Radcliffe 1993).

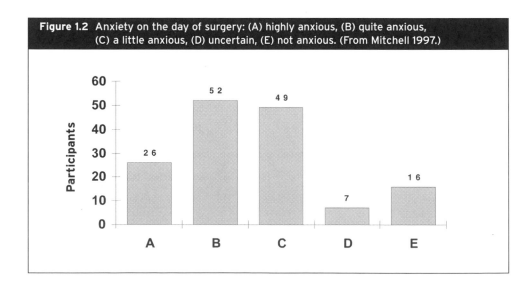

Figure 1.2 Anxiety on the day of surgery: (A) highly anxious, (B) quite anxious, (C) a little anxious, (D) uncertain, (E) not anxious. (From Mitchell 1997.)

Spitzer (1998, p. 790) states: 'Providing quality nursing care means actualising all four aspects of *care* [physical, emotional, social and managerial]. Often, however, under the pressure of a work overload and/or a high turnover of patients, the physical components of care tend to take over'. In a literature review regarding psychological intervention in nursing itself many studies were uncovered (mainly from the medical field), concerning specific physical problems and their consequent psychological issues, e.g. loss of body part, function or dependence (Priest 1999). Thereby, psychological care was viewed as necessary only because of a physical ill-health problem and not, regrettably, as an implicit aspect of nursing intervention. In addition, in an analysis of nursing textbooks concerning psychological care five main themes emerged – information provision (largest theme), emotional care, assessment, counselling and support (Priest 1999). However, it is stated that guidance regarding the application of such aspects of care is not provided.

An American analysis of perioperative nursing practices (Kleinbeck 2000) also demonstrated the strong prevalence of the physical components of care. Four aspects of perioperative nursing practice were identified:

(1) patient and family behavioural responses to surgery
(2) perioperative patient safety
(3) perioperative physiological responses to surgery
(4) the health systems required to deliver perioperative care.

It could be argued the psychoeducational elements of care appear in the first aspect, i.e. patient and family behavioural responses to surgery, although it clearly states 'behavioural responses', suggesting that gaining a compliant patient is the overall aim. The physical domination of care was also evident in a later survey of 239 theatre nurses concerning perioperative care (Kleinbeck 2000). In a further perioperative study it is stated that 'only rarely are psychological notices of patients documented' (Junttila et al. 2003, p. 104). Leinonen et al. (2001) surveyed 874 surgical patients regarding satisfaction with care establishing that physical nursing activities were deemed excellent whereas the educational aspects of the nurses' role received many negative comments.

Many studies have recommended that preoperative programmes should not merely involve information provision, as is frequently the case (Waisel and Truog 1995, Knudsen 1996, Ruuth-Setala et al. 2000). Numerous studies have stressed the need for effective programmes of psychosocial support (Mitchell 1994, Linden and Engberg 1995, 1996, Stengrevics et al. 1996, De Groot et al. 1997b, Heikkila et al. 1998, Shuldham 1999a, 1999b) and many have highlighted the benefits to be gained from such programmes (Garden et al. 1996, Klafta and Roizen 1996, Royal College of Surgeons of England and Royal College of

Psychiatrists 1997, Salmon and Hall 1997, Mott 1999). Moreover, many studies have emphasized the various aspects of psychosocial care and information provision required alongside modern surgical practices (Gould and Wilson-Barnett 1995, Motyka et al. 1997, Bradshaw et al. 1999, Fellowes et al. 1999).

Although frequently recommending psychological improvement in care, few studies provide explicit insight. One study recommended improved communication and patient control although it placed the emphasis for change on the medical profession (Horne et al. 1994). In an opinion paper, effective communication and medical assessment were stressed as important factors (Price and Leaver 2002). Heikkila et al. (1998, p. 1234), as with many studies, advocate improved assessment although they merely state: 'Patient fears could be diminished by developing individualised care'. Stengrevics et al. (1996, p. 475) state only that 'interventions aimed at improving surgical outcomes by reducing negative psychological states may lead to decreased post-operative complications'. In a review of the literature on recovery from surgery (Kiecolt-Glaser et al. 1998), a purely biobehavioural model was put forward. This merely advocates encouraging healthy preoperative behaviour and effective pain management to prevent delayed wound repair. Others have argued that group therapy and counselling are required in the preoperative phase by the more neurotic patient, but provide no indication as to what this involves or indeed the practical application of such a service in the modern surgical environment (Duits et al. 1999). A report by the Royal College of Nursing and Society of Orthopaedic Nursing concerning patient preassessment (hospital appointment before the day of admission primarily to check medical fitness for surgery and anaesthesia) recommends that psychological care should involve assessing coping with the demands of surgery (Fellowes et al. 1999). However, the only suggestion put forward is to provide adequate information – exactly what Volicer (1973), Hayward (1975), Boore (1978) and Wilson-Barnett (1984) suggested two or three decades ago! A comprehensive study of surgical inpatients by De Briun et al. (2001, p. 268) also yielded little specific guidance. 'The reduction of patients' subjective distress is surely one important goal that justifies the development and employment of these [psychological] programmes.' However, what constitutes a preoperative psychological programme of care is again not detailed.

A small number of studies have fortunately provided some indication as to the practical care required – aside from information provision. In a review of the literature (Salmon 1992a) it is suggested that to focus purely on the patient may be very difficult. Therefore, the focus may have to change to the ward environment as a potential mediator of stress, i.e. the level of health control and the provision of wider emotional support.

Salmon et al. (1994, p. 345) state that the main aspect of satisfaction concerning colonoscopy was 'the perception that staff were warm, interested and informative'. In a survey of inpatients (Webb and Hope 1995) participants were asked to rank the nursing activities deemed most important. They rated listening, relieving pain and the instructional aspects of the nurses' role as the most important. Crumlish (1998) interviewed 124 patients before and after general anaesthesia. Here participants rated their main pre- and postoperative behaviour as 'Getting professional help and doing what is recommended' (Crumlish 1998, p. 275).

The Royal College of Surgeons of England and the Royal College of Psychiatrists (1997) put forward a number of broad strategies concerning psychological management, e.g. varying degrees of information provision, emotional support, privacy, listening to patients' fears, providing a sense of control and good written communication between staff. This report greatly improves the search for tangible psychoeducational care because it specifically states the areas in which nursing intervention is required. It also recognizes the need for a more formal approach to preoperative psychological care. A research study by Clipperley et al. (1995) also highlighted a specific intervention by clearly identifying the need for different levels of information and different kinds of psychological support. Indeed, this study provides the only brief formal preoperative psychological nursing plan. Unfortunately, however, on closer inspection, even this plan does not precisely state what the nurse must do to secure effective psychoeducational support. It merely states: 'The psychological component includes interventions which explore the patient's attitudes and feelings' (Clipperley et al. 1995, p. 203). More recently, a preoperative day-surgery teaching guide outlined the most important educational information, although even this does not state the specific psychosocial interventions required on the day of surgery (Bernier et al. 2003).

A principal reason why greater attention to psychoeducational intervention may not have occurred thus far is therefore the absence of a formal preoperative psychological programme of care, i.e. no contemporary plan of the most effective way in which nurses can deliver the appropriate psychological interventions (Johnston 1987, Linden and Engberg 1996), e.g. the physical nursing interventions required by a breathless, unconscious or immobile patient have been well documented, exist in formal programmes of care, and can be easily taught and replicated whenever necessary (Mallett and Bailey 1996, Nettina 1996, Alexander et al. 2001). Nurses do not have to guess what care to provide for the breathless, unconscious or immobile patient. However, the lack of effective psychoeducational management plans both in general surgery and in day-case surgery has resulted in this very process, i.e. nurses guessing what psychological care to provide and delivering these well-meaning interventions on an ad hoc basis. When such care is detailed most texts refer to information provision, loss and grieving or spirituality, which may be appropriate for major surgical intervention but could be considered somewhat inappropriate for modern, elective day surgery (Priest 1999, Alexander et al. 2001, Rosdahl and Kowalski 2003). The lack of an explicit preoperative psychoeducational programme is also clearly evident in a number of nursing texts specifically concerning day surgery (Markanday 1997, Hodge 1999, Meeker and Rothrock 1999, Burden et al. 2000, Malster and Parry 2000). These texts deal only very briefly with the nurses' role in anxiety management and also contain no tangible elements of intervention other than recommending the provision of information, i.e. recommendations put forward in the last century by Hayward (1975) and Boore (1978). In addition, no mention is made of the growing body of evidence concerning the amount, level and type of information that patients might require (see Chapters 4, 5 and 6).

Ultimately, a formal preoperative psychological programme of care does not exist because the interventions necessary to create such plans remain under-used both in nurse education and in clinical practice (Priest 1999). The actions required to ensure effective preoperative psychoeducational support have not been systematically assembled and presented in a clinically acceptable manner. The development of a more formalized approach to psychoeducational management in day surgery is crucial for the comprehensive management of patients and the future success of day surgery (Domar et al. 1987). Without good preparation patients cannot effectively care for themselves at home, either before or after surgery. Without the ability to achieve a good level of self-care, day-surgery expansion will always remain limited. Completely eliminating all anxiety for all patients and providing precise psychoeducational care before day surgery may be an unrealistic aim. However, helping all day-surgery patients manage their anxiety more effectively in the twenty-first century is a very realistic and obtainable goal. Therefore, a first step in the development of a formal preoperative psychoeducational plan of care is to examine patient experiences of modern, elective day surgery.

Summary

- The level of day-surgery activity and the number of surgical procedures acceptable for inclusion into day surgery continue to rise as a result of advances in surgical and anaesthetic practice.
- The British government has set a target of 75% of all elective surgery to be undertaken in day-surgery facilities. As the number of patients undergoing

ambulatory surgery grows, the amount of self-preoperative preparation and self-postoperative recovery will likewise grow.
- The reduced amount of time inherent with day surgery has somewhat marginalized the psychoeducational aspects of care in favour of essential medical tasks.
- Preoperative psychological preparation has remained static during the considerable rise and expansion in day surgery, i.e. informal and uncoordinated management dominates. However, day-surgery patients remain highly anxious.
- Preoperative anxiety has been well documented for many decades and much care has been recommended although unfortunately little has been implemented.
- Such recommendations may have remained dormant because the identified components for effective psychoeducational support have not been systematically assembled and presented in a clinically acceptable manner.

Further reading

Audit Commission for Local Authorities and the National Health Service in England and Wales (1991) Measuring Quality: The patient's view of day surgery, No. 3. London: HMSO.
Audit Commission for Local Authorities and the NHS in England and Wales (1997) Anaesthesia under Examination. London: HMSO.
Audit Commission for Local Authorities and the NHS in England and Wales (1998) Day Surgery Follow-up: Progress against indicators from 'A Short Cut to Better Services'. London: HMSO.
Audit Commission for Local Authorities and the NHS in England and Wales (2001) Day Surgery: Review of national findings, No. 4. London: HMSO.
Mitchell, R.B., Kenyon, G.S. and Monks, P.S. (1999) A cost analysis of day-stay surgery in otolaryngology. Annals of the Royal College of Surgeons of England 82(suppl): 85–92.
Royal College of Surgeons of England and Royal College of Psychiatrists (1997) Report on the Working Party on the Psychological Care of Surgical Patients (CR55) London: RCS and RCP.

Websites

British Association of Day Surgery: www.bads.co.uk
International Association of Ambulatory Surgery: www.iaas-med.org
NHS Modernisation Agency: www.modernnhs.nhs.uk/theatre

Chapter 2

Day surgery: patients' perceptions

Advancements in surgical practice

A dramatic shift in medical and nursing intervention has had, and is increasingly having, a major impact on the delivery of surgical health care, as highlighted in Chapter 1. Implicit to modern surgical practices are inherent time restrictions, which habitually ensure that medical aspects of care, e.g. assessing fitness for anaesthesia, must take preference over many other aspects of care, e.g. psychoeducational nursing intervention. Advances within day surgery are increasingly reducing direct patient contact with hospital personnel and progressively leading to a greater degree of pre- and postoperative patient self-care. In a future, modern, surgical health-care system where patient self-care is an integral component of care delivery, effective psychoeducational intervention will, by necessity, become inextricably linked with its success. A logical step during the development of greater psychoeducational awareness within day surgery is therefore a review of patients' perceptions of modern day-surgical intervention in order firmly to establish the patients' views. Few recommendations, fit for a new era of surgical intervention in the twenty-first century, can be confidently made without a thorough evaluation of patient experiences of day surgery.

On examination of the literature concerning patients' perceptions of day surgery, it was found that the earliest study was from 1978. Many studies were undertaken during the 1980s with a vast number in the 1990s (Mitchell 1999a, 1999b). The vast number of studies stemming from the 1990s helps to demonstrate clearly the intense interest and subsequent rapid rise in day-surgery activity in comparison with previous decades. Studies that merely asked 'Were you satisfied with day surgery?' (of which some did) were far too brief and were therefore not considered. In addition, opinion papers (of which there are a considerable number) were also excluded. Data specifically had to be collected from, or related to, adult, elective, day-surgery patients experiencing general, local or regional anaesthesia and general surgery (e.g. no ophthalmic surgery), and be expressly concerned with the patients' self-reported experiences. From the literature, five main themes emerged and relate to preassessment and patient teaching, information provision, patient experiences on the day of surgery and patient recovery.

Preassessment and patient teaching

The need to attend for a preassessment check was a strong theme in order to (1) help to assess the patient's fitness for surgery adequately, (2) provide instructions about care and recovery at home, and (3) help increase the nurse–patient contact time in order to allay fears. In an evaluation of the preassessment clinic (Harju 1991), data were collected using a small questionnaire 3 months after surgery. The survey revealed that 74% of patients were satisfied with day surgery. This was attributed, in part, to good patient selection and adequate preoperative teaching within the preassessment clinic. A medical audit (Bottrill 1994) also revealed the preassessment visit to be beneficial because nurses had more time to explain care and treatment with prospective patients. This in turn led to a reduction in the junior doctors' workload because it delegated some of the responsibilities of explaining care and treatment to the nursing team. A further medical audit highlighted the strengths and weaknesses of day-surgery preassessment clinics (Rudkin et al. 1996). Dedicated day-surgery facilities (designated ward and theatre used only for day-case patients) and mixed day-surgery facilities (no separate ward or theatre) were compared in eight Australasian day-surgery centres. It was concluded that information provision, waiting time and general satisfaction within dedicated day-surgery units were superior to mixed inpatient facilities.

In a 2-year retrospective study (Rai and Pandit 2003), the preassessment clinic was viewed to have reduced the 'did not attend' (DNA) rate and cancellation rate from 9% to 5%. Nurse-led preassessment units were therefore recommended because they were viewed as highly effective and financially viable. In a similar study of a nurse-led preassessment clinic (Clark et al. 1999), the nurses helped to filter out patients who were unsuitable for day surgery. This contributed to the waiting list being reduced from 12 months to 3 months. In a more recent study 30 patients were interviewed 7–10 days after surgery specifically about their preassessment preparation (Gilmartin 2004). The preassessment clinic was viewed as very efficient and provided essential information. Although not a main theme, the interpersonal skills of the nurses were demonstrated to be highly relevant on several occasions in compensating for the lack of adequate information and formalized psychological aspects of care. Cancellation of surgery, however, created a problem for many patients because social arrangements had to be postponed and rearranged.

Discussions during the preoperative visit about recovery from surgery at home were viewed as an essential part of the preassessment visit (see also 'Recovery behaviour'). Discharge from a day-surgery facility is largely based on medical criteria, i.e. conscious patient with a lack of postoperative morbidity (medical complications in the postoperative period) (Thapar et al. 1994, Chung 1995, Marshall and Chung 1997). A distinction between 'home readiness' and 'street fitness' is also drawn because patients may be ready for discharge home but not necessarily ready to go out onto the street alone and immediately resume 'normal' activities (Cheng et al. 2003). 'It is important to recognise that home-readiness is not synonymous with street fitness. Therefore, patients should be given clear instructions and cautioned against performing functions that require complete recovery of cognitive ability' (Joshi 2003, p. 170). In a small early survey (Stephenson 1990) it was uncovered that no patient was fully alert after 30 minutes and 57% experienced drowsiness within the first 24 hours. This indicated that less than half of the patients reached an adequate level of consciousness at the time of their discharge. In a later study to examine surgical repair of a hernia (Bahir et al. 2001) patients' reaction times in an emergency stop situation while driving a car were noted. It was revealed that there was no significant difference in driver reaction times between day surgery patients (24 hours after surgery) and non-surgical patients. It was therefore recommended that patients could return to normal activities within a few days of such surgery.

In a study specifically concerning teaching in day surgery (Brumfield et al. 1996) both patients and nurses were interviewed about the provision of patient information. Most patients preferred teaching to take place before admission. However, this conflicted with the nurses' views because they thought it should take place on the day of admission. In a similar study employing patients undergoing laparoscopic surgery, inpatient and day-case patient outcomes were compared (Wallace 1986c). Day-case patients were more anxious on the morning of surgery and 47% had to remain in hospital overnight after surgery. It is suggested that this increase in overnight stay may have resulted, in part, from a lack of adequate preparation. However, patients were given no choice as to whether they underwent day surgery or inpatient surgery. Therefore, some patients may have covertly desired to remain in hospital to recuperate.

Otte (1996) revealed that most patients preferred an early discharge from day surgery, although only when provided with adequate information. In a study investigating patient preference for anaesthesia when undergoing knee arthroscopy two areas of concern were highlighted (Martikainen et al. 2000). Although this quasi-experimental research study explored anaesthetic drug preference and not being able to speak with the surgeon before discharge, lack of information emerged as a key source of dissatisfaction. In a qualitative study by Kleinbeck and Hoffart (1994), patients were unsure of which activities they could perform around the house in the initial postoperative period. They would have preferred more information about recovery at home, e.g. what activities could be undertaken and when, to help in this process. The issue of unsatisfactory information provision for home recovery was also revealed following the in-depth interview of 21 day-surgery patients (Donoghue et al. 1997). Many patients reported that they were satisfied with the information received although the lack of details about the possible problems encountered at home was a disadvantage. In a survey by Guilbert and Roter (1997) and a large audit by Hawkshaw (1994) it was stated that patients coped well at home when discharge information provision was good, e.g. explanations given for simple daily activities.

In summary, it has been demonstrated that day surgery is highly reliant on good medical selection. Attendance at the preassessment clinic is therefore viewed as very positive. It benefits both the patient in terms of information provision and the health-care providers because patients' fitness to undergo anaesthesia and surgery can be verified. This can save time and resources on the day of surgery because the number of cancelled operations is reduced. Dedicated day-surgery units continue to be regarded as more effective because patients are less likely to experience cancelled operations and more likely to be discharged from the day-surgery unit as planned.

Information provision

The largest theme implicit in virtually all day-surgery studies relates to information provision (such is the impact of limited hospital contact within modern elective day surgery), e.g. the different quantity and quality of information required and the mode of provision. Information provision is an extremely challenging aspect for day surgery and much has been written (Edmondson 1996, Cahill and Jackson 1997). In a survey by Reid (1997, p. 23), 15 nurses within a day-surgery unit completed a questionnaire and it was documented that 'pressures of time and/or patient choice are reported as the main factors that inhibit the sharing of information with patients'.

Quantity and quality of information provision

A plethora of studies throughout this book has highlighted the inherent dilemma with information provision in that both too much and too little can cause an increase in anxiety (see Chapters 5 and 6). In an extensive survey by the Audit Commission (1991) of approximately 800 day-surgery patients. The main complaints were the lack of privacy, lack of parking, lack of telephones, poor information (especially written) and poor postoperative pain control. The study went on to state: 'Only 50% of day case patients reported having received an explanation of their operation prior to admission, but 84% had received one once they had been admitted' (Audit Commission for Local Authorities and the NHS in England and Wales 1991, p. 6). In a wide-ranging study by Pollock and Trendholm (1997) for *Which* (an independent consumer guide magazine – such was the public interest in day surgery), information provision was revealed to be a major issue. 'It was clear from our survey that people who were given the least information were the most dissatisfied with day surgery' (Pollock and Trendholm 1997, p. 16). In a comprehensive study by the Royal College of Surgeons of England and East Anglia Regional Health Authority (1995), data were collected on both a regional and a local basis from 10 day-surgery units, 30 consultant surgeons and 1434 patients. Patients expressed many concerns about their forthcoming surgery, although information provision was of most concern. The study went on to state that, although 75% of the patients were satisfied with the care and information that they had received, 'This overall appraisal conceals significant levels of dissatisfaction in certain areas' (Royal College of Surgeons of England and East Anglia Regional Health Authority 1995, p. 2).

In a further survey of information provision for day-case patients it was revealed that 31% of patients had received no information before the day of surgery and the standard letter sent to patients before admission lacked much information (Inglis and Daniel 1995). In a study of 116 day-surgery patients to assess the value and type of information required (Bernier et al. 2003), it was recommended that improved psychosocial support should be provided and an increase in information about pain management. However, what constitutes tangible psychosocial support on the day of surgery was not stipulated. In a qualitative study, eight patients were interviewed 3 weeks after day surgery (Otte 1996). Patients preferred the convenience of day surgery, because it was less disruptive to their lifestyle although they experienced major problems with communication. All patients stated that they were unprepared for their surgery in terms of the information received and the educational support provided. However, all patients underwent surgery in a mixed day-surgery facility. As previously stated, mixed facilities have been viewed as far less efficient than dedicated facilities (Rudkin et al. 1996).

In a survey exploring patients' experiences of laparoscopic surgery, 29% of patients were unhappy with the level of information that they had received (Nkyekyer 1996). However, this figure may be misleading and may be even higher because data were collected 2 weeks after surgery in the hospital outpatient department. Asking patients to comment about their care while still undergoing medical treatment has been observed to give rise to inaccurate responses (Fitzpatrick and Hopkins 1983). In a medical survey (Menon 1998) 78 patients were interviewed before surgery and this phenomenon was again demonstrated. It was revealed that 66% of patients would have preferred more information and yet they stated that the quality of service received was good. However, all patients were to undergo vasectomy, which may carry a higher emotive value and consequently a greater degree of information may have been required. In an attempt to circumvent the possible issues of under-reporting while still undergoing medical treatment, a number of studies have used postal questionnaires after discharge. In a comprehensive day-surgery study in which 105 patients undergoing various types of surgery were examined, information provision was again found to be problematic (Linden and Engberg 1995, 1996): 36% of patients thought the information provided was insufficient and a reduced level of information was positively associated with an increase in postoperative morbidity.

Sigurdardottir (1996), in a postal survey, compared satisfaction with care between two day-surgery facilities. The main areas of concern stemmed from the lack of adequate information because 'The patients were least satisfied with items related to the educational sub-scale [patient's knowledge regarding their operation and treatment] as they seldom received any booklets or pamphlets relating to the surgery' (Sigurdardottir 1996, p. 73). Again, however, one of the day-surgery facilities within this study was a mixed facility, i.e. not a dedicated day-surgery unit. In a brief survey examining satisfaction with anaesthesia 1 week after surgery (Buttery et al. 1993), it was established that most patients were satisfied with day surgery. However, the main criticisms centred on the long preoperative waiting period, lack of postoperative privacy and the provision of insufficient information. In a similar postal survey (Willis et al. 1997), positive correlations were documented between receiving written information and the level of satisfaction, and receiving an explanation and recommending day surgery to a friend.

In a medical survey 30 patients undergoing surgery and general anaesthesia were interviewed about their care (Fung and Cohen 2001). To compare the results, 15 senior anaesthetists were also surveyed using the same questionnaire. Both patients and anaesthetists were requested to rank in order of importance the care they valued the most. In each phase of their care, i.e. preoperative, intraoperative, pre-discharge and post-discharge, patients ranked information provision and communication as the most important. The anaesthetists, although able to state what patients required on discharge, were unable to predict what was required the most – both in the preoperative phase and immediately before surgery.

In a medical audit to examine patient satisfaction and general practition-er involvement in care (MacAndie and Bingham 1998), 20% of patients stated that their discharge information was excellent and 50% good, whereas the remainder were dissatisfied. In an earlier medical audit it was revealed that 30% received no written information about their care, although 97% were happy with their discharge information (King 1989). In a small telephone survey (Fitzpatrick et al. 1998), the need for specific information in the postoperative period was established. However, this sur-vey, as with a considerable number of other medical surveys, maintained a heavy postoperative morbidity focus. Donoghue et al. (1998, p. 195) con-cluded that patients preferred day surgery because it caused minimum disruption to their lifestyle, although 'Men who received information about the day surgery procedure were less anxious than their peers who said that they had received insufficient information.' However, all patients in this study underwent a cystoscopy (tube passed via the urethra to view prostate and bladder), which may carry a higher emotive value and therefore may possibly require a greater level of information provision.

As stated earlier (and inherent in a number of the studies above), it is not necessarily a lack of information but the possibility of receiving too much or too little information that causes dissatisfaction for patients (see Chapters 5 and 6). Following a telephone survey of almost 300 patients by Oberle et al. (1994, p. 1024) it was stated:

> Although 25% of patients indicated that they had received little or no information about their surgery and post-operative course, some of them were satisfied with that; they indicated that they simply preferred not to have any details about their upcoming surgery, because the more they knew, the more frightened they would become.

In a quasi-experimental design by Goldmann et al. (1988), the effects of hypnosis and information provision on anxiety were examined. Immediately before surgery patients received an 8-minute structured interview about knowledge of surgery followed by either a neutral dis-cussion about social aspects of surgery ($n = 27$) or 3 minutes of hypnosis ($n = 25$). A mean significant difference in anxiety scores was achieved for patients who had undergone 3 minutes of hypnosis before surgery. This may indicate that, for some patients, anxiety may not be aided by infor-mation provision alone. In addition, it was established that not all patients desired the same amount of information – some required more, others less (Goldmann et al. 1988). In a further study 150 patients sched-uled for day surgery were interviewed immediately before surgery and general anaesthesia with the aim of establishing a possible link between individual information requirements and health locus of control (Mitchell

1997). No link was established, although again the need for different levels of information was recognized: 41% of patients would have preferred a detailed information booklet and 53% a simple information booklet. However, the data were collected from gynaecological patients only and at a very anxious period, i.e. approximately 60–90 minutes before surgery. In a survey by Macario et al. (1999) in which both day-case patients and inpatients were surveyed about their anaesthetic, vomiting was rated as the most unwelcome aspect followed by gagging on the endotracheal tube and incision pain. However, a number of patients refused to take part in the study: 'some patients did decline to participate in the study because of their concerns about making adverse outcomes more explicit' (Macario et al. 1999, p. 657). Again, it can therefore be concluded that some patients simply wished not to have any details about their upcoming surgery conveyed to them.

In a postoperative telephone survey by Hawkshaw (1994), 1008 patients were contacted to gauge their satisfaction with treatment. Patients' desire for information varied because 72% reported satisfaction with the information, although the survey included 27% who received no information but were happy. A patient satisfaction survey (De Jesus et al. 1996) revealed dissatisfaction with information because of its lack of adaptation to home recovery and, again, it was established that not all patients required the same level of information. Two extensive surveys (Caldwell 1991a, 1991b) concluded that patients might have different information requirements because those who had a greater need for information and received extra information experienced less preoperative anxiety. However, 43% of the patients within this study were uncertain of a diagnosis of malignancy, which may also have strongly influenced the desire for information. In a study of 197 patients undergoing general anaesthesia for a variety of day-surgery procedures, the aim was to determine what information patients required from their anaesthetist in the preoperative period and to identify which patients wanted more information (Kain et al. 1997). Implicit in this study, therefore, was the general assumption that some patients may require more information than others. It was concluded (in this American study) that a generally higher level of information was wanted by female patients and divorced patients. However, it has also been suggested that the desire for information may be influenced by culture, e.g. patients in the USA may require and expect a far greater level of information possibly than patients in other countries (Lonsdale and Hutchison 1991).

In a qualitative study by Moore et al. (2002), 33% of patients did not want to know about any possible complications after their surgery whereas 66% did want to know about the risks. Female patients wanted to know the major complications in order to help with coping and making contingency plans. In addition, patients had obtained their information from a number of sources. 'Women in this study had gathered their information about risk from a number of different sources, such as the hospital, personal and family experiences, work colleagues and the media' (Moore et al. 2002, p. 307). In a further study concerning the introduction of a new surgical technique to day surgery (septorhinoplasty), 29 patients were surveyed to assess their experiences (Georgalas et al. 2002). Approximately 57% stated that they did not receive any written information on the day of surgery. However, of the information that was received, 61% stated that it was about right whereas 14% stated that it was less than they had wanted. Other main areas of dissatisfaction were parking (19%), attitude of the doctors (14%), lack of privacy (10%) and boredom while waiting (10%). Unfortunately, such aspects of dissatisfaction, e.g. waiting and parking, have remained a constant problem for day surgery for almost two decades (Williams et al. 2003).

Mode of information provision

Virtually all the studies throughout this book that have reported the need for improved information have been referring to written information provision. However, some inpatient studies have suggested that written information may have little impact and have thereby recommended verbal information. In a study of 30 women undergoing inpatient hysterectomy one group received written information whereas a second group received verbal information only (Young and Humphrey 1985). Using a combination of behavioural and psychological outcome measures, it was concluded that a booklet was of no more benefit than verbal information. In a further inpatient study of 38 women also undergoing hysterectomy one group of patients received a booklet before admission whereas a second group received no booklet (Young et al. 1994). Behavioural measures of physical recovery in hospital were recorded and patients were asked to complete satisfaction, stress and social recovery questionnaires. Again, no significant differences were established between the two groups.

The quality of leaflet production within hospitals can be poor, which has the potential to reduce any positive effects that the written information may provide (Audit Commission for Local Authorities and the NHS in England and Wales 1993, Scriven and Tucker 1997, Coulter et al. 1998, Walsh and Shaw 2000). Scriven and Tucker (1997) examined 184 educational leaflets from 97 hospitals in England regarding information for women undergoing hysterectomy. The leaflets from 27 hospitals were found to be illegible, mainly as a result of being hospital-produced photocopies. In addition to such problems, inaccurate information or patients failing to remember the information can also occur. Williams et al. (2003) surveyed 107 day-surgery patients and documented that there was a general lack of information and that some of the information provided by the nurses was inaccurate. In a qualitative medical study of seven day-surgery patients undergoing general anaesthesia for laparoscopic fundo-plication (Barthelsson et al. 2003a), four main themes emerged: living with gastro-oesophageal reflux before surgery, anxiety and memory loss, pain and returning to normal. Forgetting postoperative instructions and the lack of information were negative aspects although all were still happy to have had day surgery. In a literature review specifically to examine the information needs of day-surgery patients (Bradshaw et al. 1999), a lack of medical agreement about general patient advice was demonstrated. The absence of evaluation of information provided to patients was also evident, although some key areas for informational content were identified, e.g. postoperative pain, wound problems, bathing, stretching and heavy exercise, return to work, driving and sex. In a further review of the literature (Mitchell 2001), a methodical approach to the required level of information, a guide to the construction of information booklets and suggestions for their application within day surgery were provided.

A number of studies have demonstrated the need for patients not only to receive verbal and written information but also to have the chance to view/hear, or take home to view/listen to, a videotaped/audiotaped presentation about the surgical procedure (Baskerville et al. 1985, Wicklin and Forster 1994, Zvara et al. 1994, Lisko 1995, Done and Lee 1998). A study by Wicklin and Forster (1994) employing a quasi-experimental design was conducted to establish whether the modelling of behaviours from a videotaped presentation was of greater benefit to patients than the provision of written information. The only conclusion from the study was, however, that women reported a greater level of preoperative anxiety than men. The number of times the presentation was viewed and the duration of the presentation were not detailed, although such factors could have influenced the outcomes. Lisko (1995) conducted a small pilot survey in which gynaecological patients viewed a short videotaped presentation. The purpose was to encourage greater autonomy of health care although no significant results were established. This may, in part, have been the result of the videotaped presentation being only 8 minutes in duration. Done and Lee (1998) demonstrated that the knowledge level of patients could be increased if they were able, on the day of surgery, to view a short videotaped presentation about anaesthesia. Knowledge scores were indeed better in the videotaped presentation group in comparison to the control group, although no difference in anxiety was established. In a survey by Mitchell (1997) 150 day-surgery patients undergoing general anaesthesia for gynaecological surgery established

LIVERPOOL
JOHN MOORES UNIVERSITY
AVRIL ROBARTS LRC
TEL. 0151 231 4022

that 83% would also have preferred to view a videotaped presentation about their surgical experience.

In a quasi-experimental study by Zvara et al. (1994), patients were divided into two groups, 2 weeks before surgery, where one group received a preoperative videotaped presentation and the other no video-taped presentation. Using a post-video test only, knowledge in one area was deemed to have been significantly improved, i.e. what to do if feeling ill on the proposed day of surgery. In an audit by Baskerville et al. (1985) over a 9-month trial period, patients were provided with an audiotaped presentation about their operation. The information was well received and highlighted the need for information before the day of surgery. In a similar day-surgery study by Coslow and Eddy (1998), 30 patients undergoing general anaesthesia for laparoscopic sterilization were randomly assigned into one of two groups. The control group received information an hour before surgery whereas the experimental group received an individual 20-minute structured programme of information 1–2 weeks before surgery. This included a tape–slide demonstration, a six-page booklet, answers to questions and a quiz to test knowledge. The aim of the study was to demonstrate that patients who receive a structured programme of preoperative education before admission would recover more quickly and be more satisfied. Requests for and consumption of analgesia in the postoperative period were significantly less in the experimental group, indicating that well-informed patients might experience less pain. The study therefore recommended that patient education in day surgery must be a central nursing responsibility and more studies about information provision within day surgery were required. However, the vast difference in information provision between the two randomized groups may indicate, for some, considerable bias and cast doubt on the veracity of the outcomes.

As a result of the lack of time on the day of surgery, a number of studies have recommended the use of the telephone as a further mode of communication (Noon and Davero 1987). In a study by Barthelsson et al. (2003b), 12 patients undergoing laparoscopic cholecystectomy were interviewed to investigate their experiences of day surgery. Many patients forgot important information about the operation given to them by the surgeon and therefore additional telephone follow-up calls were requested by them. In a study by Heseltine and Edlington (1998), of 976 day-surgery patients regarding postoperative complications, data were collected by telephone and the study recommended the continued use of such a helpful service. A number of studies have also recommended a telephone helpline be to established after discharge to contact patients routinely within the immediate postoperative period in order to check progress (see 'Recovery behaviour' p. 38). In a telephone follow-up survey conducted to evaluate satisfaction with care (Hawkshaw 1994), one of the unforeseen benefits resulting from this form of data collection was that patients viewed the telephone interview as a valuable part of their continued care and a chance to ask questions.

Finally, the timing of information provision must be considered when discussing the mode of provision and a number of studies have made recommendations specific to day surgery (Oberle et al. 1994, Brumfield et al. 1996, Mitchell 1997). Before the rise in elective adult day surgery, timing of information delivery was not a problematic issue because patients were routinely admitted to hospital 1 or 2 days in advance of surgery. This has now changed and greater resources may now be required to ensure the early delivery of information. In a study by Brumfield et al. (1996), 30 patients undergoing general anaesthesia for laparoscopic surgery were surveyed together with 29 day-surgery nurses. Both patients and nurses were given a questionnaire and asked to return it by post within a week. Data revealed that patients wanted teaching to occur before admission whereas the nurses thought some teaching should occur after admission. Brumfield et al. (1996) document that if teaching took place before surgery, e.g. videotapes, written information and preoperative visits, nurses would experience less pressure on the day of surgery. Mitchell (1997), in a survey of 150 day-surgery patients, revealed that 48% of patients would have preferred to receive some written information at least a few days before their operation. Likewise, in a survey of 294 surgical patients by Oberle et al. (1994), a large number of patients were dissatisfied with the timing of information provision, because the bulk of it occurred on the ward immediately before surgery.

In summary, information provision is a major issue for day surgery. If patients are to care for themselves effectively during the pre- and post-operative phases, adequate information provision is essential. Many studies have suggested that telephone services improve communication and it has also been suggested that patients should be routinely called 1–2 weeks before their planned admission date to verify attendance (Cook et al. 2004). Although videotaped presentations have enjoyed some success as a means of information provision, the preoperative visit where written information can be provided and questions answered by the nurse remains the optimum method of communication.

Patient experiences on the day of surgery

A vast number of studies over many decades have highlighted the public's general satisfaction with, and preference for, day surgery (Clyne and

Jamieson 1978, Jennings and Sherman 1987, Read 1990, Harju 1991, O'Connor et al. 1991, Buttery et al. 1993, Chung et al. 1994, Fenton-Lee et al. 1994, Ghosh and Sallam 1994, Gupta et al. 1994, Sigurdardottir 1996, Lawrence et al. 1997, Pollock and Trendholm 1997, Bhattacharya et al. 1998, Fitzpatrick et al. 1998, Gnanalingham and Budhoo 1998, Stockdale and Bellman 1998, Willsher et al. 1998, Kangas-Saarela et al. 1999, Yellen and Davis 2001, Cox and O'Connell 2003). However, some aspects within day surgery are not always expected or wanted and continue to be a considerable source of dissatisfaction.

Lack of privacy and inaccurate expectations

Privacy within the day-surgery facility continues to be a source of much complaint, e.g. personal details being discussed in an open ward, patients waiting in public areas while wearing only a theatre gown, rectal suppositories being given intraoperatively without prior discussion and little privacy in the recovery area (Buttery et al. 1993, Greenwood 1993, Ghosh and Sallam 1994, Royal College of Surgeons of England and East Anglia Regional Health Authority 1995). In a survey by Ghosh and Sallam (1994, p. 1636) 953 patients were given a prepaid envelope on discharge with a questionnaire about satisfaction with day surgery: 'Negative comments were mainly about insufficient information, about preoperative and postoperative information, about waiting too long in the day surgery unit before the operation, inadequacy of postoperative pain relief and lack of privacy'. In a extensive survey of 800 day-surgery patients the main complaints concerned the lack of privacy, lack of parking, lack of telephones, poor information (especially written) and poor postoperative pain control (Audit Commission for Local Authorities and the NHS in England and Wales 1991). In a study to assess the incidence of postoperative complications 976 patients were contacted by telephone 24 hours after surgery (Heseltine and Edlington 1998). Although 72.4% reported no problems after their surgery two common complaints were the lack of privacy and waiting before surgery.

In an extensive survey incorporating 13 hospitals in six health board areas in Scotland during 1995–1996, 5069 day-case patients were invited to complete a questionnaire within 2 weeks of their operation (Bain et al. 1999). Patients who received information before admission were significantly more satisfied as were patients who received an explanation. Patients who experienced little privacy were significantly less satisfied. The study goes on to recommend that improved information should be provided and patients given realistic expectations about the possible pain and course of their recovery. In a qualitative study, which gathered data via telephone discussion, 16 patients were interviewed after day surgery (Stevens et al. 2001). The main themes to emerge were pain management, anxiety and lack of privacy. Privacy was a strong concern because most patients were aware that they could hear personal details of other patients being discussed and therefore all their personal details could be heard. Williams et al. (2003) surveyed 107 patients and established that the long waiting period after admission and the lack of privacy were negative issues highlighted by the patients. Patients had to sit in a public area wearing nothing more than a theatre grown and slippers while waiting for theatre.

A further aspect, which surprised many patients, was walking to the operating theatre. In an audit by MacAndie and Bingham (1998) it was revealed that a number of patients assumed day surgery to be minor surgery although they were surprised at having to walk to the operating theatre. In a survey by Birch and Miller (1994) of patients' attitudes towards 'walk-in/walk-out' surgery, it was established that 98% expressed satisfaction for this approach. However, this was a urology clinic in which patients were all still attending the hospital outpatient department at the time of data collection. In a telephone survey by Markovic et al. (2002), 315 women were interviewed within 2 days of hospital discharge to explore their experiences. It was revealed that 93% of the women preferred day surgery both for family reasons and because it allowed other, more seriously ill patients to benefit from a hospital admission. In addition, 'Many valued the opportunity to be in control of recovery at their own pace, rather than submitting to a hospital regime' (Markovic et al. 2002, p. 56). However, the disadvantages included exclusion of a support person during their stay, walking to theatre, lack of contact with the surgeon, lack of medical supervision at home and recovery with domestic responsibilities. In a large survey by Read (1990) patients were sent a postal questionnaire 2–3 weeks after surgery. Most patients (74%) were satisfied and stated no disadvantages. This was largely because of the minimal disruption to their lifestyle, no overnight stay and the convenience of rapid treatment. However, some negative comments included the early admission time and subsequent delay before surgery, delayed discharge and not knowing the time of discharge (Read 1990, p. 370).

Patient and nurse behaviour

In an in-depth study to examine participation in decision-making in day surgery (Avis 1994), it was revealed that patients expected the doctors and nurses to make their choices for them as they viewed them as the experts. However, they also realized that such expectations limited their involvement in the decision-making process. In a medical survey it was established that, when allowed to make a choice, 91% of suitable patients preferred day surgery (Gnanalingham and Budhoo 1998). However, only 33% chose to undergo local anaesthesia whereas 47% chose general anaesthesia. A greater proportion opting for general anaesthesia obviously demands a greater clinical and financial commitment. The reasons for preferring general anaesthesia were the increased anxiety associated with being conscious and experiencing the operation, e.g. some patients perceived general anaesthesia as less anxiety provoking because they were unconscious while the surgical procedure took place. Similarly, a survey about the use of local anaesthesia for foot surgery revealed that, although scheduled for local anaesthesia, 23% of patients expressed a preference for general anaesthesia on the day of surgery (Rees and Tagoe 2002). Wanting general anaesthesia but receiving local anaesthesia was associated with decreased satisfaction, with common reasons given being discomfort from the injection and disliking being conscious during surgery.

A number of studies revealed that some patients were not happy to go home after their surgery because they were anxious about self-care and would therefore have preferred an overnight stay (Pineault et al. 1985, O'Connor et al. 1991, Michaels et al. 1992, Ratcliffe et al. 1994, Nkyekyer 1996). In a comparatively older survey by Pineault et al. (1985), 54% of day-case patients believed their stay to be too short, as opposed to 21% of the inpatients who also believed their stay was too short, i.e. even a few nights in hospital was considered too short by some patients. Michaels et al. (1992) revealed that 74% of patients would have preferred an overnight stay and, in a survey by Ratcliffe et al. (1994), 8% of day-case patients would have preferred an overnight stay. O'Connor et al. (1991) concluded that male patients might prefer day surgery more than female patients because 16% of female patients preferred an overnight stay. This figure increased further in a study by Nkyekyer (1996) – 52% of female patients would have preferred an overnight stay because of the pain and associated anxiety. However, all the patients in the study by Nkyekyer (1996) had undergone surgery with intravenous sedation and local anaesthesia. Such a method of anaesthesia and surgery may have influenced the level of discomfort because an increased degree of pain was reported.

In a survey of 150 patients (Icenhour 1988) the aim was to gauge: (1) the nurses' support of patients' feelings; (2) the physicians' emotional support; (3) the staff willingness to listen; (4) the staff understanding; and (5) sufficient time with the nurses and physicians. Patient interviews were conducted before discharge and 96% said that they had received good care and were very satisfied. Nurses who demonstrated caring and concern were viewed as providing a better quality of care. In a study by Vogelsang (1990) the impact of continued contact with a familiar nurse during the day-surgery experience was investigated. Patients were divided into two groups: continuous contact with a familiar nurse or non-continuous contact. All 40 patients from both groups were contacted 3–5 days after surgery by telephone. It was revealed that 80% of the continuous contact group were satisfied with their care whereas only 40% of the non-continuous contact group were. 'Continued contact with a familiar nurse may have eased the women's transition through the surgical stay, resulting in higher satisfaction with the nursing care received and in promoting earlier discharge from the Unit' (Vogelsang 1990, p. 320). In an audit by Mitra et al. (2003) of 260 GPs it was established that the provision of information for home recovery was insufficient. Therefore, a named nurse spent longer with each patient providing them with information about care once home. 'They [patients] had access to a telephone helpline and selected patients were visited on the first post-operative day by the day surgery community nurse from the day care unit' (Mitra et al. 2003, p. 12). Thereby, the building of a therapeutic relationship and the increased time available for greater information exchange were deemed to be highly beneficial.

In a similar study to examine nursing behaviours day-surgery patients were asked to categorize the most desired nursing behaviours from a list of 63 nursing actions (Parsons et al. 1993). The most desired actions were the nurse's reassuring presence, verbal reassurance, expression of concern and attention to physical comfort. The least important behaviours were encouraging self-belief, knowing when the patients have had enough, teaching about illness and asking patients what they most prefer to be called. In a further study, 16 day-surgery patients were interviewed about their experience of day surgery (Costa 2001). Fear of the loss of physical and emotional control, and being cut and seeing blood were main issues, although such fears were all eased by the presence and interpersonal skills of the nurses, i.e. the building of a therapeutic relationship. Similarly, in an in-depth interview with 16 day-surgery patients in the postoperative period by Stevens et al. (2001), patients' perceptions of day surgery were dominated by the nurses' work and their interaction with the patient. In a further study of patient satisfaction 63 adult day-surgery patients were surveyed and two major concerns were highlighted (Malster et al. 1998): waiting up to 4 hours on the day of surgery caused much anxiety as did the lack of patient insight into the correct identification of staff. When unable to identify members of staff correctly an immediate barrier to effective communication was formed.

In summary, patients' experiences of day surgery were, in the vast majority of cases, very positive. Most patients want day surgery because the interruption to their lifestyle is minimal and the inconvenience of many hours spent waiting or recovering in a hospital bed is avoided.

Nevertheless, challenges to the patients' experience exist. The lack of privacy was a common theme for many patients and this complaint has spanned almost two decades, e.g. communication being overheard, waiting in public areas in theatre gowns, etc. Conversely, the interaction and relationship established with the nurse in the brief time available were viewed as one of the most positive experiences within the day-surgery unit. Although the time was brief the interpersonal skills of the nurse and the continued contact with a familiar nurse were of great benefit.

Patient recovery

The final theme relates to the first few days and weeks at home and concerns morbidity, recovery behaviour and involvement of community health-care professionals. The first issue concerns the plethora of studies examining postoperative morbidity. The huge level of interest in postoperative morbidity helps to demonstrate vividly how the advancements in day surgery, outlined in Chapter 1, have had a strong medical focus. Nevertheless, such issues are clearly central to patient satisfaction and therefore to the continued success of day surgery. Numerous studies highlight the issue of postoperative morbidity, although they focus mainly on the degree and duration of pain and to a lesser extent on postoperative nausea and vomiting. Such aspects are major determinants of hospital admission after day surgery.

Pain management

Ineffective pain management is a long-standing issue in many areas of surgical intervention (Royal College of Surgeons of England and Royal College of Psychiatrists 1997, Kain et al. 2000, Manias 2003) and day surgery is no exception (Yellen and Davis 2001, Munafo and Stevenson 2003, Coll et al. 2004a, 2004b). Many patients expect to experience pain after surgery although 'The popular assumption that serious pain after surgery is unavoidable is misplaced' (Audit Commission for Local Authorities and the NHS in England and Wales 1998a). Effective pain management is frequently not achieved because (Audit Commission 1998a):

- effective pain relief is not reached (inadequate analgesia prescribed; nurses administer less than prescribed)
- patients do not tell staff they are in pain

- nurses underestimate patients' pain experience
- there is a delay in administering pain relief
- pain is not monitored.

Ghosh and Sallam (1994) reported one of the main sources of dissatisfaction in the postoperative period to be inadequate pain relief. In one of the earliest day-surgery studies (Towey et al. 1979), no significant difference between two methods of induction of anaesthesia – Althesin versus induction by Thiopental (formally known as Thiopentone) – was established although a generally high level of postoperative abdominal pain was uncovered (Thiopental is a fast-acting barbiturate mainly used intravenously for the induction of anaesthesia; Althesin is an older anaesthesia induction agent – now largely obsolete). In three additional early audits, 50% of patients experienced pain while at home (Clyne and Jamieson 1978, Cundy and Read 1981, Birch and Miller 1994). Although only a short questionnaire within the audit process was used, it was revealed that 25% of patients were awake and in pain during their first postoperative night with 31% gaining no relief or only partial relief when using the prescribed drugs (Firth 1991). In a study in which 317 day-surgery patients were sent a postal questionnaire after surgery, 90% of the patients required more analgesia than prescribed (Jennings and Sherman 1987). Pain was therefore considered a major problem during recovery at home. In addition, 8% felt that their surgeon had not spent a sufficient amount of time with them after surgery and 19% felt that they were given contradictory advice. Nevertheless, as with many such studies, patients still preferred to undergo day surgery because 95% of patients were satisfied with their care. Fraser et al. (1989, p. 194), in a comprehensive survey, interviewed 50 gynaecological patients and established that the greatest amount of pain was experienced on the first postoperative day: '51.6% of the women utilised at least 50% of their prescribed number of tablets – prescription range 10–30 tablets.' A further two studies also reported that the recommended or prescribed analgesia did not always provide adequate pain relief after surgery (Thatcher 1996, Callesen et al. 1998).

In one study it was noted that most female patients did not expect the severity and duration of the pain experienced (Donoghue et al. 1995). Numerous studies have reported higher pain levels after gynaecological surgery and therefore made specific recommendations for this group, e.g. greater use of analgesia and improved information provision (Codd 1991, Edwards et al. 1991, Agboola et al. 1998, Haldane et al. 1998, Mackintosh and Bowles 1998, Horvath 2003). In a more recent study it was uncovered that severe pain was experienced by 3% of patients – all of whom had undergone laparoscopic sterilization, i.e. gynaecological surgery (De Beer and Ravalia 2001). In contrast, it has been stated that overall pain intensity in patients undergoing termination of pregnancy was low (Hein et al. 2001) In an extensive report by the Royal College of Surgeons of England and East Anglian Regional Health Authority (1995, p. 20) many women with household duties stated they would have preferred the choice of inpatient surgery: 'These patients tended to have higher levels of worry pre-operatively and greater levels of dissatisfaction post-operatively. They were also less likely to recommend day surgery to others'. In a medical survey it was further revealed how gender roles in European society may contribute to the level of pain experienced after day surgery (Jakobsen et al. 2003). The level of domestic activity immediately after surgery was high and may well have exacerbated the degree of pain experienced. Beauregard et al. (1998, p. 309) also identified a pattern concerning pain management: 'The study revealed that the best predictor of severe pain at home was inadequate pain control in the first few hours following the surgery; the more pain the patients experienced during this period, the more likely they were to report severe pain on the first and second day after discharge.' Three recommendations were therefore put forward: (1) aggressive analgesic treatment to be initiated during the hospital stay, (2) the severity and duration of pain after day-surgery should not be underestimated, and (3) patient education and the use of take-home analgesia protocols were essential.

In an orthopaedic day-case survey by Bhargava et al. (2003) of 41 patients, 10% stated that their pain was not under control while in hospital whereas 17% experienced mobilization problems and had to remain in hospital overnight. The study therefore concluded that 'The main problem in the study was inadequate post-operative pain control experienced by 18% of the patients' (Bhargava et al. 2003, p. 153). In a telephone survey 24 hours after surgery (Claxton et al. 1997) it was established that morphine (long-acting opioid) was more effective than fentanyl (short-acting opioid), although many anaesthetists are very reluctant to use morphine because of its slow onset and long duration (Cahill and Jackson 1997). It was concluded that patients who were administered intravenous fentanyl during surgery may have a greater need for supplementary oral analgesia in the first 24 hours after surgery. However, patients underwent different surgical procedures, which may present a somewhat less than accurate picture of the individual levels of pain experienced. In a study to investigate the effective of pre-emptive analgesia (Jackson and Sweeney 2004), 56 patients undergoing orthopaedic day surgery were randomized into two groups – tramadol i.m. (opioid) 1 hour before surgery or physiological or 0.9% saline i.m. (placebo) 1 hour before surgery. No significant differences were established in the level of pain experienced. A similar study was designed to determine whether the more advantageous effects of remifentanil justified the extra expense because cost savings could be made elsewhere, e.g. postoperative complications, recovery times, hospital admission (Beers et al. 2000). (Remifentanil is a rapid-acting opioid with shorter half-life than fentanyl, although it is much more expensive.) In this study 34 patients undergoing gynaecological day surgery were randomly assigned to receive either fentanyl (bolus dose) or remifentanil (continuous infusion). However, the remifentanil group did not prove to be more cost-effective; indeed this group had a significantly greater degree of postoperative nausea and vomiting. It was therefore concluded that no cost savings could be made from the use of a more rapidly acting opioid.

Uncontrolled pain followed by nausea and vomiting are the main medical reasons for day-surgery patients being admitted as inpatients after surgery (Leith et al. 1994, Ratcliffe et al. 1994, Chung 1995, Lewin and Razis 1995, Hedayati and Fear 1999, Mitchell et al. 1999). However, the unanticipated admission rate within the UK after day surgery remains low, although it could rise if certain conditions prevail, e.g. surgery performed later in the day (Hedayati and Fear 1999, Junger et al. 2001). In a retrospective study by Junger et al. (2001), the progress of 3152 day-surgery patients was documented. It was established that 5.4% of patients were admitted (36.7% had bleeding and 19.5% high pain scores, 32.6% other surgery-related reasons, 5.3% lack of vigilance with care, 4.1% experienced postoperative nausea and vomiting, and 2.4% wanted to remain in hospital). 'Furthermore, we found that patients with the longest preoperative waiting times had the shortest postoperative day-case monitoring times. These data suggest that patients who are scheduled late, and in whom the remaining postoperative time until closure of the day-care unit is insufficient for discharge in an adequate physical status, are likely to be admitted to hospital' (Junger et al. 2001, p. 321). In a further study of day-surgery readmission rates (Morales et al. 2002) an audit of 3502 was undertaken. The readmission rate was 4.1% and caused by bleeding ($n = 23$), more extensive surgery than anticipated ($n = 22$), pain ($n = 18$) and drowsiness ($n = 10$). In addition, poor pain management is one of the most common reasons for unanticipated contact with a GP after discharge from day surgery (Ghosh and Sallam 1994, Kennedy 1995, Agboola et al. 1998, Haddock et al. 1999) (see 'Recovery behaviour' below).

Increased pain and postoperative nausea and vomiting are therefore frequently the most common reasons for patient dissatisfaction with day surgery (Parlow et al. 1999, Habib and Gan 2001). In a review of the literature by Habib and Gan (2001) the people deemed most susceptible to postoperative nausea and vomiting were female patients, obese patients, patients with a previous history of postoperative nausea and vomiting, patients undergoing long surgical procedures and patients experiencing certain types of surgery, e.g. intra-abdominal (70%), gynaecological (58%), laparoscopic surgery (40–77%), breast surgery (50–65%), and eye and ear, nose and throat surgery (71%). In an international study to examine patients' experiences of postoperative nausea and vomiting, data from 561 patients undergoing general anaesthesia for a variety of surgical procedures were examined (Pfisterer et al. 2001). Patients were invited to maintain a diary of their recovery for the first 5 postoperative days. Postoperative nausea and vomiting were revealed to be highest in patients undergoing gastrointestinal surgery (32%), gynaecological surgery (15%) and general surgery (17%). It was concluded that postoperative nausea and vomiting were not adequately recognized or antiemetic agents were inadequately administered. A questionnaire to measure postoperative nausea and vomiting reliably in ambulatory surgery is currently under development, although it does not identify susceptible patients preoperatively (Fetzer et al. 2004). In a quasi-experimental study by Parlow et al. (1999), patients were randomized, before laparoscopic surgery and general anaesthesia, into two groups. Group 1 received a prophylactic intramuscular injection of promethazine (antiemetic) whereas the second group received an intramuscular placebo injection (physiological saline). No differences were established between the two groups concerning the level of nausea, vomiting or rescue antiemetics administered. However, patients identified as experiencing higher levels of nausea and vomiting in the recovery room continued to experience higher levels throughout the first 24-hour period. It was therefore recommended to target the highly nauseated patients in the recovery room for prophylactic antiemetic therapy.

In a trial to determine whether withholding oral fluids before discharge would decrease nausea and vomiting, 726 patients undergoing general anaesthesia for a variety of day-case procedures were included (Jin et al. 1998). Patients were randomly assigned into drinking (mandatory 200 ml fluid provided once initial recovery phase completed) and non-drinking groups before discharge from the day-surgery unit. All patients were contacted by telephone 24 hours after surgery to complete a questionnaire about nausea and vomiting, and the level of eating and drinking. No significant difference in nausea and vomiting was established between the two groups before discharge although the drinking group had a significantly longer stay before discharge. The drinking group also took significantly longer to recover physically before their discharge. In the non-drinking group 64.4% stated that they would go without drinking again after such surgery. In addition, while travelling home, no significant differences emerged between the two groups regarding the level of nausea and vomiting. Jin et al. (1998) therefore recommended that withholding early postoperative fluids did not decrease the incidence of nausea and vomiting but might reduce the length of stay in the day-surgery unit before discharge.

In a quasi-experiment (Alkaissi et al. 1999), the effectiveness of nausea-relieving pressure wristbands (SeaBands®) was evaluated: 60 women undergoing a variety of gynaecological day surgery were randomized into three groups – one group received acupressure with bilateral stimulation, a second group received bilateral placebo stimulation (SeaBands® not placed in the correct position) and a third group received no acupressure wrist bands but served as a control. The patients wearing the correctly sited SeaBands® reported significantly less nausea and vomiting over a 24-hour period in comparison to the other two groups. In a further study to investigate the effectiveness of complementary therapy (Anderson and Gross 2004), patients who had undergone day surgery were divided into three groups in the recovery area: aromatherapy with isopropyl alcohol, oil of peppermint or saline (placebo) gauze pad inhalations. Patients were assisted in taking deep breaths with the gauze pad held near their nostrils on three occasions: 0, 2 minutes and 5 minutes. No significant differences were established for the three groups and 52% required rescue intravenous antiemetics. However, the entire sample was selected because they were already reporting postoperative nausea and vomiting. It has been suggested further that increased oxygen during anaesthesia is advantageous in combating postoperative nausea and vomiting (Purhonen et al. 2003); 100 patients were therefore randomly allocated into two groups – 30% oxygen or 80% oxygen while anaesthetized. However, no significant differences were established in the experimental group receiving supplementary oxygen.

A number of studies have highlighted the link to an increased demand for analgesia when not provided with sufficient information (Frisch et al. 1990, Coslow and Eddy 1998, Haddock et al. 1999, Barthelsson et al. 2003b, Dewar et al. 2003, Watt-Watson et al. 2004). A quasi-experimental study by Coslow and Eddy (1998) noted that a greater number of patients demanded analgesia when not provided with information in the preoperative phase. However, the experimental group within this study had a planned programme of education spanning 1–2 weeks. This is in sharp contrast to the control group who received information only 1 hour before surgery. A planned 1- to 2-week programme of education may be considered by some as somewhat clinically unrealistic or, at best, a poor group from which to gain realistic comparisons. Limb et al. (2000) surveyed 62 patients undergoing day surgery for haemorrhoidectomy. A multimodal analgesia technique was employed, i.e. combination of two or more drugs and/or two or more methods of delivery, to improve pain management and minimize the side effects. Of the patients 95% were satisfied with their pain management, although implicit within this method of pain control (as it was a new day-case procedure) was the added information provided to patients about pain management (Limb et al. 2000). Frisch et al. (1990) employed both written questionnaires and postoperative telephone interviews to establish patient satisfaction with day surgery for 16 couples, i.e. patients and their carers. It was concluded that improved teaching about pain management, recovery rates and a greater emphasis on general education would be beneficial. In a quasi-experimental design study, 59 patients were randomly assigned to one of two groups: postoperative analgesia and foot massage or just postoperative analgesia (Hulme et al. 1999). The patients in the group who received 5 minutes of foot massage from the nurses during the immediate postoperative period stated that they experienced less pain. However, the experimental group gained extra time with the nurse during the foot massage treatment, which may have enhanced information provision and self-efficacy appraisal. The control group received no additional attention. Watt-Watson et al. (2004) surveyed 180 patients undergoing day surgery and a large number were still experiencing severe pain on the seventh postoperative day. However, a considerable number of patients did not receive clear information about taking their medication (45%) or changing medications that were ineffective or causing adverse effects (56%). 'Several patients commented that they did not fill their analgesia script or stopped taking the analgesia because of previous or current experiences with constipation and/or nausea. It was significant that half of the patients stopped taking analgesia at 72 hours despite moderate pain' (Watt-Watson et al. 2004, p. 159).

Several audits concluded postoperative pain management to be a considerable problem and recommended prepacked analgesia plus the relevant information to be provided at discharge (Lewin and Razis 1995, Marquardt and Razis 1996, Beauregard et al. 1998, Haddock et al. 1999). This was deemed necessary because it became clear that although some patients experience considerable pain after day surgery others have very little pain. One audit established that 96% of patients were satisfied with their postoperative pain management, although a community liaison nurse visited during the immediate postoperative period to attend to the wound and provide advice, e.g. additional information (Fenton-Lee et al. 1994). In a further audit using a community liaison nurse (Ismail 1997), it was documented that 94% of patients did not require analgesia on the first night and 60% used the 5-day supply provided at discharge. In an earlier audit of 145 patients undergoing both general and local anaesthesia for a variety of surgical procedures, it was revealed that 69% of patients experienced little or no pain in the postoperative period (Ramachandra 1994). Likewise, in a telephone survey by Kangas-Saarela et al. (1999) of 217 randomly selected day-surgery patients, it was established that 31% of patients had no pain 24 hours after their operation.

A number of studies have strongly recommended the use of non-steroidal anti-inflammatory drugs (NSAIDs) to pre-empt pain and thereby help to manage it more effectively (Edwards et al. 1991, Leith et al. 1994, Ratcliffe et al. 1994, Aasboe et al. 1998, Callesen et al. 1998, Kangas-Saarela et al. 1999, Limb et al. 2000, Lau et al. 2002). The effects of celecoxib (an NSAID) were evaluated in a group of patients undergoing general anaesthesia for minor ear, nose and throat day surgery (Recart et al. 2003). Patients were randomized into a control group (placebo), celecoxib 200 mg group and celecoxib 400 mg group. The drugs were administered preoperatively and the group who received celecoxib 400 mg experienced significantly less pain postoperatively, although this did not affect the time to discharge or the recovery process once at home. In a descriptive study of 34 patients undergoing herniorrhaphy, pain was assessed postoperatively to gauge the demand for analgesia (Morris 1995). No difference in the degree of pain experienced was established between patients given either diclofenac sodium (an NSAID) or bupivacaine hydrochloride (local anaesthesia for wound infiltration) intraoperatively, although the results demonstrated a reduction in the recovery time when bupivacaine hydrochloride was used. However, it has been stated that non-selective NSAIDs, e.g. ketorolac or diclofenac, can increase bleeding at the operation site because of their effect on platelet function, whereas more specific NSAIDs, e.g. celecoxib and rofecoxib, may not affect platelet function (Issioui et al. 2002). To demonstrate this, Issioui et al. (2002) randomly assigned patients to four treatment groups: group 1 or control (500 mg vitamin C); group 2 (2 g acetaminophen or paracetamol – a non-selective NSAID); group 3 (50 mg rofecoxib); or group 4 (2 g acetaminophen/paracetamol and 50 mg rofecoxib). 'In this study involving an adult ambulatory surgery population, the oral administration of rofecoxib (50 mg) prior to surgery was effective in reducing pain after ear, nose and throat surgery and led to improved satisfaction with their pain management and quality of recovery compared with acetaminophen (2 g)' (Issioui et al. 2002, p. 934).

Conversely, a few studies have examined the effects of steroidal anti-inflammatory agents in day-case surgery. Aasboe et al. (1998) administered betamethasone 12 mg (steroidal anti-inflammatory) for pain management before surgery in a double-masked experimental study investigating postoperative pain. Positive results were established using this technique and it was recommended that more studies should be conducted to gauge the beneficial effects of corticosteroids. In a further randomized controlled trial of steroid administration, patients were either given 1 ml intravenous saline or 4 mg dexamethasone intravenously following induction of anaesthesia

(Coloma et al. 2002). Both groups also received 12.5 mg intravenous dolasetron (antiemetic) at the time of gallbladder removal. The results revealed that patients receiving dexamethasone recovered more quickly and left the unit earlier, were more satisfied, and had fewer episodes of nausea and vomiting in the first 24 hours.

Other studies have examined more modern, innovative antiemetic agents known as the 5-HT_3 (serotonin or 5-hydroxytryptamine) receptor antagonists, e.g. ondansetron and dolasetron (a cheaper version of ondansetron). A randomized controlled trial was undertaken to determine whether postoperative nausea and vomiting were controlled more effectively with the use of ondansetron 8 mg (disintegrating tablets) for the first 3 postoperative days (Thagaard et al. 2003). The two groups received either ondansetron 8 mg or a placebo. However, no significant differences were established between the two groups. Two further randomized studies were also undertaken to determine the beneficial effects of 5-HT_3 receptor antagonists, e.g. dolasetron or ondansetron (Darkow et al. 2001, Tang et al. 2003), although again no significant differences were established. It was therefore recommended that traditional antiemetics should form the core of postoperative nausea and vomiting prophylaxis in ambulatory surgery. In a study to determine the greater effectiveness of timing of the administration of dolasetron (Chen et al. 2001) 150 patients undergoing gynaecological day surgery were randomly divided into three groups: group 1 dolasetron 12.5 mg i.v. 10–15 min before the induction of anaesthesia; group 2 dolasetron 12.5 mg i.v. at the end of the laparoscopy; and group 3 dolasetron 12.5 mg i.v. at the end of anaesthesia. However, no significant differences were established between the groups. The study therefore concluded that dolasetron 12.5 mg i.v. administered before the induction of anaesthesia is as effective as dolasetron given at the end of surgery or at the end of anaesthesia in preventing postoperative nausea and vomiting after day-case laparoscopic surgery.

It has been reported that severe surgical pain affects only a small number of day-case patients once discharged (Ramachandra 1994, Mackintosh and Bowles 1998, Tong and Chung 1999, De Beer and Ravalia 2001). However, in a study by McHugh and Thoms (2002, p. 272), severe pain was a problem for 21% of patients after discharge: '17% of patients reported having severe pain immediately following day-case surgery, and a significant number continued to experience pain at home for up to 4 days following discharge.' It was also reported that day-case staff did not always ask patients whether the patients were in pain before discharge. In a review of the literature on day-case pain management by Coll et al. (2004b, p. 61), pain after day surgery was established to be high even on the third postoperative day: 'The high levels of pain reported in the literature suggest that many pain management policies [protocols] have been overlooked.' In an audit by Firth (1991), pain was also identified as a considerable problem once patients were at home. Patients had expected to have some pain but had not purchased any analgesia before admission. This was either because they had expected the hospital to provide analgesia or they had not been adequately instructed before admission. To improve the problem of postoperative pain management it was suggested, in audits by Lewin and Razis (1995) and Marquardt and Razis (1996), that prepacked analgesia or analgesia packs with the relevant accompanying information be provided. These packs could vary according to the operation type and help establish a more effective programme of pain management (Robins et al. 2000). However, such a system may involve the nursing staff establishing which pack to administer, explaining the accompanying information and possibly, in some instances, securing payment. Thatcher (1996) in a qualitative study interviewed four patients 2–4 days after surgery. It was established that patients expected to experience some pain on discharge but, when the recommended or prescribed analgesia did not bring relief, they found it difficult to cope. One patient was required to pay for the prescribed analgesia while in hospital and subsequently refused the medication.

In a survey to evaluate the incidence of the most common side effects of day surgery once home and their relationship to anaesthetic technique employed (Ture et al. 2003), pain was revealed to be the most common problem. The second most common side effect was muscle weakness and this was twice as high in patients experiencing inhalation anaesthesia. It was therefore concluded that central or peripheral neural blockade and total intravenous anaesthesia (TIVA) should be the anaesthesia of choice because the incidence of side effects was much lower with this group. Kelly et al. (1994) collected data from 143 patients in a postal survey 1 week after surgery. The questionnaire contained 11 items requiring mainly yes/no responses or tick box of possible postoperative problems. During the first night of discharge 42.7% reported feeling drowsy and 38.8% had a headache, although 50% took no analgesia. 'There was a wide distribution in the time to recover to full normal daily activity, ranging from the day of operation in four patients, one to two days in 45, three to five days in 33 and six days or more in 21 patients' (Kelly 1994, p. 29). In a similar study to evaluate the incidence of postoperative complications (Heseltine and Edlington 1998), patients were telephoned and a questionnaire completed 24 hours after surgery. Almost 1000 patients were surveyed and 15% required more information over the telephone during data collection. Advice about pain management was the most commonly requested aspect of information. The study therefore recommended the continued use of a postoperative telephone service.

Recovery behaviour

The second recovery issue concerns patient recovery behaviour. Once they were discharged from the hospital, Gupta et al. (1994) discovered that some patients drove home (4%) and many went home unaccompanied by an adult; 25% were home alone during the first 24 hours and 8% alone during the first 24 hours without an adult to look after the children. An audit by Birch and Miller (1994) also revealed that 13% of patients drove their car the same day and the majority returned home alone. Kelly (1994), using a short questionnaire, reported that 7% drove their car on the first night of discharge, 42.7% reported feeling drowsy and 38.8% had a headache. In a telephone survey of compliance with postoperative instructions (Correa et al. 2001) 24 hours after surgery, it was revealed from a sample of 750 patients that 1.8% of patients had consumed alcohol within 24 hours, 4.1% had driven a vehicle and 4% did not have an adult to care for them. In a survey of 60 patients after day surgery (Rawal et al. 1997), it was documented that tiredness was experienced by 20% of patients and 28% of patients were home alone after surgery. In a study by Jakobsen et al. (2003) many patients booked their surgery before a weekend or a vacation to avoid time off work. The study surveyed 76 female patients after laparoscopic surgery and revealed that driving was resumed on the first postoperative day. Child care, climbing stairs, cooking, cleaning and shopping were also resumed on the same day as the surgery.

In a comprehensive postal survey of 1511 day-surgery patients (Philip 1992), it was documented that the main postoperative problems were muscle aches, sore throat and drowsiness. For all patients, such problems lasted 1 day for 59%, 2 days for 28% and 3 or more days for 14% of patients, although 32% of patients resumed normal activities the next day, with a further 62% after 3 days. In a survey of 100 day-surgery patients regarding postoperative morbidity by Willsher et al. (1998), muscle ache, malaise, drowsiness and hoarseness of voice were also commonly reported although, again, 95% preferred day surgery and would opt for day surgery again. In a comprehensive survey of 5264 day-surgery patients (Higgins et al. 2002), a sore throat was found to be 12 times more common in patients having an endotracheal tube and 5 times more common in laryngeal mask airway, compared with patients receiving a facemask or no airway management. It was concluded that a sore throat was a common adverse outcome in ambulatory patients especially for female patients, younger patients and patients undergoing gynaecological surgery. However, a sore throat has been viewed as an inevitable consequence after endotracheal intubation (Thomson et al. 2003). An audit by Clyne and Jamieson (1978) reported that 52% of patients surveyed stayed off work for more than a week. However, postoperative recovery rates may differ widely because Ratcliffe et al. (1994) established that 75% of patients still had problems 3 days after their operation. Similarly, in a survey of 588 day-surgery patients (Wilkinson et al. 1992), 84% had problems after 3 days – the main issue being pain. One in ten patients made appointments to visit their GP as a result of their discomfort. Conversely, in an earlier audit by Stephenson (1990) it was reported that almost 50% of day-surgery patients were active on the second postoperative day.

In a survey by Donoghue et al. (1995), 31 patients were divided into different data collection groups, e.g. semi-structured interview at either 1 week or 3 weeks, telephone interview or face-to-face interview. Many challenging aspects of recovery were reported and 'Many of the participants reported that there were experiences they had not anticipated, surprises that they did not welcome and things that they would have liked to have known before the operation' (Donoghue et al. 1995, p. 173, 1997). Again, in two large surveys about coping at home after surgery (Guilbert and Roter 1997, Ruuth-Setala et al. 2000) the most important determinant of satisfaction was patient preparation, e.g. effective communication and instruction. In a further study using in-depth interviews, data were collected from 19 patients by telephone for approximately 20 minutes on two occasions in the postoperative period (Kleinbeck and Hoffart 1994). Patients stated that they felt quite vulnerable when going home and were unsure about what activities they could perform around the house because clear instructions had not been received preoperatively. This led to trial-and-error learning of everyday activities around the home. Similarly, in a study of 21 day-surgery patients, telephone contact was established in the postoperative period (Fitzpatrick et al. 1998). It was concluded that, although 90% were satisfied with the information provided, unexpected situations during recovery demonstrated their lack of knowledge. In a comprehensive survey of 585 women to evaluate their experience of gynaecological day surgery, almost 33% of women visited their GP during the first 3 weeks and 33% required 'quite a lot' of care from relatives or friends (Petticrew et al. 1995). In an in-depth interview of 112 patients after recovery from a termination of pregnancy, an increase in self-efficacy was recognized as a strong predictor of good adjustment and recovery from surgery (Cozzarelli 1993).

Frisch et al. (1990) conducted one of the few surveys that also asked the carers to complete a questionnaire about their experiences of tending for a relative after day surgery. More than 30% of the patients required help with activities of daily living during the first 7 days, although 'Helpers tended to overestimate the patients' need for assistance' (Frisch et al. 1990, p. 1006). This was mainly evident in the increased level of help believed to be required during bathing and the amount of pain believed to be experienced. However, some of the morbidity issues may have resulted from the patients all undergoing orthopaedic surgery. In an Australian survey of 150 day-surgery patients, 62% of patients required a carer for 1 day or less and 20% for 1–2 days (O'Connor et al. 1991). Female patients required more assistance than male patients with 3% of female patients paying someone to help with child care and housework. However, no consideration was given to the different types of surgery undertaken. In a comprehensive survey by the Royal College of Surgeons of England and East Anglia Regional Health Authority (1995) more than one-third of patients required a great deal of support from helpers at home, 20% of whom had to take time off work. Willis et al. (1997) established that 21% of patients required help from carers, 10% of whom had to take an average of 3 days off work with 7% of carers losing earnings. In a brief review of the literature about discharge from day surgery, the increase in the amount and complexity of day-case surgery currently being undertaken in the UK is discussed (Mitchell 2003a). The continued increase in day surgery has led to a corresponding rise in patient and lay-carer involvement throughout the pre- and postoperative period. The main challenges identified for the lay-carers were pain management, patient recovery behaviour and community health-care provision.

In a survey of day-surgery patients undergoing both local and general anaesthesia, 252 carers were surveyed during the discharge of their relative/friend from the day-surgery unit (Knudsen 1996). Approximately 90% of carers were concerned about their relative, with pain management, wound care, sleep disturbance, nausea and general information being the most common issues. After this survey and others, a leaflet especially constructed for carers was recommended (Ruuth-Setala et al. 2000). In a further carer survey, 200 questionnaires were received from relatives attending nine different day-surgery units (Hazelgrove and Robins 2002). The lack of adequate parking, lack of written information, lack of instructions about medications and absence of any telephone helplines were all problematic issues.

Although wound management is an issue for many patients and carers after discharge, the overall wound infection rate according to one study is only 3.5% (Grogaard et al. 2001). Gastroenterological surgery resulted in the highest rate of wound infections, i.e. laparoscopic cholecystectomy. However, it is suggested that, with the increase in the level of surgery being undertaken in day-case facilities, this figure may increase. Nevertheless, Grogaard et al. (2001) suggest that individual factors associated with the practices of surgeons and nurses may also influence infection rates. In an inpatient study of stress before surgery (Broadbent et al. 2003), the impact of wound healing was assessed in 47 patients undergoing hernia repair. The results revealed that increased anxiety levels were associated with lower cellular wound repair processes in the early postoperative period. In addition, patients who smoked also experienced significantly reduced wound-healing abilities. In a further study of wound infection (Minatti et al. 2002), a comparison of wound infection rates between inpatient and day-surgery patients was surveyed. The inpatient infection rate was 21% (*n* = 123) whereas the day-surgery infection rate was 11% (*n* = 238). Therefore, an advantage of day surgery is the reduced risk of hospital-acquired infections.

Primary health-care professionals

The final aspect of recovery concerns the involvement of primary health-care professionals. To enable both patients and their carers to gain much needed advice after discharge, a number of studies have strongly recommend the use of a telephone service, e.g. nurse-initiated telephone call from the day surgery unit 24 hours after surgery and the establishment of telephone helplines (Kempe and Gelazis 1985, Kleinbeck and Hoffart 1994, Lewin and Razis 1995, De Jesus et al. 1996, Wedderburn et al. 1996, Willis et al. 1997, Heseltine and Edlington 1998, MacAndie and Bingham 1998, Challands et al. 2000, Horvath 2003). In an in-depth study by Donoghue et al. (1995), data collection partially involved a telephone interview during the postoperative period. The telephone interview was viewed in itself to be a positive experience for patients as the study states: 'There seemed to be a therapeutic factor embedded within the interview process for some women' (Donoghue et al. 1995, p. 176). In addition, some day-surgery units have a telephone service where patients can initiate the calls. In an audit of an unlimited telephone access line after day surgery over a 12-month period (Mukumba et al. 1996), the most frequent reason for contact (40%) was for further information. The second largest group was 16% for pain management.

Increasingly, as new surgical techniques are introduced into day surgery, the telephone is becoming a primary source for patient communication. In a randomized controlled trial, 60 patients scheduled for hand surgery underwent the procedure using an axillary plexus blockade (Rawal et al. 2002). After the procedure, the axillary plexus catheter was connected to an elastomeric, disposable 'homepump', containing 100 ml of either 0.125% bupivacaine or 0.125% ropivacaine. When patients experienced any pain while at home, they could self-administer 10 ml of the drug via a patient-controlled analgesia device. The aim of the study was to compare the effectiveness of 100 ml 0.125% bupivacaine versus 0.125% ropivacaine for pain relief. Although the patients recorded some data, e.g. level and degree of pain experienced, a 24-hour telephone call was made to enquire about progress and offer advice. Although patient satisfaction was high, numbness and persistent motor function block were problematic, e.g. patients could not use an arm effectively. Nevertheless, the telephone call was viewed as an essential monitoring tool. In an earlier study to evaluate the progress of 40 patients recovering from day-case laparoscopic cholecystectomy, all patients received a visit by a district nurse during the first postoperative night and for a further 2 days (Singleton et al. 1996). Patients were also telephoned on the first postoperative day with an enquiry about their experience of pain, nausea and satisfaction with care. In addition, they were contacted via telephone 2 weeks later by an anaesthetist to ask about pain relief, antiemetic use and the need for community support services. Of the patients 50% were mobile on the first postoperative day, 42% required a carer for an average of 2 days and 79% rated their management as 'very satisfactory'.

Conversely, in a similar study to examine the experiences of 101 patients after laparoscopic cholecystectomy (Blatt and Chen 2003), 20% of patients were readmitted and 22% stated that they would have preferred an overnight stay. Problems occurred because patients were unhappy with the ward and with the care and treatment provided by the nursing staff. However, an inpatient surgical ward was used for this study and not a dedicated day-surgery unit, i.e. day-case patients on an inpatient ward. The 80% of patients who were successfully discharged home the same day as their surgery were telephoned during the first evening and again the following morning by nursing staff. It was recommended that this telephone contact was a sufficient source of help and advice, and thereby there was no need for any additional community staff involvement. Likewise, in a small survey after nasal surgery (Agha et al. 2004) many patients stated that they would have preferred a hospital visit after the day of surgery as a means of checking progress or a telephone call the following day from the day-surgery unit because 22% of patients had to seek help and support from primary health-care professionals as a result of bleeding or infection.

Many studies have examined the involvement of the GP and district nurse after day-surgery intervention because it is widely assumed that the increase in day surgery has increased the workload for such community health-care professionals (Russell et al. 1977). In a survey by Kennedy (1995), 93% of the patients, although having undergone a moderate surgical procedure and general anaesthesia, did not seek community-based help during the first 3 postoperative days. Birch and Miller (1994) found that only 19% of patients had contacted their GP within the first 2 weeks, and in an audit by King (1989) it was documented that only 5% of day-surgery patients required help from the community health-care professionals during the first 48 hours. A survey by Wedderburn et al.

(1996), using a very brief questionnaire, established that 19% of day-surgery patients had to visit their GP at least once regarding pain or wound management. In an Australian survey by Singleton et al. (1996), it was revealed that 21% of patients contacted their GP within the first 2 weeks about pain management or wound care, and the district nurses were required to visit patients an average of two or three times in the post-operative period. In a further audit, it was discovered that 18% of patients had visited their GP for either a medical certificate or wound care advice (Woodhouse et al. 1998). However, GPs were also included in the survey and 70% stated that day surgery had not caused a significant increase in their workload. An audit by Thomas and Hare (1987, p. 447) reported that GPs were satisfied with day surgery and gave 'wholly favourable comments'. Many patients remained self-sufficient although a number of patients contacted their GP or community nurse for additional help or information.

In a more recent study by MacAndie and Bingham (1998), the GPs of patients who had undergone nasal surgery were sent a questionnaire to gauge their involvement with patient care in the postoperative period. The study recommended the improvement of information, analgesia provision, sick leave certificate provision and the provision of a telephone helpline. A further study also highlighted the issue of sick leave certification, stating that an insufficient recovery period was given on the medical certificates issued by the hospital (Cox and O'Connell 2003). Consequently, many women thought that they were experiencing problems longer than the doctors had expected which led to concern over their progress. Information about what is considered 'normal' symptoms of recovery were lacking, although the majority (88%) were glad to have had day surgery. In a study to compare inpatient with day-case patient workload placed on the primary care staff, Lewis and Bryson (1998) collected data from patients admitted to a local hospital for elective surgery, i.e. day surgery and inpatient surgery. It was documented that 74% of GP house calls were for unexpected patient events after both inpatient and day-case surgery. In addition, 14% of all district nurse visits were for unexpected patient events. The most common contact with GPs and district nurses was therefore about unexpected patient events. 'Problems relating to the operation wound (infection and bleeding) were the most frequent reason for unplanned contact with the health care team and accounted for 45% of all recorded unexpected events' (Lewis and Bryson 1998, p. 202). Visits to day-surgery patients were deemed to be very low with inpatients requiring the highest number of visits. The study therefore suggested that the present level of day-surgery activity does not create a greater workload for primary care and community health-care services, although this could change with the further expansion of day surgery.

LIVERPOOL JOHN MOORES UNIVERSITY
LEARNING SERVICES

Conversely, in an extensive survey by Kong et al. (1997) support for the increased demands placed on GPs as a result of day surgery is provided. About 1800 questionnaires were sent to patients who had been treated by the local day-surgery unit over a 6-month period: 16% ($n = 247$) of patients consulted their GP after day surgery – the main reason being pain management. The majority who visited their GP did so within the first 24 hours of surgery whereas the rest visited between 1 and 7 days. The study concludes by stating that 'An increase in workload for general practitioners is inevitable when more ambitious procedures are performed on less fit patients on a day case basis' (Kong et al. 1997, p. 294). These sentiments are reiterated in other day-surgery studies, e.g. as more complex surgical procedures are undertaken on a greater number of day-surgery patients, the level of community activity concerning day surgery patients will inevitably increase (Singleton et al. 1996, Jarrett 1997).

A number of studies have specifically examined the workload for district nurses during the rise in the level of day-surgery activity. In an early study (Ruckley et al. 1980), 118 district nurses were surveyed to gauge the effects of day surgery on their workload. Preoperative visits were favoured by 86% of nurses to give advice, help establish a relationship and assess the home environment for postoperative care. However, 25% of nurses stated that such intervention had increased their workload. In a study to determine the feasibility, patient acceptability and potential safety of tonsillectomy in adults within day surgery, 25% of the sample of patients ($n = 50$) were telephoned during the postoperative period (Mehanna et al. 2001). Of this number 82% reported they would have day surgery again, although implicit within this study was a visit from a day-surgery liaison nurse who visited all the patients during the first 24 hours. In a Canadian study of a new procedure to day surgery (shoulder surgery), four patients were sent home with a brachial plexus blockade infusion pump for pain management which administered 0.2% ropivacaine (patient-controlled analgesia) (Nielsen et al. 2003). A day-surgery liaison nurse, together with the anaesthetist, visited patients once a day for 2–3 days. However, the anaesthetist visited only because this was a new surgical procedure. Patients were also telephoned at 24 hours, 48 hours, 72 hours and 7 days. As there were no complications associated with the local anaesthetic or catheter use, it is suggested that considerable cost savings can be achieved by the use of this method of anaesthesia and pain management. However, the visit from a day-surgery liaison nurse may become an inevitable and much-desired aspect of such future surgical intervention. Similarly, in a further study of a relatively new day-surgery procedure (haemorrhoidectomy) (Hunt et al. 1999), 86% of patients were very satisfied with day surgery, although a registered nurse visited all patients after discharge with some patients requiring nine separate visits.

A number of studies have suggested that improved information provision about what to expect after day surgery would reduce patient need to contact the primary health-care professionals. In a postal survey of 244 patients by Willis et al. (1997) a significant correlation between information and satisfaction was established. Of this sample, 27% consulted their GP, with 78% of this number arranging a visit for sick-notes, sutures out, etc. 'The bulk of the primary care workload was in the form of a visit to the GP or a treatment room nurse' (Willis et al. 1997, p. 73). It is therefore suggested that much of the work would have been carried out regardless of any day-surgery increase, i.e. changing surgical practices in the form of earlier discharge from hospital had increased the workload and not merely the increase in day surgery as such. Conversely, in a survey by Michaels et al. (1992) the attention required by patients undergoing inpatient surgery was compared with that needed by patients undergoing day-case surgery. Employing a single-page questionnaire, it was documented that day-surgery patients required more medical attention after discharge. Likewise, in studies by the Royal College of Surgeons of England and East Anglia Regional Health Authority (1995) and Willis et al. (1997), almost half of the day-surgery patients required help from one community health-care agency.

As a result of changing surgical practices and the discharge of patients from day-case beds, the lack of information and minimal collaboration between community services and local ambulatory surgery units have been perceived as problematic (Robaux et al. 2002). GPs were largely not informed about pain management protocols and, despite experiencing severe pain, patients did not take their prescribed medication. In a brief survey undertaken by Oxfordshire Community Health Care Trust, closer collaboration between the day-surgery units and the Trust was recommended in order to improve communication once patients have been discharged from hospital (James 2000). In an audit to determine the processing of patient information between day-surgery units and community services after day surgery considerable differences were documented (Gui et al. 1999). It took an average of 73 days for the community services to receive a patient discharge summary sheet (range 1–512 days). Most patients were therefore fully recovered before the community services were even formally informed of the surgical treatment undertaken. In a survey of 40 GPs and 45 district nurses, an increase in workload was not deemed to have arisen from the increase in the level of day-surgery activity (Kelly et al. 1998). However, the minimal level of communication between hospital and community was a challenging issue because only 67% of community services received a final discharge letter and this was 2 weeks after the patient had been discharged from the day-surgery unit. In addition, both GPs and district nurses desired training about current surgical techniques employed in day surgery, together with common post-operative complications.

In summary, recovery from day surgery has given rise to many issues, e.g. pain management, patient recovery behaviour and community health involvement. Pain management is a considerable issue and a small but significant number of patients experience a high level of pain during the first 24–48 hours after day surgery. Accurate postoperative assessment and pain management protocols have been strongly recommended, e.g. use of prepacked analgesia together with NSAIDs. In addition, patients should be contacted by telephone 24–48 hours after surgery to enquire about their recovery pattern. In turn, this may also reduce the number of occasions patients need to contact their community health-care team because most such patient contacts concern pain management, wound infection and sickness certification. A small number of patients appear to avoid medical advice and drive their car, drink alcohol or are home alone after day surgery for the first 24 hours. However, the lack of information and subsequent lack of knowledge for the correct course of action to be taken in the event of an unforeseen circumstance dominate the recovery behaviour for many patients. The lack of information provided for carers has also been highlighted as a challenging issue. Finally, the increase in primary health-care team involvement as a result of the increase in day surgery has received mixed reviews. However, it appears to be generally accepted that, if the level of day surgery continues to grow together with a surgical population who possess increased co-morbidities, this situation may change (Kuusniemi et al. 1999, Ansell and Montgomery 2004, Cook et al. 2004, Watt-Watson et al. 2004).

Conclusion

A review of the literature revealed the satisfaction within day surgery to be very high although five main themes emerged and relate to preassessment and patient teaching, information provision, and patient experiences on the day of surgery and recovery. Within preassessment and patient teaching, there was a strong requirement for the establishment of preassessment clinics to increase patient contact time, improve communication and help allay fears. Day surgery is highly reliant on good medical selection and attendance at the preassessment clinic is therefore viewed as very positive for both patient and health-care providers. Dedicated day-surgery units continue to be regarded as more effective because patients are less likely to experience cancelled operations and are more likely to be discharged from the day-surgery unit as planned.

Information provision is major issue for day surgery because virtually every aspect of the patient's experience is influenced by information provision. The influence of information provision cannot be over-emphasized. A general lack of information was a common element, especially within mixed day-surgery facilities, e.g. day-surgery patients within inpatient wards. However, not all patients wanted the same level of information, because some were made more anxious when provided with too much information and others more anxious with too little information. If patients are to care for themselves effectively during the pre- and postoperative phases, the correct level of information provision is essential. Pre- and postoperative nurse-initiated telephone services have the ability to improve communication and videotaped presentations have enjoyed some success as an alternative means of information provision. However, the preoperative visit where written information can be provided and questions answered by the nurse remains the optimum method of communication.

Patients' experiences of day surgery were, in the vast majority of cases, very positive. Most patients want day surgery because the interruption to their lifestyle is minimal and the inconvenience of many hours spent waiting or recovering in a hospital bed avoided. Nevertheless, there are challenges to the patient experience. A great deal of recovery now takes place at home and the instant access to help and advice once available to the traditional surgical patient has been lost. Improved information provision to facilitate home recovery may now be urgently required. Information provision designed to aid recovery and provide explanations about the handling of perceived problems at home was strongly recommended. Some patients encountered events for which they felt unprepared, because they had not been informed of what to do should such an unforeseen event occur. Unforeseen events caused many problems for patients struggling to regain full fitness as a result of the limited information available, e.g. how best to proceed in the event of an unforeseen occurrence. Trial-and-error learning frequently took place, therefore, because patients were uncertain of how best to proceed. In addition, unforeseen events contributed to the increased contact with community health-care professionals. The opportunity to speak with a health-care professional from the hospital or day-surgery unit was of considerable benefit. The lack of privacy was a common theme for many patients and this complaint has spanned almost two decades. However, the interaction and relationship established with the nurse in the brief time available were viewed as one of the most positive experiences within the day-surgery unit. Although the time was brief the interpersonal skills of the nurse and the continued contact with a familiar nurse were of great benefit.

Recovery at home from day surgery has given rise to a number of other related issues, e.g. pain management, patient recovery behaviour and community health involvement. Pain management is a considerable issue and accurate postoperative assessment and pain management protocols have been strongly recommended. This was a particular problem for gynaecological patients because ineffective pain management generated much dissatisfaction and increased anxiety. This may be indicative of a lack of adequate preparation and information provision. A small number of patients do not follow medical advice although the lack of information and subsequent lack of knowledge for the correct course of action to be taken in the event of an unforeseen circumstance dominate. The lack of information provided for carers and an increase in primary health-care team involvement have also received much attention. It is broadly accepted that, as the level of day surgery grows and patients with co-morbidities feature more widely, the need for greater community health-care resources will increase. The number of patients at home caring for themselves and attempting to gain a full recovery with limited information is clearly evident. If in the future additional inpatient surgery is to be converted into day-case surgery, the need for improved information provision will be a pressing issue. Moreover, the continued expansion of day surgery clearly depends on willing and able laypeople to care for their relatives/friends. This is frequently at some financial and emotional expense to themselves. In such an uneasy domestic situation a dearth of information provision may seek only to exacerbate such problems.

Summary

- Effective day surgery depends greatly on accurate patient assessment and selection. This can be most effectively achieved within a nurse-led preassessment clinic.
- Dedicated day-surgery units are deemed to be more effective and efficient than inpatient day-surgery facilities.
- The lack of adequate information or an adequate level of information is a considerable source of dissatisfaction to many patients. Not only is this the most central patient issue but information provision influences virtually all other aspects of patients' experiences. Effective information provision must therefore be positioned at the core of any effective preoperative psychoeducational programme of care for modern, elective surgery.
- Patients' experiences on the day of surgery are broadly good. However, issues of privacy, lack of knowledge and accessing the day-surgery units remain problematic.
- For a small but significant number of patients, pain management after day surgery can be a considerable issue. Effective protocols must therefore be

developed and followed in order that all patients exper
pain, nausea and vomiting.
- Once discharged some patients require continued support in th.
  telephone contact, a day-surgery liaison nurse visit or a visit to the p.
  health-care team. When communication between the day-surgery unit ana .
  patient continues for 24–48 hours, contact with the primary health-care team is
  diminished.
- As the level of day-surgery activity increases the need for day-surgery liaison
  nurse visits may increase because the primary health-care team may have
  insufficient knowledge and expertise to assist patient recovery. This may be the
  case especially when new procedures are undertaken using different forms of
  pain management.
- The influence of satisfactory information provision cannot be over-emphasized.

Further reading

Cahill, H. and Jackson, I. (1997) Day Surgery: Principles and nursing practice. London:
　Baillière Tindall.
Hodge, D. (1999) Day Surgery: A nursing approach. London: Churchill Livingstone.
Malster, M. and Parry, A. (2000) Day surgery. In: Manley, K. and Bellman, L (eds), Surgical
　Nursing – Advancing practice. London: Churchill Livingstone, pp. 286–310.
Markanday, L. (1997) Day Surgery for Nurses. London: Whurr.
Penn, S., Davenport, H.T., Carrington, S. and Edmondson, M. (1996) Principles of Day Surgery.
　London: Blackwell Science.

Websites

Association of Anaesthetists of Great Britain and Ireland: www.aagbi.org
Patient information:

　　www.transformationstrategies.co.uk
　　www.informedhealthonline.org
　　www.cfah.org/factsoflife

Royal College of Anaesthetists: www.rcoa.ac.uk
Royal College of Surgeons: www.rcseng.ac.uk

Chapter 3

Patient anxiety and elective surgery

Patient anxiety

To establish recommendations confidently for effective psychological management that is fit for a new era of surgical intervention, a thorough evaluation of patient experiences of anxiety when undergoing modern elective surgery is required. Again, as highlighted in Chapter 2, few recommendations fit for the twenty-first century can be confidently made without an evaluation of patient experiences. A separate evaluation is required because:

(1) a large number of studies have examined the issue
(2) anxiety before day surgery is a considerable issue for many patients
(3) the current recommended interventions to aid anxiety management require full discussion.

Studies between 1980 and 2004 (aside from a few classic studies) directly concerning patients' anxiety before intermediate surgery, i.e. excluding studies about major surgery (principally cardiac surgery) or surgery for a malignancy, will be considered in this section. In addition, this overview deals only with studies that embrace surgical intervention, i.e. not invasive medical procedures or investigations. During the early 1980s day surgery began to expand dramatically and highly relevant studies therefore began to appear during this period. Anxiety management strategies extracted from studies beyond 1980, which principally employ inpatients undergoing traditional surgical techniques, e.g. extensive surgical wounds, extended hospital admissions, etc., are no longer appropriate for modern, elective, day-surgery practices (Mitchell 2003b). Although such a wide search inevitably embraces some studies in which traditional surgery has been employed, day-surgery studies receive greater prominence. From the literature three main themes concerning patient anxiety emerged: anxiety-provoking events, anxiety and safe anaesthesia, and anxiety management.

Anxiety-provoking events

Anxiety experienced by patients undergoing hospitalization for surgery has been viewed as a normal human response to a stressful event (Royal College of Surgeons of England and Royal College of Psychiatrists 1997, Ridner 2004):

> One can understand the apprehension of the best prepared patients before an operation: they not only allow a surgeon they have met only briefly to explore their body with no guarantee of a successful outcome, but also accept a degree of scarring and discomfort. Indeed, it would be unusual not to be anxious about the prospect of surgery and all that is involved in the preparation for and recovery from an operation.
>
> Royal College of Surgeons of England
> and Royal College of Psychiatrists (1997, p. 1)

Studies over five decades have established that many patients are indeed fearful before surgery and four recurring aspects have commonly emerged (see Chapter 4). These aspects are the anaesthetic (commonly the main aspect concerned with waking during surgery or not waking up after surgery), followed by the possible pain and discomfort, the operation itself and being unconsciousness (Egbert et al. 1964, Ramsay 1972, Ryan 1975, Male 1981, Johnston 1987, McCleane and Watters 1990, Mitchell 1997, Chew et al. 1998, McGaw and Hanna 1998, Calvin and Lane 1999, Costa 2001) (Figure 3.1). Studies have also suggested that anxiety has not

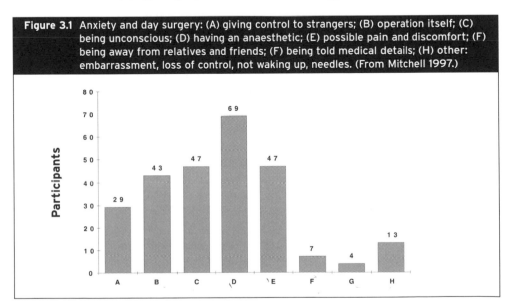

Figure 3.1 Anxiety and day surgery: (A) giving control to strangers; (B) operation itself; (C) being unconscious; (D) having an anaesthetic; (E) possible pain and discomfort; (F) being away from relatives and friends; (F) being told medical details; (H) other: embarrassment, loss of control, not waking up, needles. (From Mitchell 1997.)

diminished with the advent of modern day surgery (Caldwell 1991a, Mitchell 1997, 2000); indeed it may even be increasing because many patients become anxious about the wait on the day of surgery (Cobley et al. 1991, Mitchell 2000) (Figure 3.2).

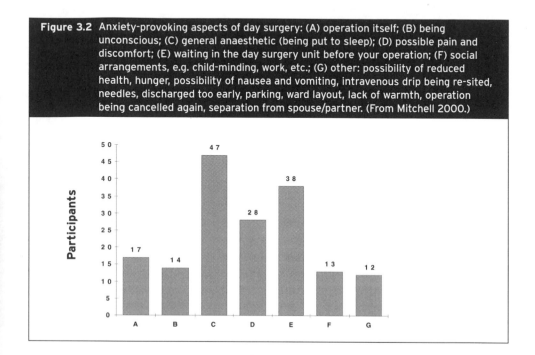

Figure 3.2 Anxiety-provoking aspects of day surgery: (A) operation itself; (B) being unconscious; (C) general anaesthetic (being put to sleep); (D) possible pain and discomfort; (E) waiting in the day surgery unit before your operation; (F) social arrangements, e.g. child-minding, work, etc.; (G) other: possibility of reduced health, hunger, possibility of nausea and vomiting, intravenous drip being re-sited, needles, discharged too early, parking, ward layout, lack of warmth, operation being cancelled again, separation from spouse/partner. (From Mitchell 2000.)

Conversely, a few studies have demonstrated patients' desire for general anaesthesia rather than local or regional anaesthesia (Gnanalingham and Budhoo 1998, Rees and Tagoe 2002). The dislike of being conscious, needle phobia and previous adverse experiences of local anaesthesia are common reasons provided. It has therefore been suggested that patients with low-trait anxiety are more suitable for local/regional anaesthesia than high-trait anxiety individuals because they have a greater ability to preserve their emotional stability during stressful events (Papanikolaou et al. 1994). In one study 162 patients were surveyed in order to determine the causes of preoperative anxiety (Voulgari et al. 1994). Although reporting of the causes of anxiety was limited, 10% of patients were anxious for several days postoperatively and 16% were also depressed during the postoperative period. Personality traits, e.g. an anxious predisposition, were put forward as the most probable cause for such a response. In a similar survey (Zvara et al. 1994), 200 day-surgery patients were asked to note their main concerns about anaesthesia. Of most concern was the method of induction and the anaesthetic drugs to be used. The second concern involved the possible side effects followed by the length of time to recover. It was suggested that such details could therefore form the basis of the information provided by the anaesthetist to the patient on the day of surgery.

Female patients have been consistently reported to experience a greater level of anxiety before surgery in comparison to male patients (Wolfer and Davies 1970, Nyamathi and Kashiwabara 1988, Van Wijk and Smalhout 1990, Shevde and Panagopoulos 1991, Wicklin and Forster 1994, Butler et al. 1996, Shafer et al. 1996, Caumo et al. 2001, Nishimori et al. 2002, Karanci and Dirik 2003). In a study (Badner et al. 1990) to establish a possible link between anxiety 12 hours before surgery and anxiety on the day of surgery, 84 patients were surveyed. Anxiety was revealed to be higher in female patients and novice patients. In addition, anaesthetists were deemed to be poor predictors of anxiety within the time frame available, i.e. brief visit 12 hours before surgery. However, no additional intervention for the anxious patient was suggested. In a day-surgery study employing 124 patients undergoing local anaesthesia (Birch et al. 1993), the Hospital Anxiety and Depression (HAD) questionnaire (Zigmond and Snaith 1983) was administered together with a visual analogue scale (VAS) for anxiety during the postoperative period. These data from day-surgery patients were then compared with data from general surgery inpatients and no significant differences in anxiety were established. However, it was again demonstrated that female and novice patients experienced greater anxiety, although not at a significant level. It is suggested that the administration of premedication may help patients manage their anxiety more effectively.

Several studies have attempted to examine specific anxiety-provoking events (Cobley et al. 1991, Jelicic and Bonke 1991, Calvin and Lane 1999, Canonico et al. 2003). A mask placed over the face during induction of anaesthesia can give rise to considerable anxiety because of the real or perceived sensation of claustrophobia associated with any type of mask (Oordt 2001). In addition, enduring apprehension can arise from previous experiences of the facemask (Moerman et al. 1992). However, in a day-surgery study of 190 patients (van den Berg 2003) about induction of anaesthesia patients were asked if they preferred needle induction or 'breathing a new anaesthetic gas – sevoflurane – via a fruit-scented mask'. Intravenous needle induction was chosen by 26% and inhalation (mask) induction by 53%, with 22% having no preference. Therefore, the majority of patients (75%) either had no preference for induction of anaesthesia or preferred a mask. However, 49% of all patients requested a premedicant to help manage their anxiety.

To determine what events surgical patients found most distressing (with particular reference to denture removal), Cobley et al. (1991)

studied 124 inpatients undergoing general anaesthesia. The five most distressing events were revealed to be waiting to be collected for theatre, not being allowed to drink, not being allowed to wear dentures, entering the theatre and being taken on a trolley to theatre. Women were significantly more distressed than men at having to remove their dentures. It was therefore recommended that dentures could be worn to the operating theatre. Jelicic and Bonke (1991) surveyed 40 inpatients in an effort to determine the possible difference in anxiety between voluntary and non-voluntary surgery, e.g. reduction (voluntary) and general surgery (non-voluntary). Using just the State–Trait Anxiety Inventory (STAI – Spielberger et al. 1983), a significant difference was established between the two groups, e.g. breast reduction patients were less anxious. However, the survey states that it is most unlikely that this was the sole reason because only the level of anxiety was measured and not the specific cause.

In a survey by Calvin and Lane (1999), a slightly different approach to the study of preoperative anxiety was undertaken, although its rationale is not clearly determined, e.g. anxiety and its association with the adult stages of development. STAI (Spielberger et al. 1983) and Mishel Uncertainty in Illness Scale (MUIS – Mishel 1981) were employed as subjective measures of anxiety and ill-health. Moderate levels of uncertainty and anxiety were recognized in all patients, although no differences between the adult stages of development were established. Increased communication and programmes of psychoeducational management were, however, recommended. In a retrospective study of day-surgery patients by Canonico et al. (2003), data from 2032 surgical patients were examined to determine the feasibility of day surgery for older patients, e.g. patients over 65 years. Of the study sample, 98 patients aged over 65 years were treated in a day-surgery facility and 1036 were treated as inpatients. No significant differences were established between the over-65s and under-65s. However, anxiety about not wishing to undergo day surgery was identified as an issue for the over-65s in 18% of patients – because of the balance between wanting a short hospital stay and the fear of possibly being unwell at home and far from medical attention. Canonico et al. (2003) conclude that adequate preassessment is required in order to obtain good results because many older patients have concurrent pathologies.

In summary, for many decades preoperative anxiety has been strongly associated with four main aspects: the anaesthetic, possible pain and discomfort, the operation and being unconsciousness. However, a fifth aspect is emerging with the advent of modern-day surgery – the preoperative wait. Nevertheless, the anaesthetic remains the most anxiety-provoking event because of the thought of either waking during surgery or not waking afterwards. Conversely, some patients prefer to have general anaesthesia because of their anxiety about medical equipment, needles or past poor experiences. Female patients have repeatedly either been willing to report more anxiety or actually experienced more anxiety. Finally, studies undertaken with older adults have established no differences in the degree of anxiety, although undergoing day surgery and being at home that night far from medical attention were identified as stressful.

Anxiety and safe anaesthesia

The measurement of preoperative anxiety in modern, elective surgery is becoming very difficult to administer, mainly as a result of the imposed time restrictions (Mitchell 2004). Many measures of anxiety have been used and are available, although their widespread use in clinical practice is very limited (Volicer 1973, Volicer and Bohannon 1975, Swindale 1989, Shuldham et al. 1995, Moerman et al. 1996, Mitchell 1997, Reid 1997, Krohne et al. 2000, Boker et al. 2002). Several reviews of the literature in previous decades have reported a plethora of studies employing clinical measures to gauge psychological recovery, e.g. length of hospital stay, analgesics consumed while in hospital, level of postoperative mobility, blood cortisol level, etc. (Wilson 1981, Mathews and Ridgeway 1984, Vogele and Steptoe 1986, Miller et al. 1989, Rothrock 1989, Suls and Wan 1989, Johnston and Vogele 1993). However, in modern, elective, intermediate day surgery, such methods of gauging recovery and anxiety are now obsolete and other measures are required because patients remain in hospital only for a very brief period (Salmon et al. 1986, Salmon 1993, Munafo and Stevenson 2003).

As a result, in a small study to examine anxiety levels in hospitalized patients undergoing laparoscopic cholecystectomy (Storm et al. 2002), the skin conductance of 11 patients was monitored intraoperatively, the purpose being that increased sympathetic nervous activity is detectable as electrical changes within the skin. Palmar electrodes were employed to monitor anxiety at specific intraoperative intervals. Such monitoring revealed positive correlations between the amplitude of skin conductance, an increase in adrenaline (epinephrine – a hormone that plays a central role in the short-term physiological stress reaction) levels and an increase in blood pressure. Therefore, from a physiological perspective, anxiety had increased because the biochemical changes associated with the 'fight-or-flight response' were mirrored by the rise in skin conductance. It was recommended that such intraoperative monitoring could be used to help gauge intraoperative anxiety. In an earlier study (Miluk-Kolasa et al. 1994), saliva was sampled for a rise in cortisol (corticosteroid hormone produced by the adrenal glands in response to a stressful situation).

Thirty-four inpatients were divided into three groups: (1) patients not awaiting surgery; (2) patients awaiting surgery; and (3) patients awaiting surgery who were randomly selected to undergo music therapy. Music was played via headphones for 60 minutes on the day before surgery for group 3 only. Saliva samples were then taken from all groups at six intervals during the day before surgery. Both groups 2 and 3 experienced a sharp increase in cortisol 15 minutes after being informed of their surgery. Although the music group experienced a more rapid decline in their level of cortisol, no significant differences were established between the groups, i.e. music therapy did not aid anxiety management.

The focus on the physiological monitoring of anxiety is indicative of the medical concern about the impact of anxiety on safe anaesthesia. Therefore, a number of studies have examined patient anxiety because of its potential to influence safe anaesthesia (McCleane and Watters 1990, Lydon et al. 1998, Daoud and Hasan 1999, Maranets and Kain 1999, Hahm et al. 2001). Daoud and Hasan (1999) observed 94 day-case patients to evaluate the effects of anxiety on induction of anaesthesia. It was revealed that an increase in anxiety was associated with an increased time for the jaw to relax, a higher incidence of coughing and thereby more anaesthetic interventions during insertion of the laryngeal airway. However, although demonstrating a link between anxiety and an increase in anaesthetic interventions, no recommendations about anxiety management were suggested. In a similar study by Maranets and Kain (1999), 57 inpatients undergoing general anaesthesia were surveyed. Using the STAI (Spielberger et al. 1983), the Monitor–Blunter Style Scale (MBSS) (Miller 1987), and monitoring the depth of anaesthesia, an increase in STAI anxiety was associated with an increased intraoperative anaesthetic requirement, e.g. patients with a predisposition to anxiety required increased anaesthesia. Previous poor experiences of light anaesthesia (although rare; Myles et al. 2000) can also have a considerable psychological impact (Schwender et al. 1998, Spitellie et al. 2002). However, because they are so rare it has been suggested that they may not warrant additional intervention (Sandin et al. 2000). Nevertheless, such events are unfortunately commonly reported in the media, reinforcing such negative views within society, e.g. scare, scandal and breakthrough are the three main health-care narratives constantly reported by the media (Hawkes 2004).

In an experimental design by Lydon et al. (1998), 21 inpatients were observed in order to examine the association between anxiety and gastric emptying. This was undertaken because it was believed that gastric emptying could be reduced when a patient was experiencing an increase in anxiety. Patients fasted preoperatively for 8 hours and then a paracetamol solution was ingested. Intravenous blood was taken at certain intervals over a 90-minute period to gauge the absorption rate of the paracetamol solution. It was concluded that gastric emptying was not adversely delayed by anxiety, e.g. the highly anxious patient did not experience slower emptying of the stomach. However, it is emphasized that, as a liquid preparation was used, the conclusions could relate only to liquids. Similar, non-significant results were also reached in a comparable study using 40 dental day-surgery patients (Schwarz et al. 2002).

Hahm et al. (2001) studied 44 inpatients to determine whether clonidine (a premedicant) could minimize an increase in plasma adrenaline and thereby prevent a decrease in serum potassium (hypokalaemia can result from increased adrenaline and lead to life-threatening cardiac arrhythmias during general anaesthesia). Patients were randomly assigned preoperatively into two groups: (1) clonidine 300 μg 2 hours before induction of anaesthesia and (2) the same dose and administration of a placebo. The clonidine group had higher potassium levels immediately before induction and these levels were higher than the control group, although not significantly higher. However, the use of clonidine was recommended as a premedicant to avoid potential intraoperative hypokalaemia. McCleane and Watters (1990) surveyed 200 inpatients to determine the relationship between anxiety and serum potassium. Blood was taken 12 hours before surgery and again immediately before anaesthesia. Again, only modest, non-significant changes were established between serum potassium and anxiety. However, 60% of patients who received an anxiolytic premedication (temazepam 10–30 mg) and a visit from their anaesthetist 12 hours before surgery were significantly less anxious before surgery in comparison to the previous day. Therefore, a visit from the anaesthetist combined with the use of a premedicant helped reduce anxiety for most of the patients surveyed.

In summary, safe anaesthesia is of vital importance with any surgery. It is also the aspect of surgery that generates the greatest amount of apprehension. Anaesthetists are therefore very concerned with any aspect, such as anxiety, that has the potential to influence the smooth induction, maintenance and recovery from anaesthesia. However, mixed results have been achieved regarding the influence of anxiety over physiological processes. Muscle relaxation may be a problem although biochemical imbalance appears to be less so.

Anxiety management

Studies about the specific management of preoperative anxiety have been extensively investigated in four main areas: anxiolytic premedication, distraction, communication and hospital environment. Each aspect is examined in greater detail and the relevant studies discussed.

Anxiolytic premedication

In a review of the literature from 1980 to 1999 (Smith and Pittaway 2002) specifically concerning premedication in day-case surgery, it was revealed that premedication is not widely used in day-surgery practice. Such agents are not widely employed because (1) of fear of delayed discharge (benzodiazepines can have a slow onset and long duration), (2) day-case patients are required to remember important information on discharge, and (3) day-case patients are required to be able physically to walk out of the day-surgery facility. Smith and Pittaway (2002) identified 29 reports and 14 studies with data from 1263 patients. Although the three main drugs employed were benzodiazepines, β-adrenoceptor blockers and opioids, no difference was established in the discharge time between premedicated and non-premedicated patients. However, the authors add a note of caution because anaesthetic techniques and day-surgery practices have developed enormously over the given search period, i.e. 1980–1999. Therefore, inferences for current practice should be viewed with care.

Many patients experience anxiety before day surgery and a large number (49%) want management of their anxiety with an anxiolytic preparation (van den Berg 2003). In a Swedish study by Gupta et al. (1994) to evaluate satisfaction with day surgery and patient experience of anxiety, 290 patients were surveyed. Two simple questionnaires with mainly yes/no items were administered during both admission and the postoperative period: 62% of patients were nervous about their operation and almost 50% expressed a desire to have premedicant to relieve their anxiety. In addition, this number was not restricted to general anaesthesia patients because 27% were to undergo local or regional anaesthesia. As many patients experienced anxiety, recommendations were made about their care.

> Emphasis should be laid on relieving preoperative anxiety, and the problem of patients being sent home without a responsible adult should be looked at very closely. Written instructions should also be provided to the patient and this should also include the telephone number to be used in case of problems.
>
> Gupta et al. (1994, p. 112)

In a day-surgery study by Mackenzie (1989), 200 adult patients were assessed for anxiety levels on the day that their operation was booked and then again on the day of surgery. No gender differences were established on the day of booking surgery, although a significant difference was established on the day of the surgery, e.g. women were more anxious. In addition, patients undergoing surgery for the first time were very anxious:

> Anxiety scores of the 'novices' were greater than those of
> 'experienced' patients. Those with previously unpleasant experience
> displayed more anxiety than those who had had an uneventful
> experience.
>
> Mackenzie (1989, p. 440)

Moreover, anxiety level at the time of booking could accurately determine which patients would be more anxious on the day of surgery:

> The anxiety scores at booking were the prime determinants of the
> scores on the day of operation. Thus anxiety detected at the time of
> booking could alert medical staff to the need for reassurance, and if
> necessary anxiolytic pre-medication on the day of operation.
>
> Mackenzie (1989, p. 440)

In a survey also concerned with the use of premedication (Hyde et al. 1998), 184 inpatients were provided with a brief questionnaire to determine the required level of sedation and preferred preoperative activities. Light sedation was preferred by 54.1% of patients and listening to music or reading by 56.5%. Many preferred not to watch general videotaped presentations (62%) or a videotaped presentation about their operation (76.6%). Although a number preferred light sedation other patients preferred to be alert although distracted. The study therefore recommended that patients be provided with alternatives to mere sedation.

Two main aspects of anxiolytic premedication have been repeatedly examined, e.g. patient-controlled administration and the drugs employed. Two studies have investigated the possibility of patient-controlled premedication (Bernard et al. 1996, Murdoch and Kenny 1999). Bernard et al. (1996) randomly assigned two groups of day-surgery patients to receive a fixed dose of midazolam 4 mg (benzodiazepine) or a patient-controlled pump containing midazolam. No significant differences were established between the groups and, for the highly anxious patient, anxiety decreased whichever method was employed. Murdoch and Kenny (1999) studied 20 day-case patients all of whom received a patient-controlled anxiolytic premedication of propofol (intravenous sedative/anaesthetic induction agent). Although no control group was used for comparison, the postoperative satisfaction questionnaire revealed that all patients rated their care as excellent (70%) or good (30%). In a further day-surgery study to examine the effects of propofol on patient anxiety (Winwood and Jago 1993), 25 patients were randomly assigned into two groups. Group 1 received a propofol induction and group 2 received a Thiopental induction (barbiturate agent causing sedation). Anxiety fell in most patients in the postoperative period, although patients who had received propofol had significantly lower anxiety scores.

With regard to the sedative agents employed, the efficacy of diazepam (a benzodiazepine) on preoperative anxiety has been investigated with both day-case patients (Wittenberg et al. 1998, De Witte et al. 2002, Duggan et al. 2002) and inpatients (Wikinski et al. 1994, Martens-Lobenhoffer et al. 2001). In a day-case study of 202 patients, Wittenberg et al. (1998) randomly assigned patients into one of two groups: (1) oral diazepam 5 mg 30 minutes before surgery and (2) the same dose and timing of placebo. Both groups demonstrated an improvement in anxiety 30 minutes after surgery. However, again the diazepam group was significantly less anxious. Duggan et al. (2002) randomly assigned 60 day patients into three groups: (1) oral diazepam 0.1 mg/kg 60 minutes preoperatively, (2) oral diazepam 0.1 mg/kg 90 minutes preoperatively and (3) placebo premedicant. No significant differences were established when employing self-rated measures of anxiety and urinary cortisol monitoring. However, a significant difference in the level of catecholamines (adrenaline and noradrenaline/norepinephrine) was established between groups 1 and 3 (control), although not between groups 2 and 3. The results may therefore demonstrate some benefit for the reduction of anxiety in day-surgery patients who are prescribed oral diazepam 60 minutes before surgery.

In a study by De Witte et al. (2002) of 45 day-surgery patients undergoing general anaesthesia for laparoscopic gynaecological surgery, patient psychomotor performance and the side effects to alprazolam and midazolam (benzodiazepines) as premedicants were assessed. The study aimed to compare alprazolam and midazolam because an oral formulation of midazolam is not approved in certain countries. The patients were randomly assigned into one of three groups: (1) alprazolam 0.5 mg 60–90 minutes preoperatively, (2) midazolam 7.5 mg 60–90 minutes preoperatively and (3) placebo. Measures of anxiety were undertaken both pre- and postoperatively together with postoperative psychomotor skills, e.g. joining dots, matching numbers with symbols and clinical measures relating to anaesthesia. No difference in anxiety for any of the groups was established after discharge from the recovery area. Postoperatively, the group who had received no premedication was able to perform the psychomotor tests effectively in comparison to the other two groups. Learning and remembering were worse in the midazolam group because 33% remembered little about their time in the recovery room. Alprazolam was therefore recommended as an alternative to midazolam for anxiety reduction, although caution must be taken postoperatively because it may cause greater impairment of psychomotor function in the early postoperative period. In a study to examine the ability of propranolol 10 mg (β-blocking agent) to reduce anxiety (Mealy et al. 1996), 53 day-surgery patients were surveyed. Patients were randomly assigned into one of two groups: (1) propranolol 10 mg at 7.00am before admission and (2) same dose and timing of placebo. A VAS for pain and satisfaction and a HAD scale (Zigmond and Snaith 1983) were all completed before discharge and again the next morning (returned by post). No significant differences were established before discharge using physiological measures, although the propranolol group experienced significantly lower scores on the HAD scale. A low dose of propranolol on the morning of day-case surgery was therefore recommended to help reduce patients' anxiety.

Wikinski et al. (1994) randomly assigned 30 inpatients into two groups: (1) oral diazepam 10 mg 2 hours before surgery and (2) same dose and timing of placebo. Self-rated emotional measures (STAI – Spielberger et al. 1983 – and VAS) demonstrated no significant differences, although the mean arterial blood pressure was significantly lower in the diazepam group. In a further survey of 26 inpatients by Martens-Lobenhoffer et al. (2001), the oral midazolam absorption rate and personality traits were explored, the assumption being that patients with a predisposition towards raised anxiety, in such a situation, may have a slower gastric absorption rate. Patients were assigned to either the high-anxiety or the low-anxiety group with respect to their self-rated anxiety and personality scores. However, no significant differences were established between the two groups. In a similar study about absorption rate and premedication (Hosie and Nimmo 1991), 100 patients were enrolled to receive temazepam 30 mg (benzodiazepine) either in elixir or capsule form as a premedicant. Again, the individual level of anxiety had no influence on the absorption of the preparations. Using a researcher-designed questionnaire Leach et al. (2000) surveyed 116 inpatients about their anxiety: 45% of patients stated that they were anxious and that their anxiety varied depending on the type of surgery scheduled. In addition: 'Patients who had no prior surgery were more likely to be anxious than patients who had undergone surgical procedures in the past' (Leach et al. 2000, p. 31). However, patients having a premedication, although it had reduced their anxiety, still experienced some anxiety during the perioperative stages. The study therefore recommended an increase in information provision and alternative forms of anxiety management such as relaxation.

In summary, the above studies demonstrate the medical profession's considerable concern with safe and effective anaesthesia, and their customary employment of rigid, objective measures to obtain such evidence, e.g. physiological indices. Subsequently, the main treatment to emerge is frequently the maintenance of physiological equilibrium in order to avoid possible complications before and during anaesthesia. However, such an approach is very restrictive. First, the mere provision of a premedication agent is restricted to a select number of patients who have been perceived as highly anxious. Second, in the brief time available accurate assessment of all patients is unreliable. Third, such intervention will influence the physiological response to anxiety immediately only before anaesthesia, e.g. anxiety during the days before and after surgery will remain problematic. Finally, such intervention is not available to most day-surgery patients because premedication agents can delay discharge after surgery and are not widely employed. Therefore, although premedication is an effective method of preoperative anxiety reduction and preferred by many patients, its effectiveness in modern-day surgery is very limited.

Distraction

The second specific anxiety management issue concerns the employment of distracting interventions, e.g. listening to music, watching television, relaxing or having visitors. Such studies, for the purposes of this exposition, have been subdivided into three categories: (1) preoperative distraction techniques, (2) intraoperative distraction techniques and (3) recovery room distraction techniques.

Preoperatively

Music therapy, as a distracting technique within the preoperative period, has received considerable attention. Literature reviews concerning the value of music therapy in hospital itself suggest an overall positive influence, although various types of music were employed over different time periods that encompassed many aspects of nursing (Snyder and Chlan 1999, Biley 2000, Evans 2002). In a study by Hyde et al. (1998) concerning preferred preoperative activities, 184 inpatients admitted for elective surgery were surveyed. It was revealed that 54% wanted to be sleepy preoperatively whereas 72% preferred not to be asleep. Reading (57%), listening to music (57%) and chatting with other patients (40%) were the preferred activities. The physiological effects of listening to music before surgery were also evaluated using 100 inpatients (Miluk-Kolasa et al. 1996). On the day of surgery, after receipt of information about their operation, patients were randomly assigned into two groups: (1) listening to music via headphones for an hour before surgery and during recovery, and (2) routine care. Anxiety in both groups increased once the information about their surgery had been provided. However, no significant difference was established using physiological measures, e.g. blood pressure, heart rate, cardiac output, skin temperature and glucose levels. Augustin and Hains (1996) further evaluated the effectiveness of music on preoperative anxiety: 41 day-case patients were randomly assigned into two groups: (1) 15–20 minutes of listening to music of choice via headphones and (2) routine care. Patients in the experimental group had significantly lower heart rates immediately before surgery. However, there appeared to be an element of selection bias in the sample as the authors state: 'Some of the patients wanted to be aware of every-thing going on around them and they did not want to be distracted by listening to music' (Augustin and Hains 1996, p. 756).

In a similar study (Gaberson 1995) 46 day-surgery patients were ran-domly divided into three groups: (1) 20-minute music audiotape before surgery; (2) 20-minute comedy audiotape before surgery; and (3) no audiotape (control group). Although the patients who listened to music reported lower levels of anxiety, the difference was not significant. In two further day-surgery studies (Mok and Wong 2003, Lee et al. 2004), patients were randomized into two groups: (1) headphones with broad choice of music and (2) no music group. It was revealed that the experi-mental group (broad choice of music via headphones) was significantly less anxious, although it was acknowledged that it might not necessarily have been the music that helped and any distraction may have been equal-ly effective. In a slight variation (Wang et al. 2002), 93 day-surgery patients were randomly assigned into two groups: (1) music of choice via headphone for 30 minutes and (2) control group who also wore head-phones although with no music for 30 minutes. Patients who listened to 30 minutes of music of their own choice experienced lower self-reported anxiety than the control group. However, such results could have been obtained because the experimental group were being treated differently, i.e. Hawthorne effect.

Second, a number of studies have examined television watching (Friedman et al. 1992, Wicklin and Forster 1994). Friedman et al. (1992) observed the effects of television viewing on preoperative anxiety in 69 inpatients. Patients were randomly assigned into two groups: (1) televi-sion watching and (2) routine care. Only patients who were observed to spend more than an hour watching television were included. Using the STAI (Spielberger et al. 1983) the television-watching group were signifi-cantly less anxious than the control group. However, this may be somewhat biased because the more relaxed patients may choose to be dis-tracted more by viewing the television, i.e. these patients may have been less anxious irrespective of watching television. The researchers did not allocate the groups, and patients merely chose their individual activities. The assumption that anxiety reduction was merely the result of watching television may therefore be an erroneous one. In a day-surgery study by Wicklin and Forster (1994), 91 patients were divided into three groups

1 week before day surgery to view a videotaped presentation about their surgery. The videotaped presentations differed in their approach, e.g. factual approach and personal approach via patients' personal experiences. It was hypothesized that those patients who viewed the personal approach videotape programme would have lower levels of preoperative anxiety than those who viewed the factual videotape programme. However, no significant differences were established.

Third, in a related method to achieve lower anxiety, positive imagery has been examined. Eller (1999) conducted a review of the literature about the use of positive imagery in hospital. The review encompassed a wide range of hospital treatments and concluded: 'It appears that state anxiety may be amenable to modification with imagery techniques' (Eller 1999, p. 68). In a study of 51 inpatients undergoing abdominal surgery patients were randomly assigned into two groups: (1) listening to a 30-minute audiotape of positive ways in which they could deal with the problems they might encounter during hospitalization and (2) listening to background information about the hospital (Manyande et al. 1995). Although the experimental group expressed more positive sentiments, no significant differences in anxiety were established using physiological measures. In a further study to examine guided imagery (Tusek et al. 1997), 139 patients were randomly divided into two groups: (1) routine perioperative care and (2) listening to guided imagery tapes for 3 days before their surgical procedures, during anesthesia induction, intraoperatively and in the recovery room, and for 6 days after surgery. Although anxiety was determined to be lower in the experimental group, the difference again was not significant.

Fourth, the utility of relaxation techniques and the employment of hypnosis have also been reported. A group of 24 inpatients were randomly assigned into two groups: (1) taught by a clinical psychologist to use biofeedback to aid relaxation (use of positive self-talk, positive feelings of self-efficacy and pleasant images) and (2) routine care only (Wells et al. 1986). Although the experimental group had significant positive outcomes, the considerable extra attention provided to the experimental group may again have contributed to the more positive conclusions. In a complex study by Levin et al. (1987) to assess the effectiveness of two different relaxation methods, 40 female patients undergoing inpatient cholecystectomy were randomly divided into four groups: (1) experimental group receiving a tape-recording of a rhythmic breathing exercise, (2) a second experimental group receiving a tape-recording of a further relaxation technique, (3) an attention–distraction control group receiving a tape-recording of the history of the hospital and (4) a standard control group receiving routine perioperative care. No significant differences in pain or anxiety were established among the groups, although 'Subjects' responses to exit interviews suggest that some people find relaxation techniques very helpful for diminishing post-operative pain while others do not' (Levin et al. 1987, p. 470). In a day-surgery study to examine the impact of anxiety on intraoperative outcomes (Markland and Hardy 1993), 24 patients were divided into three conditions: (1) relaxation (21-minute relaxation tape), (2) attention (control) and (3) no-treatment control group. Both the relaxation group and the attention (control) group required significantly less time to induce anaesthesia and less anaesthetic agent was used to maintain anaesthesia. However, the study states that a reduction in anxiety could have resulted from the fact that the groups were merely 'distracted' rather than relaxed. Further inpatient studies have examined vigilant and avoidant coping styles and the use of different methods, e.g. guided relaxation, although they have not established differences (Daltroy et al. 1998, Miro and Raich 1999a, 1999b). One study employing acupuncture (Wang et al. 2001) established a significant difference in preoperative anxiety, although some of the patients used were to undergo surgery for suspected malignancy.

Preoperative hypnosis has been examined in two studies, both within the field of day surgery (Goldmann et al. 1988, Faymonville et al. 1997). In both studies patients were randomized to receive either hypnosis or routine care. Goldmann et al. (1988) established no differences between the groups although they concluded that patients required different levels of information. Conversely, Faymonville et al. (1997) established that the hypnosis group required significantly less sedation: their postoperative anxiety was lower, intraoperative control reported as higher, and comfort and satisfaction were higher. However, anxiety in the hypnosis group was significantly higher before surgery, e.g. these patients were much more anxious and may have appreciated additional psychological interventions because they were initially very anxious. Faymonville et al. (1997) also highlighted the issue of patients who catastrophize all events, e.g. have a tendency to display, focus on and exaggerate the negative aspects of the noxious situation, and thereby have a propensity to feel overwhelmed and unable to cope with or control the situation.

The final preoperative aspect frequently examined concerns the positive effects of a visitor, fellow patient, spouse or partner. Johnston (1982, p. 259) suggests that: 'The results show that other patients are more accurate in estimating the number of worries a patient has and tend to be more sensitive in detecting which worries a patient has than are nurses with responsibility for the patient.' She therefore goes on to suggest that relatives may have the time and the relationship to be more responsive to the patients' wishes and thereby act like 'therapists' towards the patient. In a study of 60 patients undergoing cholecystectomy, participants were randomized to receive reassuring information, self-care information or neutral information (description of a general hospital and admission with no specific information about the operation) (Hartsfield and Clopton 1985). No significant differences were established among the groups, although contact with visitors, including the researcher performing the interviews, led to a significant reduction in patient anxiety. Likewise, in a study to evaluate the effect of preoperative visits by theatre nurses on pre- and postoperative levels of anxiety (Martin 1996), a visit from a theatre nurse before surgery had a significantly positive influence on patient anxiety.

Intraoperatively
Three studies have examined the use of music immediately before surgery (Kaempf and Amodei 1989, Winter et al. 1994, Lepage et al. 2001). In a study of 62 inpatients undergoing gynaecological surgery by Winter et al. (1994), patients were randomly assigned into two groups in the surgical holding area: (1) music of their choice via headphones and (2) no music. Although no significant differences were established, the study recommends a choice of music for all patients to aid anxiety immediately before surgery. In a study by Lepage et al. (2001), 50 day-surgery patients undergoing spinal anaesthesia were randomly assigned, in a preoperative waiting area, to two groups: (1) listening to music of their choice via headphones and (2) routine care. During this period patient-controlled sedation (midazolam) was administered to all patients, although none had received any premedication. No significant difference in anxiety was established using self-rated questionnaires, although the experimental group required less midazolam to achieve the same relaxed state. The study therefore recommends that anxiety before day surgery could be managed in a non-pharmacological manner. In a very similar experimental study by Kaempf and Amodei (1989), a significant reduction in respirations was achieved in the experimental group, although researchers state that this may be of little clinical significance.

A number of studies have used headphones and music during surgical procedures under local anaesthesia (Steelman 1990, Stevens 1990, Heiser et al. 1997) and general anaesthesia (Nilsson et al. 2001). Although only one study established a significant difference between groups (Nilsson et al. 2001), music was broadly viewed as a positive means of distraction. Increasingly, technological advances in audiovisual equipment are expanding the range of devices available to aid patient distraction during local anaesthesia (Man et al. 2003). In the study by Man et al. (2003), an experimental design was employed to evaluate whether watching the playing of a compact disc intraoperatively via a liquid crystal display aided anxiety (similar to wearing a pair of glasses and earphones where the inside of the lenses provide the screen). Using the STAI (Spielberger et al. 1983) the experimental group were significantly less anxious than the control group (no intervention) immediately after the surgical procedure.

Two studies have specifically examined the noise level for the conscious patient in theatre (Cruise et al. 1997, Liu and Tan 2000). Liu and Tan (2000) discovered that during induction of anaesthesia the mean number of staff present was 6.6, of whom 2.7 need not have been present. Of the conversations during this period, 88% were not with the patient and not patient related. In the study by Cruise et al. (1997), there was no significant difference in patient satisfaction as a result of the noise heard via headphones, e.g. relaxing suggestions, white noise (normal level of noise in a quiet environment), operating room noise or relaxing music. The most satisfied patients were those who had experienced the relaxing music followed by the relaxing suggestions. In a similar experimental study (O'Neill 2002), again no differences were established between two groups of patients provided with music/no music at the end of their stay in the recovery room.

In a further study of the theatre environment and the conscious patient (Kennedy et al. 1992), 115 women experiencing elective caesarean section under regional anaesthesia were surveyed. Arrival at theatre was the most stressful aspect, although not necessarily because of the environment – the imminence of the surgical procedure dominated. Helplessness was a strong sensation although patients found the music, and the support of their partner and members of the theatre team, the most helpful aspects. Leinonen et al. (1996), in an extensive survey, uncovered similar results, e.g. the most effective anxiety-reducing aspect was the availability of nurses and their interpersonal skills. In this study, 246 inpatients were surveyed preoperatively and 158 surveyed postoperatively about their experiences of intraoperative care. Both pain and failure of the anaesthetic were the main causes of their anxiety; 60% of patients underwent local anaesthesia and were therefore not fully unconscious during the surgical procedure: 'the best experiences of care giving was the good quality of nursing care and the fact that they were available to the patient at all times.'

> In their open-ended responses, the patients said the best thing about their care had been the personnel (and particularly their professional competence, friendliness and sense of humour).
>
> Leinonen et al. (1996, p. 848)

In addition, mere handholding during a surgical procedure has been observed to be of benefit for day-surgery patients undergoing local anaesthesia for ophthalmic surgery (Moon and Cho 2001). However, selective sampling took place in this experiment, which could have resulted in biased reporting, e.g. only patients who were observed to be anxious received physical contact.

LIVERPOOL JOHN MOORES UNIVERSITY
LEARNING SERVICES

Some studies have also considered the well-being of relatives during surgery. In a study to survey the experience of 40 relatives during the period spent waiting while their family member was in theatre (Trimm 1997), a number of problem-focused and emotionally focused strategies were put forward for relatives to consider (Jalowiec et al. 1984) (see Chapter 5). Overall, relatives employed problem-focused coping strategies (using formal support systems and dealing directly with any problems) and broadly remained optimistic throughout. In a literature review (Dexter and Epstein 2001) of relatives' wishes for those undergoing day surgery, provision of an in-person progress report specific to the individuals' relatives was the most effective method. It was deemed that relatives became very anxious if a delay in proceedings occurred and, therefore, providing an approximate minimum–maximum time in theatre was recommended.

Postoperatively

In a study to examine the effect of visitors to the post-anaesthetic recovery unit, i.e. stage 1 recovery (Poole 1993), 40 inpatients, admitted on the day of surgery, were randomly assigned into two groups: (1) visitor for 15 minutes in the post-anaesthetic recovery unit (once vital signs were stable) and (2) no visitor; 75–80% of patients could recall their stay in the post-anaesthetic recovery unit the next day. In addition, the patients who received a visitor were significantly less anxious 24 hours postoperatively. The study therefore recommended that patients who wished to have visitors in the recovery room immediately after surgery should be granted their request. In a further postoperative experimental study (Shertzer and Keck 2001), 97 patients were assigned to one of two groups: (1) listening to music while staff kept extraneous noise at a minimum in the recovery room and (2) typical recovery room noise (the control group). When asked to recall aspects of comfort during their recovery room stay, the experimental group reported significantly less noise caused by staff voices, equipment and a greater perception of nurse availability.

In summary, a number of distraction techniques have appeared to aid patient anxiety management throughout the surgical experience. However, it is clear that not all patients require distraction and that what is a helpful distraction for one patient may not be suitable for another. Distraction has largely been employed because it is quick and simple, and provides time for the staff to undertake other essential tasks. However, such distracting techniques have not demonstrated improvements significant enough to warrant their more wide-scale adoption. Such techniques are limiting and very simplistic, e.g. switching on a television/radio, and clearly not all patients require distraction. Other more central issues in anxiety management in modern day surgery, e.g. information provision, may be of greater importance. In addition, such interventions may be considered to have little practical application because of the restrictions within the clinical environment, e.g. music via headphones, noise in theatre, visitors in the recovery room, hypnosis or acupuncture before surgery for all day-surgery patients.

Information provision

Many studies have endeavoured to deal with the issues surrounding information provision and anxiety. As can be viewed throughout this book, a major emphasis has been placed on information provision, largely as a result of the lack of time inherent in day surgery for personal communication and the need for patients to have information once home in order to manage their recovery effectively (see Chapters 2, 5, 6 and 7). Literature reviews and full studies about information provision before surgery have deemed information to be extremely important, although some early reviews have continued to debate the most effective method of presentation, e.g. procedural, behavioural or sensory (Hathaway 1986, Rothrock 1989, Beddows 1997, Lithner and Zilling 1998, Shuldham 1999a, Lee et al. 2003) (see Chapter 5). As discussed, the method of information presentation may be of less importance with the advent of modern-day surgery, the level of information provision and the timing of delivery being vastly superior issues (see Chapters 5, 6 and 7).

In a study by Beddows (1997), 40 inpatients were surveyed to determine their level of anxiety on admission and immediately before surgery. Two weeks before admission, patients were randomly assigned to two groups: (1) home visit by the ward nurse to provide information/administer anxiety questionnaire and (2) no visit, merely a letter containing general hospital information and the questionnaire for completion. Although both groups experienced an increase in anxiety on the day of surgery, the control group were significantly more anxious. However, the study lacked an attention-control group and the observed improvement in anxiety in the experimental group could quite reasonably have happened because of the extra attention provided, i.e. being treated differently (Hawthorne effect) (Neale and Liebert 1986). Numerous studies have examined the information required most by patients once admitted to hospital before surgery. In a study by Lithner and Zilling (2000) of 50 patients admitted for cholecystectomy, information on pain was the most important aspect of personal communication. In addition: 'At admission, 94% of the patients wanted to receive information about complications after surgery' (Lithner and Zilling 2000, p. 34). In an Australian survey (Farnill and Inglis 1993), patients were questioned about their desire for information about their impending anaesthesia. The foremost aspects that patients wanted to know were when they would be allowed to eat and drink again, when they would be allowed to get up and common complications of their condition. In addition, all patients wanted to meet their anaesthetist before surgery.

In a further study of preoperative anxiety 96 patients scheduled for elective surgery were shown a videotaped presentation about their anaesthesia in the preassessment clinic followed by a survey to uncover the most valued method of information provision (Krenzischek et al. 2001). The most preferred method of information provision was the videotaped presentation (50%), instruction by staff (47%), written information (9%) and the internet (3%). In a study by Yount and Schoessler (1991), 116 patients and 159 nurses completed a questionnaire about patient information provision. Both patients and nurses indicated that psychosocial support was highly desirable before admission, although skills teaching or behavioural training was wanted mostly once the patient had been admitted (see Chapter 5).

> Patients in this study rated psychosocial support as the most important dimension of pre-operative teaching to receive from a nurse.
>
> Yount and Schoessler (1991, p. 23)

Once patients are admitted to hospital, structured teaching has been demonstrated to have no more of an impact than unstructured teaching (Siew et al. 2000), although the lack of an appropriate level of information is a major issue (Biley 1989).

Increasingly, studies examining patients' experiences of modern, elective day surgery have established information provision to be a very challenging issue because many patients frequently want more information than has been provided (Ruuth-Setala et al. 2000, Fung and Cohen 2001, Georgalas et al. 2002, Markovic et al. 2002, Moore et al. 2002, Barthelsson et al. 2003a, 2003b, Bernier et al. 2003). It has long been established that patients may want to cope with a stressful encounter, e.g. hospital admission for surgery, by seeking information about their experience or, conversely, by wanting to know very little about their impending experience, preferring to trust in the health-care professionals (Miller 1980, 1987, Roth and Cohen 1986, Krohne 1989, Krohne et al. 1996). Such a method of coping has been termed 'vigilant and avoidant coping' (Krohne 1978, 1989, Losiak 2001) (see Chapter 4). Numerous studies over many decades have examined the desire for different levels of information provision to help manage anxiety more effectively. In an early study (Ziemer 1983), 111 inpatients were randomly assigned to receive either 5 or 22 minutes of audiotape-recorded information on the eve of surgery. It was assumed that the group receiving 5 minutes of audiotape-recorded information would be less satisfied and more anxious, although this was not the case. No significant differences were established between the two groups, possibly because patients with vigilant and avoidant coping preferences had not been recognized, e.g. some patients may have wanted very little information. In a comprehensive study of information provision before surgery using 60 inpatients (Ridgeway and Mathews 1982), one of the main conclusions was that patients may have a preference for different levels of information provision in order to enhance cognitive coping.

As a result, many studies have subsequently developed preoperative booklets containing different levels of information to assess their influence on anxiety (Wilson 1981, Levesque et al. 1984, Wallace 1984, 1986a, Young and Humphrey 1985, Young et al. 1994, Butler et al. 1996). However, none of these studies took account of vigilant and avoidant coping preferences so no significant differences for information provision were established, e.g. detailed and standard information booklets were sent at random to patients. However, studies that have recognized vigilant and avoidant coping when distributing information, e.g. detailed and standard information booklets sent to specific patients, have had greater success (Martelli et al. 1987, Kerrigan et al. 1993, Miro and Raich 1999b). Such recognition is, however, not widespread because Breemhaar et al. (1996, p. 39) documented that such a method of information distribution may have so far failed to be provided at discharge, e.g. detailed and standard information booklets provided for specific patients about discharge information: 'Many patients said they were not informed about the proper behaviour after discharge in order to facilitate recovery.'

In summary, information provision remains a challenging issue for modern, elective day surgery and inadequate information can greatly influence the level of preoperative anxiety. Different levels of information are deemed most appropriate, although ensuring that the correct patient receives the correct amount of information may ultimately be achieved only when a more formal psychoeducational nursing assessment is undertaken before hospital admission (see Chapters 7 and 8).

Hospital personnel

Studies have indicated that the physical surroundings of the hospital environment can give rise to anxiety (van Balen and Verdurmen 1999), although it is the interpersonal skills of the hospital personnel that demonstrate the greatest impact. The limited time available in which to develop a relationship between doctor and patient or nurse and patient can give rise to anxiety (Carnie 2002). Therefore, a preoperative visit from the theatre staff and anaesthetist has been deemed to be very important

(Lonsdale and Hutchison 1991, Caunt 1992, Carter and Evans 1996, Rudolfsson et al. 2003a, 2003b). Such visits extended the window of opportunity (although still very brief) in which the patient might benefit from the interaction with the hospital personnel (Mitchell 1997, 2000, Gilmartin 2004).

Sitting and talking to a patient has traditionally been viewed as the hallmark of effective psychological nursing intervention. Such preoperative intervention has historically been labelled as 'reassurance'. In a study by Teasdale (1995b, p. 79) reassurance is defined as 'the attempt to communicate with people who are anxious, worried or distressed with the intention of inducing them to predict that they are safe or safer than they presently believe or fear'. He divides nursing actions of reassurance into four categories: (1) uncertainty reduction (provision of information), (2) patient control (accepting individual wishes and acting as the patients' advocate), (3) cognitive re-framing (discouraging unjustified fears and suggesting that events may be less stressful than feared) and (4) attachment (the assuring presence of the nurse as with young children and the presence of their parents/guardians). Such implicit verbal and non-verbal actions have also been recommended by others and are frequently termed 'therapeutic use of self'. In a study in which 30 inpatients were surveyed after surgery (Leino-Kilpi and Vuorenheimo 1993), patients wanted the nurse to be near to them during the perioperative period for assurance in the way highlighted by Teasdale (1995b), i.e. attachment. Likewise, Rudolfsson et al. (2003a, 2003b) referred to core categories of perioperative care of the patient as 'making time for me' and two main categories: 'comforting me' and 'becoming involved'.

In an experimental study (Schwartz-Barcott et al. 1994), 91 inpatients were divided into three groups to receive preoperative relaxation therapy: tape-recorded information about sensations, provision of information by a nurse and routine intervention. However, no significant differences in anxiety were established between the information groups and the routine care group. It is suggested that the different experimental designs were greatly influenced by the interpersonal skills of the nurse, e.g. she or he was able to facilitate a reduction in, or improved management of, anxiety. Therefore, the interpersonal skills of the nurses effectively overcame the manufactured groups within the experimental design. As stated previously (see Chapter 2), nurses who demonstrate care and concern were viewed as providing a better quality of management (Icenhour 1988, Parsons et al. 1993, Costa 2001, Stevens et al. 2001) and were more likely to be chosen by the patients for communication (Teasdale 1995a, 1995b). In addition, in further studies, continuous contact with a familiar nurse during the preoperative period was determined to help patients manage their anxiety more effectively (Vogelsang 1990, Mitra et al. 2003).

Conclusion

Preoperative anxiety has been strongly associated with four main aspects: the anaesthetic, possible pain and discomfort, the operation and being unconsciousness; now, with the advent of day surgery the preoperative waiting is a further major influence. Anaesthesia remains the most anxiety-provoking event because of anxiety associated with either waking during surgery or not waking afterwards. Conversely, some patients prefer to have general anaesthesia because of their anxiety about medical equipment, needles or past poor experiences.

Safe anaesthesia is of vital importance with any surgery and is also the aspect of surgery that generates the greatest amount of apprehension. Anaesthetists are therefore very concerned with any aspect, such as anxiety, that can influence the smooth induction, maintenance and recovery from anaesthesia. The main concern appears to be associated with patient relaxation and the gaining of an acquiescent patient on whom the anaesthetist can work.

A number of distraction techniques have appeared to aid patient anxiety management throughout the surgical experience. However, not all patients want to listen to music, watch television or experience guided imagery. Indeed, all the techniques have gained a little success but none has proved to be singularly effective. Distraction, although sometimes effective, is very limiting, very simplistic and not always possible, e.g. switching on a television/radio, nurse talking to a patient when able, handholding during surgery, etc. Hospital personnel and the relationship they establish with the patient in the very brief period available have been observed to be a highly effective method of anxiety management. However, as opportunities to undertake such interventions may be extremely restricted in modern day surgery, other more sophisticated measures of nursing intervention are required. A combination of adequate information provision and the interpersonal skills of the nurse may have the potential to become the basis of a formal psychoeducational nursing plan fit for the twenty-first century, and able to replace the now largely obsolete physical nursing interventions.

Summary

- Patients are anxious before day surgery and little or no formal anxiety intervention has been documented.
- The reliance on previous methods of preoperative anxiety measurement and intervention are now obsolete in the modern day-surgery setting.
- Many anxiety management studies have physiological equilibrium as their focus and thereby employ largely physiological measures of anxiety assessment.

- The main interventions recommended for preoperative anxiety management are anxiolytic premedication and distraction.
- Although there can be sound physiological justification for anxiolytic premedication, the application of such a practice in day surgery is very limited, e.g. it is restricted to a select number of patients who have been perceived as highly anxious, does not influence anxiety during the days before surgery and after surgery, and is not available to most day-surgery patients because the use of premedication is not encouraged.
- Although pharmacological treatment for preoperative anxiety has clearly demonstrated many benefits, more subtle and therapeutic interventions are required in this new era of modern elective day surgery.
- Distraction has largely been employed because it is quick and simple, and leaves time for the staff to undertake other essential tasks. However, such distraction techniques have not demonstrated improvements that are significant enough to warrant their more wide-scale adoption. Such techniques are limiting and very basic, e.g. switching on a television, and not all patients require distraction.
- A great deal of recovery now takes place at home after day surgery and the instant access to help and advice once available to the traditional surgical patient has been lost. Patients can become very anxious because they are unaware of the best course of action.
- Different levels of information are deemed most appropriate, although ensuring that the correct patient receives the correct amount of information may ultimately be achieved only when a more formal psychoeducational nursing assessment is undertaken before hospital admission.
- The presence and behaviour of hospital personnel have demonstrated many benefits for patient anxiety. Therefore, the challenge for the nursing profession is to harness such behaviour, provide adequate information and assemble helpful therapeutic strategies fit for this new surgical era.

Further reading

Baum, A., Newman, S., Weinman, J., West, R. and McManus, C. (eds) (1995) Cambridge Handbook of Psychology, Health and Medicine. Cambridge: Cambridge University Press.

Broome, A. and Llewelyn, S. (eds) (1995) Health Psychology Process and Applications, 2nd edn. London: Chapman & Hall.

Cahill, H. and Jackson, I. (1997) Day Surgery: Principles and nursing practice. London: Baillière Tindall.

Pitts, M. and Philips, K. (1991) The Psychology of Health: An introduction. London: Routledge.

Websites

www.transformationstrategies.co.uk
www.informedhealthonline.org
www.cfah.org/factsoflife

Chapter 4

Psychological approaches to coping

Broad psychological approaches

Psychology, or the study of human behaviour, is not an exact science because it deals with individuals who, by definition, can display or experience many different thoughts and emotions, e.g. it has been established that many people prefer to spend their time immediately before surgery in different ways, e.g. talking to a relative, listening quietly to music or being given light sedation (Poole 1993, Wang et al. 2002), as highlighted in Chapter 3. Therefore, suggesting that ALL people prefer to listen quietly to music before surgery would be inaccurate. A number of psychological theories or assumptions are therefore presented here to help explain such diversity of human behaviour. Three competing theories have historically been put forward to help gain insight into how we endeavour to cope with a stressful episode such as day surgery. The three competing theories are the psychodynamic, transactional and convergent approaches.

Psychodynamic approach

Early in the twentieth century, Sigmund Freud, Alfred Alder and Carl Jung first put forward the psychodynamic approach. This perspective provided the initial understanding of how people might cope with adversity. The management of anxiety was considered to be part of unconscious defensive mechanisms, which helped to protect the individual (self) from both internal and external conflicts. The type of coping behaviour, which subsequently arose from this approach, was rigid, reality distorting, unconscious cognitions, driven by past experiences (Suls et al. 1996). In short, this approach is broadly based on our past experiences (beginning in childhood), which subsequently become unconsciously embedded in our everyday thoughts and actions as we grow, i.e. personality traits (Figure 4.1).

One of the first studies into the psychological impact of surgery also pursued a psychodynamic theme (Janis 1958). Janis claimed that the

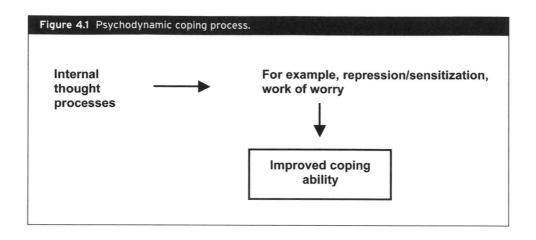

Figure 4.1 Psychodynamic coping process.

anxiety response could be reduced and recovery prospects improved if the patient thought about the adverse event and worked through their fears before surgery. He termed this type of preoperative mental process the 'work of worry' and believed it to be essential for reducing the stress associated with physical trauma. He described the 'work of worry' as a mental process, similar to mourning after bereavement, which aided adjustment to a painful situation. If a patient were to undergo a surgical procedure he or she would mentally rehearse the various situations together with their possible consequences. The benefit of this would be to have accurate expectations of the possible pain and discomfort and thereby gain greater reality-based insight. However, Janis focused on the stress resulting mainly from the physical trauma of surgery. For many decades the fear associated with surgery has been associated with four main aspects: fear of anaesthesia, pain and discomfort, being unconscious and the operation itself (Egbert et al. 1964, Ramsay 1972, Male 1981, Mathews and Ridgeway 1981, McCleane and Cooper 1990, Salmon 1993, Leinonen et al. 1996, Mitchell 1997, McGaw and Hanna 1998, Mitchell 2000). Therefore, to focus on the anxiety arising purely from the physical trauma may often provide too narrow a view because clearly other aspects of the surgical experience also generate apprehension.

A further theory of coping using this approach is a personality trait termed 'repression–sensitization' (Byrne 1961, p. 334):

> At one extreme of this continuum are behaviour mechanisms of a predominantly avoiding type (denying, repressing), while at the other extreme are predominantly approaching (intellectualising, obsessional) behaviours.

Byrne (1961) therefore suggested that individuals prefer to cope with threatening stimuli by either actively ruminating over events or completely avoiding all such thoughts. Krohne (1978) referred to the repressor–sensitizer model as an anxiety defence mechanism, i.e. a method of protecting the self from stress (Krohne 1978). More recently, this theory of coping has been referred to as 'vigilant and avoidant coping' (Krohne 1989).

Transactional approach

In the 1960s the transactional approach was put forward as an alternative to the psychodynamic approach. The psychodynamic approach focused purely on internal and largely unconscious processes, whereas the transactional model considered the interplay between the individual and their current environment (Lazarus 1966). Two constructs central to this approach are 'cognitive appraisal' and 'coping' (Figure 4.2).

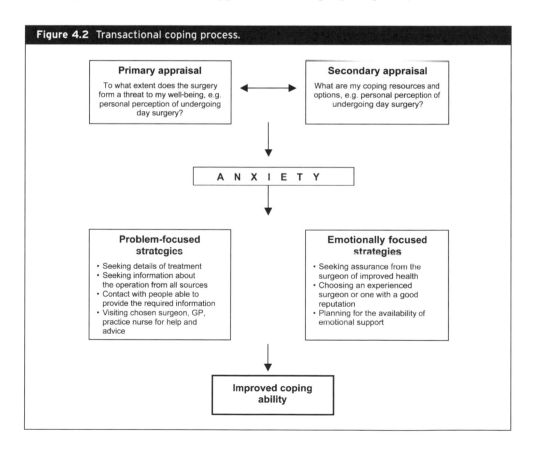

Figure 4.2 Transactional coping process.

Primary appraisal
To what extent does the surgery form a threat to my well-being, e.g. personal perception of undergoing day surgery?

Secondary appraisal
What are my coping resources and options, e.g. personal perception of undergoing day surgery?

A N X I E T Y

Problem-focused strategies
- Seeking details of treatment
- Seeking information about the operation from all sources
- Contact with people able to provide the required information
- Visiting chosen surgeon, GP, practice nurse for help and advice

Emotionally focused strategies
- Seeking assurance from the surgeon of improved health
- Choosing an experienced surgeon or one with a good reputation
- Planning for the availability of emotional support

Improved coping ability

First, cognitive appraisal (thoughts) is divided into 'primary' (initial thoughts) and 'secondary' appraisal (subsequent thoughts regarding the ability to avoid, tolerate or ameliorate the level of stress). Primary appraisal concerns our initial impressions of an event, e.g. told of the need for surgery and immediately feeling anxious because of the thought of 'needles' or 'injections'. Secondary appraisal concerns the coping resources available to help master, reduce or tolerate the internal and/or external demands created by the stressful transaction (Folkman 1984).

> The degree to which the person experiences psychological stress, that is, feels harmed, threatened, or challenged, is determined by the relationship between the person and the environment in that specific encounter as it is defined both by the evaluation of what is at stake and the evaluation of the coping resources and options.
>
> Folkman and Lazarus (1980, p. 223)

As the situation changes so too does the individual's response. Coping is viewed as a dynamic process and determined by the exchanges between the person and his or her environment, e.g.

- Primary appraisal: first informed of need for day surgery but patient knows very little about what surgery is to be undertaken and why
- Secondary appraisal: subsequent coping thoughts and actions employed to alleviate the perceived stressor, e.g. ability to uncover information about the planned surgery.

The second construct in this approach concerns 'coping'. Two broad types of coping behaviour have been put forward: problem-focused coping and emotionally focused coping (Folkman and Lazarus 1980, Folkman 1984, Folkman et al. 1986, Lazarus and Folkman 1987). Problem-focused coping includes strategies in which the person attempts to challenge the stressor directly by embarking on a physical plan of action, e.g. when faced with the prospect of day surgery a patient may wish to discover exactly what will happen to him or her, gain information about the operation, events on the day of surgery and the length of the recovery period in order to alter, circumvent or eliminate a particular stressor(s).

Emotionally focused coping refers to an individual's emotional attempts to deal with a stressor, such as the conscious thoughts and feelings associated with the prospect of admission to hospital for surgery and general anaesthesia, e.g. when faced with the prospect of an operation a patient may be able to cope more effectively if he or she is aware that the latest equipment is to be used by an experienced surgeon, in a modern prestigious hospital using the most effective anaesthetic drugs.

The type of coping strategy employed, i.e. problem-focused or emotionally focused coping, depends largely on individual appraisal of the situation (Lazarus 1966, Folkman and Lazarus 1980, Folkman et al. 1986). If the stressor is deemed susceptible to change then problem-focused coping strategies are frequently employed, e.g. gaining as much information as possible about the operation, the possible alternatives, and choosing a convenient date (Folkman et al. 1986). If the stressor is deemed less susceptible to change, then emotionally focused strategies are more likely to be employed, e.g. gaining assurance of improved health after surgery, talking with someone who has undergone a similar surgical experience. Emotionally focused coping is therefore more akin to changing the cognitive response, e.g. how an individual thinks and feels about a given situation, as opposed to the direct action associated with the problem-focused approach.

Convergent or combined approach to coping

The final approach concerns the convergent or combined approach. The psychodynamic and transactional approaches can be broadly viewed as being internally and externally orientated, respectively, with a degree of flexibility, e.g. the coping behaviour elicited by the psychodynamic approach emanates from the individual's innate responses. The coping behaviour elicited by the transactional approach emanates from the interplay between the individual and their environment, e.g. stress experience ameliorated by the availability of external resources.

This either/or approach has been considered too narrow and a combination of the two has been put forward, e.g. employing a combination of internal and external resources to reduce the stress response. It has been referred to as the 'convergent approach' (Suls et al. 1996). The need for a convergent approach has arisen as both internal and external factors have demonstrated their ability to impact, to a greater or lesser extent, on human coping behaviour, e.g. personality traits, physical environment, person–environment interaction (Byrne 1961, Folkman and Lazarus 1980, Mumford et al. 1982, Folkman 1984, Wallace 1984, Folkman et al. 1986, Lazarus and Folkman 1987, Van Balen and Verdurmen 1999). Such an approach is extremely relevant to a modern health-care situation such as day surgery where individual requirements and interaction with the environment are restricted and brief.

From a psychodynamic viewpoint, individuals may cognitively appraise day surgery as more stressful, purely as a result of their internal influences, e.g. personality, individual traits, fear evoked by the thought of hospitalization or fear of the unknown. Such individual internal influences may determine a desire to manage their anxiety in a particular manner. From a transactional viewpoint, individuals may evaluate the prospect of undergoing day surgery by their interaction with the hospital personnel/environment and knowledge of hospital resources, e.g. opportunity to discuss planned surgery, perceived sources of stress, reputation of the hospital, physical environment (Figure 4.3). Therefore, the adoption into day surgery of this combined approach to coping will be much more appropriate because it allows for both individual traits and external influences to assist anxiety reduction. Thereby, individual personality traits may be taken into consideration along with individual attempts at primary and secondary appraisal.

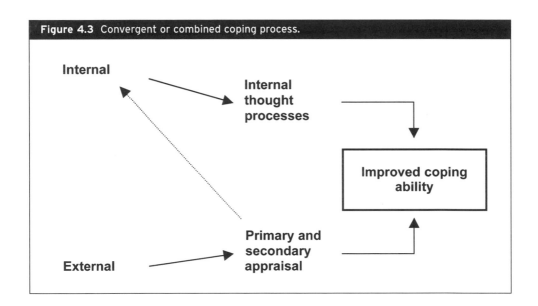

Figure 4.3 Convergent or combined coping process.

Specific psychological approaches

Over many years, a large number of studies have been undertaken in order to demonstrate how specific factors can influence postoperative outcomes (Mathews and Ridgeway 1984, Suls and Fletcher 1985, Hathaway 1986, Suls and Wan 1989, Devine 1992, Johnston and Vogele 1993, De Groot et al. 1997a). Such specific aspects have received greater attention because of their adjudged impact on recovery, e.g. a vast number of studies have employed specific psychological approaches when examining patients undergoing cardiac surgery (Gould and Wilson-Barnett 1995, Thomas 1995, Stengrevics et al. 1996, Goodman 1997,

Crumlish 1998, Lamarche et al. 1998, Walsh and Shaw 2000, Hartford et al. 2002, Koivula et al. 2002b, Mahler and Kulik 2002, van der Zee et al. 2002, van Weert et al. 2003). Cardiac surgery patients have received such attention because it is a common major surgical procedure, which carries considerable psychological implications (Tromp et al. 2004).

All the approaches used within these studies have evolved directly from the broad psychological coping approaches above, i.e. psychodynamic and transactional perspectives. However, all too frequently the broad psychological approach to coping is bypassed and a specific aspect of coping investigated. Such specific measures are usually employed simply because they are easy and convenient. However, this does not necessarily mean that they are the most appropriate or that they investigate the associated psychological paradigm (Mitchell 2004), e.g. when investigating the transactional approach to coping it may be considered somewhat inappropriate to employ measures (as many studies do) that fundamentally examine personality traits or measures more suited to the psychodynamic approach to coping. Such unsuitable combinations invariably result in multiple conclusions, many of which may be erroneous or have no clinical application. Indeed, this may be an indication of why numerous suggestions about psychological recovery have been made without subsequent progress. The specific areas that have received much attention are: (1) personality traits (neuroticism, vigilant and avoidant traits, health locus of control and self-efficacy); (2) social support (degree of assistance from friends and family); and (3) optimism (level of confidence in achieving good recovery).

Personality traits

Neuroticism (anxious predisposition)

Many earlier studies explored the link between personality and ability to cope effectively with surgery. Ridgeway and Mathews (1982) believed that the more anxious patient could be identified using measures of 'trait anxiety' and 'neuroticism'. However, no link between neuroticism and a desire for greater psychological support was uncovered, e.g. the more highly anxious patient did not require increased preoperative support. Indeed, in their study some participants declined any type of preparation. In an earlier study (Sime 1976), 57 patients admitted for abdominal surgery were provided with no information preoperatively. The participants were merely left to their own devices to gather information although their behaviour was closely observed. Some participants actively sought information from the hospital staff and it was these individuals who had a better recovery. It was therefore concluded that an unspecified personality variable associated with information seeking may have helped to ameliorate the negative effects of stress.

In a similar study 40 participants undergoing minor abdominal surgery were divided into two groups where one group received relaxation therapy and the second group procedural information, e.g. told what will happen next or the sequential order of events (Manyande et al. 1992) (see Chapter 3). The relaxation group were made worse by this type of intervention because it was concluded that their 'work of worry' had been disrupted. It is suggested that if they had been left alone their stress reaction might not have been as great. Allowing patients to pursue individual methods of pre-operative preparation more suited to their personality type was therefore suggested as a far more effective method of preparation. Manyande and Salmon (1992) also studied 40 participants undergoing minor abdominal surgery. The study was 'designed to establish whether, in the absence of explicit programmes of study, active coping is correlated with a speedier recovery' (Manyande and Salmon 1992, p. 228). It was concluded that type A personality behaviour and a feeling that one's health was independent of powerful others were related to an increased ability to cope.

In a recent study of relaxation before surgery the Eysenck Personality Questionnaire (which examines personality type) was employed (Eysenck and Eysenck 1975). No significant differences were established concerning personality although: 'in our study, about 70% of subjects experienced a high degree of situational anxiety associated with hospitalisation' (Miluk-Kolasa et al. 2002, p. 58). Therefore, the vast majority of patients were anxious although this was not related to broad personality traits such as type A behaviour. In addition, 112 inpatients undergoing various surgical procedures were studied, establishing a link between personality and recovery (Kopp et al. 2003). Using a range of measures, just one strong correlation on one aspect of a personality questionnaire was established, e.g. satisfaction with life and a more positive recovery. Personality type may therefore provide some of the answers to the question of how individuals cope with surgery. However, as suggested by Sime (1976) and Manyande and Salmon (1992), personality type may be too broad a term and other more specific personality traits may be strongly influential. Consequently, very few studies of recovery from surgery now pursue a broad personality approach.

Vigilant and avoidant coping

One of the earliest studies undertaken, concerning vigilant and avoidant personality traits, was by Byrne (1961) in which he referred to this type of coping as the 'repression–sensitization' scale. He suggested that these two characteristics were on a continuum with the extreme forms at opposite ends. Repression consisted primarily of avoiding, denying and repressing behaviours, e.g. side-stepping any information, not thinking about the event and averting any thoughts. Sensitizing behaviours consisted predominantly of confronting the problem and seeking information in an almost obsessional manner, e.g. persistent and relentless pursuit of information. Furthermore, Byrne (1961, p. 336) stated: 'Individuals are consistent in their defensive reactions to threatening stimuli over a period of time.' Hock et al. (1996, p. 1052) stated that cognitive vigilance can be defined as the 'increased intake and exhaustive processing of threatening information' and cognitive avoidance as 'turning attention away from, and inhibiting the further processing of, cues associated with threat'.

These two broad modes of coping have been referred to as an anxiety defence mechanism and termed 'cognitive vigilance' and 'cognitive avoidance' (Krohne 1978, 1989, Krohne et al. 1996). Cognitive vigilance is defined as an approach to, and an intensified processing of, threatening information. Its purpose is to help gain control over the main threat-related aspects of a situation, thereby protecting the individual from the perception of unexpected dangers, e.g. nothing surprises them because they are already aware of all the pertinent issues (Krohne 1989). Cognitive avoidance is defined as a withdrawal from threat-relevant information. Its purpose is to reduce the arousal caused by the confrontation with an aversive event (Krohne 1989) (Table 4.1).

Table 4.1 Innate coping styles   From Krohne et al. (1996).

Coping style	Description
Vigilant coping	A coping approach in which the individual has an intensified processing of threatening information. Copious levels of detailed information are frequently desired because too little will cause an increase in anxiety. Such individuals must be informed of all aspects of care so that nothing surprises them because omissions may be too anxiety provoking
Avoidant coping	A coping approach in which the individual makes efforts to withdraw from threatening information. A minimal level of simple information is frequently desired because too much will cause an increase in anxiety. Such individuals may prefer to trust in the doctors and nurses, minimize events and give positive interpretations to events
Fluctuating coping	A coping approach in which the individual has a desire for variable levels of information. Some information required may be highly detailed whereas other aspects may be only minimal, e.g. details about the operation only. Incorrect communication of the desired amount or selected areas of information may give rise to an increase in anxiety
Flexible coping	A coping approach for dealing with a stressful situation characterized by assuming an adaptable stance regarding information provision. Generally, whatever information is provided will be acceptable

Not all individuals are, however, observed to maintain such extreme forms of behaviour. Therefore, two further aspects have been put forward to create a two-dimensional model: fluctuating coping (variable information requirements) and situation-related or flexible coping (information requirements adaptable to the given situation) were added (Krohne et al. 1996). In one day-surgery study, the proportion of patients falling into these coping categories was investigated (Mitchell 2000). Almost 33% of day-surgery patients were deemed avoidant copers and 25% vigilant copers (Figure 4.4). Therefore, about a third of day-surgery patients required very little information and approximately one-quarter required a great deal of information. Other studies have found similar results (Kerrigan et al. 1993, Garden et al. 1996), although more work is required in this area before this could become a 'rule-of-thumb' guide to information provision in modern elective day surgery.

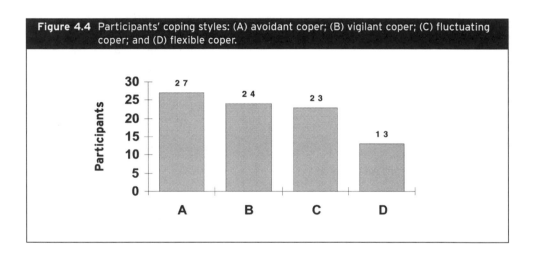

Figure 4.4 Participants' coping styles: (A) avoidant coper; (B) vigilant coper; (C) fluctuating coper; and (D) flexible coper.

In other studies by Miller, such coping methods have been referred to as the 'blunting hypothesis' and the terms 'monitors' and 'blunters' employed (Miller 1980). Miller states that blunting strategies have a positive side, e.g. distraction, self-relaxation and re-intellectualization (re-interpretation of a given situation). It is suggested that such defensive coping modes are behaviours learnt in childhood and, once learnt, could become a habitual response in stressful situations that persist over time (Averill and Rosenn 1972, Mechanic 1980, Roth and Cohen 1986, Krohne et al. 1992, King et al. 1998).

It has also been suggested that anxiety-prone individuals (vigilant copers) in acutely stressful situations might very easily activate their perception of threat-relevant cues. Vigilant copers can go into 'cognitive overdrive' in a stressful situation, extracting information from their environment and processing it constantly as negative or threatening (Mogg et al. 1990). Vigilant individuals can often make matters worse for themselves in stressful situations because they 'often impose threatening interpretations on ambiguous event descriptions' (Hock et al. 1996, p. 1062). Such cognitive activation or cognitive overdrive involving the internal and external searching for cues requires little conscious effort and highly anxious people can become extremely adept at picking up negative information with minimal conscious endeavour (Bonanno et al. 1991). Miller et al. (1996) also suggest that high monitors (vigilant copers) with a serious medical condition ruminate continually:

> This increase in intrusive ideation [invasive negative thoughts] indicates that high monitors are more likely to think about their disease status when they do not mean to do so, to dream about it, to have trouble falling asleep because of it, to be reminded of it, and to have strong feelings about it. (p. 221)

> Intrusive ideation entails recurrent, reliving of the event with intense psychological distress when exposed to symbolic reminders of the event (including self-generated cues), as well as sleep disturbance. (p. 848)

An increase in anxiety can therefore be easily triggered in such individuals because they are in a heightened state of arousal.

Cognitive avoiders, according to Bonanno et al. (1991, p. 396), do the opposite in that 'repressors are associated with a general cognitive capacity for avoidant processing that can be invoked whenever the motivation to disattend is present, regardless of the specific source of that motivation'. Such an ability has been referred to as 'attentional narrowing' (Hansen et al. 1992). This becomes an effective perceptual defence or barrier to unwanted material. Hock et al. (1996) also stated that cognitive avoiders process (unconsciously in the initial stages) far less threatening information than vigilant copers. In a dental surgery study (Baume et al. 1995), this was seen as advantageous because such patients were viewed as being less anxious during the dental procedure. However, avoidance can be a disadvantage in the long term because all too frequently health-care matters requiring attention may be ignored and health-care appointments missed or cancelled (Mullen and Suls 1982, Suls and Fletcher 1985, Kohlmann et al. 1996).

A number of older studies about preparation for surgery recognized the need to consider patients' different coping styles (Egbert et al. 1964, Andrew 1970, Mathews and Ridgeway 1981, Roth and Cohen 1986, Fox et al. 1989). A survey of 69 patients was undertaken to examine how differences in preference for information influenced stress and coping in patients undergoing outpatient surgery (Caldwell 1991a). It was revealed that some patients had a low preference for information and some a high preference. In a further study, 60 hysterectomy patients were randomly assigned to one of three groups to investigate the most effective form of preoperative psychological preparation (Ridgeway and Mathews 1982). One group received additional preoperative information, a second group cognitive coping technique (positive thoughts to draw upon) and the final group general ward information. However, as a result of the participants being able to choose the research group in which they were placed, no significant differences were established. It is therefore suggested that patients may opt for a choice of methods of preparation, e.g. individuals may demonstrate their vigilant or avoidant coping styles.

More recent studies have also examined vigilant and avoidant coping styles although with mixed results. Garden et al. (1996) conducted an experiment on 45 patients scheduled to undergo cardiac surgery. Patients were divided into three groups and provided with different levels of information: 'full' disclosure, 'standard' disclosure and 'minimal' disclosure'. However, no significant difference in anxiety was established among the groups. This may have occurred, in part, because some patients again self-selected the level of information that they required. The study goes on to recommend different levels of information and that full disclosure of information for those who want it does not give rise to greater levels of anxiety. Mitchell (2000) mailed a simple information booklet at random during the preoperative period to 60 day-surgery patients and an extended information booklet to a further 60 day-surgery patients. Participants were also sent a questionnaire to determine their coping style, e.g. vigilant or avoidant coping behaviours, the assumption being that vigilant copers would be more anxious and less satisfied when in receipt of the simple information in comparison with the vigilant copers in receipt of the extended information. Although a difference in anxiety was established, this marginally failed to reach a significant level. This may have resulted partly from information being gained by the participants from other sources. Patients who required more information but received only the simple booklet may have made further informational enquiries.

Other researches have also highlighted additional information from other sources as a confounding issue. In an experimental design (Miro and Raich 1999b), vigilant and avoidant copers were identified and place into three groups: (1) sensory and procedural information, (2) relaxation training and (3) general hospital talk. However, all patients were found to obtain information about their surgery from a variety of sources, e.g. doctors, nurses, friends and family members, thus introducing numerous confounding variables. However, low monitors (avoidant copers) trained in relaxation experienced less pain and greater mobility than the low monitors (avoidant copers) in the attention-control group. This suggests that avoidant copers (low monitors) preferred little information and more relaxation training. In a study by Daltroy et al. (1998, p. 478) similar results were also achieved: 'Patients who tend to avoid thinking about unpleasant possibilities (deniers) tend to desire less information and to have to sort out information from fewer sources before surgery, but benefit most from provision of information pre-operatively.' Vigilant and avoidant coping theories are therefore increasingly becoming the focus for many current studies, such is their ability to explain modern coping behaviour (Bar Tal and Spitzer 1999, Losiak 2001).

Health locus of control

Numerous studies suggest that an individual's desire to be included in the decision-making process with regard to health may be related to level of internal and external health locus of control (real or perceived). Rotter (1966) was one of the first researchers to examine and validate a questionnaire to help test claims of control. The theory is based on the assumption that people with an increased perception of control or 'internals' have a greater belief in their ability to shape their own destiny, whereas people with an decreased perception of control or 'externals' feel more influenced by luck, fate and powerful others (Rotter 1966) (Table 4.2).

Table 4.2 Locus of control

Locus of control	Description
External health locus of control	Strong belief that one's future is influenced more by luck, fate or powerful others, e.g. doctors, nurses, employer. Such individuals may therefore readily assume decisions will be made on their behalf
Internal health locus of control	Strong belief in one's ability to shape the future and therefore a desire to be firmly involved in the decision-making process. Control can be real or perceived, e.g. not necessarily much control granted although a semblance of control perceived

Although Rotter (1966) suggested that locus of control beliefs could be viewed as an enduring personality characteristic, other more recent studies have demonstrated the possible dynamic status of health locus of control beliefs after hospitalization. Halfens (1995) interviewed patients before, during and after admission to hospital for surgery. It was concluded that health locus of control beliefs changed when an individual was hospitalized, especially the powerful others aspect, e.g. people became far more influenced by powerful others. 'The findings of this study indicate that in new and ambiguous situations, health locus of control can react as a situation-dependent belief' (Halfens 1995, p. 165). In a survey of 12 surgical patients before day surgery similar controlling influences were also observed (Avis 1994). Expectations of involvement were limited by the professional agenda, professional knowledge and conceptions of themselves as a 'work object'.

A number of studies over many decades have indicated that, when a patient is given an increased amount of health control, adaptability and recovery are enhanced (Strickland 1978, Seeman and Seeman 1983, Peterson and Stunkard 1989, Shaw et al. 2003). In a review, Peterson and Stunkard (1989) concluded that patients with increased appraisals of control were more likely to follow medical advice and be more skilled at coping. The review also asserts that control resided in the transaction between the individual and the environment, i.e. it is context specific and thereby open to manipulation. Therefore, although health locus of control may be considered a personality trait, external factors (such as admission to hospital) can strongly influence such behaviour. Other studies have likewise indicated that more favourable outcomes may result from an increase in health control, because it has been positively associated with a reduction in the level of stress (Richert 1981, Mahler and Kulik 1990, Ludwick-Rosenthal and Neufeld 1993, Kugler et al. 1994, Litt et al. 1995). Mahler and Kulik (1990, p. 748) studied 75 men who were undergoing heart surgery, 85% of whom expressed responsibility for their own recovery: 'greater perceived control did marginally predict both lower pre-operative anxiety and fewer post-operative negative psychological reactions'.

In a later review of the literature (Duits et al. 1997), it was concluded that psychological factors of control, social support and optimism can, to a certain extent, be responsible for psychological outcomes after surgery. A greater level of control may provide a degree of predictability that removes, for some patients, the stress of the unforeseen event (Miller et al. 1989). The level of health control required may need to be only minor or 'real or perceived', e.g. in a blood donor survey, the clients giving blood were provided with a simple choice of which arm to use during the procedure (Mills and Krantz 1979). Which arm should be used mattered little to the hospital personnel but for the patient it bestowed the perception of choice. In a related study Miller and Mangan (1983, p. 232) gave different levels of information to 40 female surgical patients and concluded: 'One salient possibility is that information only decreased stress when it allows the individual to exert (or to perceive to exert) some choice or control over the situation.' In a review of the literature, greater control was associated with a more optimistic bias (Klein and Helweg-Larsen 2002), i.e. people associated being in control with being more prepared to avoid poor health or medical complications. In a more recent study, patients were divided into two groups and either provided with a CD containing information about their intended surgery for home viewing or given no additional information (Deyo et al. 2000). The CD group were found to be more informed about their treatment and the possible alternatives. The number of patients deciding to have no surgery and choosing more conservative treatment was also greater in the CD group, i.e. patients who were well informed took greater responsibility for health decisions. However, this group discussed their treatment with the doctor and also received the booklet whereas the control group merely discussed their treatment with the doctor and did not receive the booklet. Therefore, the CD group may have been considerably more informed and thereby perceived a greater level of control.

If a degree of health control is not provided, anxiety can also increase. Peerbhoy et al. (1998, p. 600), studying 30 patients undergoing orthopaedic surgery, concluded that taking control had little real meaning, because 'patient control over medical care appears to be a theoretical and professional construct'. The patients viewed control as either a right to individualized care from the nursing staff or a reliance on personal 'willpower'. Information was required because the patients wanted to know what was happening in order to reduce uncertainty and retain dignity; it was not for the involvement in the decision-making process. Other studies have also highlighted the limited opportunities to establish a measure of control within the health-care setting (Miller et al. 1989, Malin and Teasdale 1991). For the patient who wants some control in such a situation, again this can lead to an increase in stress.

Some studies have, however, recognized a mixed response to control, indicating that not all patients require such involvement. In one study (Eachus 1991), data about health locus of control were collected from 88 nurses and compared with the health locus of control beliefs of the general public. It was confirmed that patients expect to be controlled, to some extent, by powerful others while in hospital, e.g. doctors and nurses. Breemhaar and van den Borne (1991, p. 203) stated: 'Increasing the level of perceived control can lead to an increase in stress if this control brings with it demands, which the person concerned does not wish to meet or which he/she cannot (or thinks he/she cannot) meet.' Folkman (1984) suggested that having only a small amount of control did not always equate with an increase in stress, and Miller et al. (1989) and Avis (1994) state that control could involve relinquishing responsibility to another person, chosen by them as more competent. Therefore, if a choice can be made of which surgeon to consult, an element of control may have been established. It has been suggested (Smith and Draper 1994) that the hospitalized patient has a strong belief in the expertise and ability of the doctors and nurses, e.g. powerful others, and is therefore frequently very willing to relinquish control to such 'expert' hospital personnel.

Self-efficacy

Self-efficacy or confidence in one's ability to behave in such a way as to produce a desirable outcome can give rise to considerable distress if these abilities are reduced (Bandura 1977, Kurlowicz 1998).

> By conjuring up fear-provoking thoughts about their ineptitude, individuals can rouse themselves to elevated levels of anxiety that far exceed the fear experienced during the actual threatening situation.
>
> Bandura (1977, p. 199)

The perception of self-efficacy can easily be enhanced or reduced by social interaction, e.g. verbal persuasion (Bandura 1982). In a review of the literature in which the broad question of coping was examined it is stated:

> In our view, perceptions of personal efficacy are one very important source of favourable expectations for successful goal attainment.
>
> Scheier and Carver (1992, p. 223)

Cozzarelli (1993) studied 336 women undergoing termination of pregnancy under sedation. After being given a brief explanation of the operation on the day of surgery, each patient was asked to complete a questionnaire containing five sections: optimism, self-esteem, perceived health control, self-efficacy and depression. This battery of questionnaires was repeated on the second and twenty-first postoperative days. Within the conclusions Cozzarelli (1993, p. 1232) states that: 'one of the most important contributions of personality in the context of coping with stressful life events may be to help motivate individuals facing such events to exert appropriate and/or continuous coping efforts by increasing feelings of self-efficacy.' In a similar study by Litt et al. (1995), 231 patients undergoing dental extraction under local anaesthesia were studied. Participants were divided into four groups and given slightly different methods of preparation, e.g. standard preparation, premedication, relaxation, and relaxation and self-efficacy enhancement (told falsely they were able to relax well). The participants in the group where self-efficacy was enhanced had superior outcomes, e.g. lower levels of self-reported anxiety, increased feelings of self-efficacy and higher scores on behavioural adaptation (reported by the dental surgeon).

> The results indicate that this [false feedback via verbal persuasion and enactive mastery or falsely being informed of their skilful ability to relax] was an effective, and potentially clinically useful, means of enhancing self-efficacy appraisals and thereby improving coping.
>
> Litt et al. (1995, p. 445)

More recently, 120 day-surgery patients were surveyed about their coping style and assessment of self-efficacy (Mitchell 2000). The appraisal of self-efficacy for avoidant copers was significantly greater than for vigilant copers, irrespective of the level of information received. Participants deemed to be avoidant copers therefore believed that they had a greater ability to cope with their day-surgery experience compared with vigilant copers.

Some studies have employed self-efficacy training in the form of additional education, provided by the researcher (Oetker-Black et al. 1997). However, the teaching sessions in this particular study involved behavioural teaching only (see Chapter 5), e.g. postoperative mobilization, deep breathing and relaxation techniques for when pain occurs. No psychological aspects of care were used such as self-efficacy enhancement, emphasizing aspects of personal control. Merely relying on additional teaching in the form of increased information provision may not therefore always equal improved psychological preparation (see Chapter 6). Moreover, as previously stated, the benefits of improved information provision have already been established in classic nursing research (Volicer 1973, Hayward 1975, Boore 1978, Wilson-Barnett 1984) and now require expansion, not simple duplication (see Chapter 1). Again, in a study that provided different forms of preparation, e.g. various forms of videotaped information (Mahler and Kulik 1998), it was uncovered that information provision alone did not just enhance self-efficacy. Self-efficacy was enhanced because patients discovered that by employing the correct behaviours they were personally capable of speeding their recovery. Finally, 50 patients undergoing orthopaedic surgery were provided with training concerning effective postoperative leg exercising and ambulation (Moon and Backer 2000). Again, it was established that training alone was insufficient and patients with a greater degree of self-efficacy were more successful mobility wise. It was therefore recommended that patients' self-efficacy beliefs might need to be considered when planning preoperative educational programmes.

Conversely, some claims against the success of increased self-efficacy appraisals have been made (Manyande et al. 1995); 51 patients undergoing abdominal surgery were studied and divided into two groups: one group received a 30-minute audiotape instructing them in the positive ways to deal with any problems that they might encounter whereas the second group received an audiotape of general hospital information. It was concluded that, although self-efficacy appraisals had increased, anxiety had not decreased with the provision of additional positive imagery. Providing preparatory information aimed at increasing self-efficacy could therefore potentially have the opposite effect to the one intended, i.e. it could increase the stress response and potentially reduce self-efficacy.

Social support

In a classic study by Spector and Sistrunk (1979, p. 122), social support and social contact were viewed as beneficial before an anxiety-provoking event: 'The results suggest that anxiety reduction did indeed occur in the presence of other people. However, it was not the mere presence of others, but their actual statements of reassurance that caused the reduction.' Such claims have been supported within the health-care situation (Hartsfield and Clopton 1985). In this study, 60 female patients undergoing general anaesthesia for cholecystectomy were surveyed. Participants were divided into three groups: reassuring information (medical and psychological), self-care instructions (postoperative advice about diet, exercise, coughing technique, etc.) and neutral information (description of a general hospital and admission procedures with no specific information about the operation). There were no significant differences in anxiety reduction resulting from the different forms of information provided. Contact with visitors (including the researcher), however, led to a significant reduction in patient anxiety. In a similar study, 74 patients admitted for elective surgery were randomly divided into two groups: 5-minute visit by anaesthetist to discuss procedural information (see Chapter 5) or a 30-minute visit from the nurse mainly to discuss procedural and behavioural information (Elsass et al. 1987a). The vast majority of participants preferred the visit by the nurse, although there was clearly a time bias between the two groups, i.e. 30 minutes and 5 minutes! However, it was concluded that emotional support given by a 'contact person' (nurse) is more effective than either detailed information or a tranquillizer.

Gender may also contribute to the preference for social support. Sherman et al. (1997, p. 244) examined two decades of research concerning coping and gender differences: 'Women appear to have larger social networks than males, be more communicative within their networks, and be exposed to more life events via these networks.' The positive influence of increased social support for both men and women has also been recognized elsewhere (Salmon 1992a). Salmon suggested that focusing too much on the patient preoperatively could become a very difficult task and therefore the environment should become the main focus of attention, i.e. providing the facilities for the patient to maintain some control and encouraging emotional support from the relatives. Stressful everyday factors were also seen to have some bearing on the outcome of an operation (Liu et al. 1994). Lui et al. (1994) suggested that recent stressful life events had a negative influence on recovery and anxiety, additional to that of the surgery, and could be detrimental.

The social support or physical presence of a person can clearly be a duty undertaken by the nursing staff. In a survey of 103 patients undergoing an invasive medical procedure and local anaesthesia (Foulger 1997), 32% of participants stated that they would have preferred a third person to be present. The patients were in hospital only for the day undergoing cardiac catheterization (fine catheter passed into the chambers of the heart under local anaesthesia) but, because of the associated anxiety, reduced amount of time in hospital, lack of opportunity or a combination, insufficient information was gained/retained. In such situations the mere presence of the nurse has been found to provide a great deal of comfort to the patient, even if merely holding the patient's hand (Leino-Kilpi and Vuorenheimo 1993, Leinonen et al. 1996, Moon and Cho 2001). In an acute hospital setting two main themes about feelings of being reassured were identified: internal (perception of the environment) and external (nurse being near the patient) (Fareed 1996). The presence of a nurse again provided an assurance of safety. Furthermore, the concept of reassurance has been defined in three ways: (1) a state of mind – renewed confidence in something or someone; (2) a purposeful attempt to restore confidence in someone; and (3) an optimistic pledge given to someone in an attempt to guarantee safety (Teasdale 1989). Such definitions may necessitate the physical presence of a doctor or nurse. Moreover, the presence of the doctor or nurse has been compared with the assuring presence that a parent or guardian can bestow on an infant, e.g. they feel safer when the parent is nearby (Teasdale 1995b).

Such a presence has been referred to within the nursing profession as the 'therapeutic use of self' and can be an extremely powerful method of anxiety management (Leino-Kilpi and Vuorenheimo 1993, Leinonen et al. 1996, Costa 2001). In a study by Mitchell (2000) of 120 patients undergoing day surgery, patients stated that the most anxiety-reducing aspect of their stay in the day-surgery unit was 'talking to and being with the nurse'. In a study undertaken to help to re-design an information booklet for patients undergoing urological surgery, it was established that: 'Patients valued the nurses' interaction and approach and rated this higher than informational needs' (Fagermoen and Hamilton 2003, p. 289).

Finally, in a study of 84 men and their roommates after coronary artery bypass surgery, support from other patients was viewed as very positive (Kulik et al. 1996). Patients who were placed in the same room as other men who had undergone the same operation, and were recovering well, had a better recovery. Seeing someone who was less fortunate and seeing someone who was more fortunate serve different purposes (Taylor and Lobel 1989). Downward evaluations appear to make the person feel better about their personal situation, whereas upward contacts provide information valuable for potential self-survival and successful coping. In a similar study (Parent and Fortin 2000), the benefits to be gained from ex-patients visiting current patients have been demonstrated. Personal self-efficacy appraisal was increased in the group who had a visit from an ex-patient. However, these patients also experienced the highest levels of preoperative anxiety. Moreover, the participants who had contact with the ex-patients chose to be in the experimental group. This indicates that such patients wanted the contact because they were experiencing additional anxiety.

Optimism

Positive expectations or an optimistic outlook about a stressful medical event has been observed to have a considerable impact on postoperative outcomes (Carver and Scheier 1994, Schweizer et al. 1999, Mahler and Kulik 2000, McCarthy et al. 2003). In an early literature review of the association between locus of control and health-related behaviour (Strickland 1978), it was concluded that, if a match between the patient's optimistic expectations and the actual events was achieved, outcomes could be enhanced. In a later review (Scheier and Carver 1992), coping and optimism were positively correlated with a problem-solving approach to coping and the acceptance of the reality of an uncontrollable health-care situation.

In a comprehensive study of the powerful influence of expectations, 348 male patients were studied after benign prostatic surgery (Flood et al. 1993). Strong support for an optimistic view of recovery was established because patients with positive expectations before surgery had better short- and long-term outcomes. In a later study (Schroder and Schwarzer 1998), the coping resources and recovery rates of 248 patients undergoing cardiac surgery were investigated. Having an optimistic belief about the outcome of surgery was viewed as superior to all other aspects of coping. From a biological viewpoint, a number of studies have suggested that a pessimistic outlook can have a negative effect on physiological functioning, e.g. the immune response, rendering a patient more susceptible to ill-health and delayed healing (Kiecolt-Glaser et al. 1995, Scioli et al.

1997, Segerstrom et al. 1998, Raikkonen et al. 1999). Kiecolt-Glaser et al. (1995) compared 13 people caring for relatives with dementia with 13 other people matched for age and financial status. The participants encountering greater levels of stress caring for their relatives experienced significantly slower rates of wound healing. Scioli et al. (1997) also reported that lower 'hope' scores correlated with frequency and severity of illness. Segerstrom et al. (1998) found T-helper cells (phagocytic white cells) to be greater in number in more optimistic individuals, e.g. such patients had the potential for faster healing with fewer complications. Raikkonen et al. (1999) found more pessimistic and anxious patients to have elevated blood pressure and thereby to be more susceptible to increased postoperative morbidity.

Finally, in a review of the literature about immune system functioning (Miller and Cohen 2001), only modest evidence was established for improved immune system functioning when preoperative psychological programmes were employed. Notably, this review did not uncover any study with a brief surgical episode such as with modern surgery. Only more major types of illness and major surgical intervention were deemed worthy of examination. However, a more recent study of patients' experience of a brief hospital stay, e.g. 24 hours, for hernia repair demonstrated the negative effects of increased preoperative stress on wound healing (Broadbent et al. 2003, p. 867): 'This study found that higher reported psychological stress before surgery predicted lower cellular wound repair processes in the early post-operative period.' In addition, participants in the study who smoked also experienced significantly reduced wound-healing abilities.

Conclusion

When studying psychological recovery from surgery, three broad approaches are available: psychodynamic, transactional and convergent approaches. The combined approach may prove to be of greater benefit in modern elective surgery because it has the ability to focus on both individual aspects of personality and the patients' interactions with the health-care environment. In addition, a large number of studies about psychological recovery have focused on specific aspects, e.g. personality traits, social support and optimism. Such studies have helped to identify the most pertinent issues in the psychological recovery of patients from surgery. However, they have also demonstrated that patients are individuals and it cannot be assumed, as stated at the start of this chapter, that all identified aspects will be beneficial to all patients. Nevertheless, such specific psychological considerations may have the potential to be extremely useful in the construction of a preoperative psychological plan of care rooted in the combined approach to coping. Such psychological theories could form the basis of an innovative preoperative anxiety management plan fit for twenty-first century surgical nursing intervention.

Summary

- There are three broad competing psychological theories which endeavour to explain human coping: psychodynamic, transactional and convergent approaches. The psychodynamic approach is broadly concerned with unconscious drives and motives that determine behaviour, e.g. personality traits. The transactional approach is broadly concerned with the dynamic interplay between the environment (social situations) and the individual, e.g. some external influence. The convergent approach is a combination of the two, e.g. coping influenced by both personality traits and social interactions.
- Using a convergent approach to coping in the day-surgery environment will allow for greater flexibility. Individual personality traits can be considered alongside the interplay between the environment and the individual, i.e. internal and external influences.
- Specific approaches to coping, which have their roots in the above broad psychological approaches, have been studied on a large scale because of their repeated influence on coping with a surgical event, e.g. personality traits, social support and optimism.
- Some people may have a personality trait (neuroticism or anxious predisposition) that causes them to become highly anxious when confronted with the likelihood of surgery.
- When confronted with the likelihood of surgery some people prefer little information and place their trust in the doctors and nurses, e.g. avoidant copers, because too much information can increase their anxiety. Vigilant copers, although also trusting the doctors and nurses, prefer to be well informed because too little information may increase anxiety. Fluctuating copers desire a variable level of information, e.g. detailed information required in certain areas but very little in others. Flexible copers assume an adaptable stance - whatever information is provided will be acceptable.
- Many studies have determined that people do not feel that they have much control (real or perceived) over events once admitted to hospital. For many, this can lead to an increase in anxiety and/or greater dissatisfaction.
- Self-efficacy or confidence in one's ability to behave in such a way as to produce a desirable outcome or manage well at home after day surgery can be reduced in certain people, also giving rise to an increase in anxiety.
- Highly optimistic patients have been observed to experience quicker and more positive recovery experiences after surgery.

- Patients who have experienced greater social support from relatives, friends or the nursing staff (therapeutic use of self) have also been observed to have a quicker and more positive postoperative recovery.

Further reading

Audit Commission for Local Authorities and the National Health Service in England and Wales (1991) Measuring Quality: The patient's view of day surgery. No. 3. London: HMSO.
Audit Commission for Local Authorities and the NHS in England and Wales (1993) What Seems To Be the Matter: Communication between hospitals and patients. London: HMSO.
NHS Management Executive (1998) The New NHS: Modern and dependable. London: HMSO.

Websites

British Association of Day Surgery: www.bads@bads.co.uk

Chapter 5

Information selection

Information categories

Information provision has been highlighted as the most basic element of psychological care provided by nurses (Nichols 1985). Its provision before an aversive surgical or medical procedure has been studied extensively in the search for more effective methods of preparing patients for surgery (Wilson-Barnett 1984, Leino-Kilpi et al. 1993, Stengrevics et al. 1996, Goodman 1997, Lamarche et al. 1998, Shuldham 1999a, Parent and Fortin 2000, Walsh and Shaw 2000, Lee et al. 2003). As information provision is an extensive topic and implicit within the broad and specific psychological approaches to coping (see Chapters 1 and 2), it is discussed separately here. Moreover, psychoeducational care (see Chapter 1) is a combination of psychological concepts of care and the provision of information; it is an extremely important issue in modern day surgery because of (1) the limited time available for interaction with the medical and nursing staff, (2) the considerable amount of recovery that takes place at home with little recourse to professional help (Pfisterer et al. 2001) and (3) it being a major challenge to the future of effective day surgery (Bradshaw et al. 1999, Mitchell 1999a, 1999b, Dixon-Woods 2001, Mitchell 2001).

For the purposes of clarity, information provision is discussed under the terms of problem-focused coping information and emotionally focused coping information (see Chapter 4) (Table 5.1). Problem-focused and emotionally focused information provision are further subdivided into six categories: procedural, behavioural and sensory information, cognitive coping strategies, relaxation and modelling (Wilson 1981, Mathews and Ridgeway 1984, Miller et al. 1989, Rothrock 1989, Suls and Wan 1989, Johnston and Vogele 1993). Each of the six categories of information are discussed in association with preoperative preparation for surgery.

Problem-focused coping information

The most commonly used preoperative information provided in the health-care situation is problem-focused coping information, e.g. procedural,

Table 5.1 Information focus	
Information focus	**Description**
Problem-focused coping information	Problem-focused coping information aids empowerment or a person's ability to make informed decisions. It provides information to help the person directly challenge the stressful episode and assists him or her in construction of a plan of action to alter, circumvent or eliminate a particular stressor. Problem-focused coping information is commonly used when the stressor is deemed to be more susceptible to change by direct action
Emotionally focused coping information	Emotionally focused coping information helps a person to view the stressful experience in a more positive manner. It provides information to help indirectly challenge the stressful episode. Emotionally focused coping information is commonly used when the stressor is deemed to be less susceptible to change by direct action

behavioural and sensory information (Table 5.1) (Folkman and Lazarus 1980, Folkman 1984, Folkman et al. 1986, Lazarus and Folkman 1987). Problem-focused coping involves the individual attempts to challenge the stressor directly by embarking on a plan of action, e.g. when faced with the prospect of surgery a patient may wish to discover exactly what will happen to him or her, gain information about the operation, events on the day of surgery and the length of the recovery period, in order to alter, circumvent or eliminate a particular stressor. Such a method of coping is commonly employed when the stressor is deemed to be open to change. In addition, it is most helpful for the medical and nursing staff when patients make use of such information. When patients follow the recommended advice, it can result in a quicker physical recovery with fewer complications (Lindeman and Van Aernam 1971, King and Tarsitano 1982, Hathaway 1986, Yount and Schoessler 1991, Myles et al. 2002).

The terminology employed within these three categories of information provision has differed over many years so the definitions, for the purposes of this book, are outlined in Table 5.2. In addition, many studies from the USA use different terms to describe the same aspects of information provision, e.g. procedural information is described as situational information and behavioural information as role information. Many studies suggest that problem-focused coping information is the most effective form of preoperative information provision. This may result because patients perceive (or they have been informed) that they can positively influence their recovery from surgery, e.g. stopping smoking, losing weight, undertaking the recommended pre- and postoperative exercises, arranging adequate time off work, etc. If patients can therefore undertake problem-solving actions to improve their recovery prospects, problem-focused coping information will be of great benefit.

Table 5.2 Problem-focused coping information categories

Category	Description
Procedural or situational information	The sequential order of events on the day of surgery once admitted to the surgical unit, i.e. what will happen next and the order in which the events will occur. Studies in the USA often refer to this as situational information
Behavioural or role information	The behaviour(s) or action(s) the patient is required to undertake before, during or after the surgical procedure, i.e. adopting a certain position for the procedure, keeping a limb elevated, gentle movements only, deep breathing exercises, no lifting for 6 weeks, etc. Studies in the USA often refer to this as role information
Sensory information	The bodily sensations the patient is likely to experience before, during or after the surgical procedure, i.e. the likely sensations of the drugs entering the body during the initial stages of anaesthesia, degree and duration of pain, medical equipment used in the immediate postoperative phase

During the delivery of problem-focused information, some emotionally focused coping information can be gained leading to some obvious overlap, e.g. when gaining information about procedural events on the day of surgery from the nurse (problem-focused coping), a patient may benefit from the words of assurance implicitly provided (emotionally focused coping), such as high-quality care, interpersonal skills of the nurses, preoperative assessment safety measures (Leino-Kilpi and Vuorenheimo 1993, Leinonen et al. 1996, Moon and Cho 2001). However, for the purposes of theoretical explanation the following classification is employed.

Procedural or situational information

A number of studies have emphasized the importance of this form of information, suggesting that it is one of the most important. In an early study (Elsass et al. 1987b), 81 patients undergoing surgery were divided into two groups. Group 1 received routine procedural information for 5 minutes whereas group 2 received a detailed account of procedural information plus information about the various stages of anaesthesia/surgery (20 minutes). The experimental group (additional information) demonstrated lower levels of anxiety, although not at a significant level. In an early review of the literature on patient information (Rothrock 1989), it was concluded that sensory and psychological information were more effective for highly anxious patients whereas low-anxiety patients benefited more from procedural information. Schoessler (1989) studied 116 patients undergoing various types of surgery and asked them what information they most preferred. Psychological support, situational information (procedural) and role information (behavioural) were all rated as the most desirable forms.

A mixture of approaches, as highlighted above (Schoessler 1989), has also demonstrated positive effects. In an early review of the literature it was concluded that a combination of both procedural and sensory information was the most effective method (Suls and Wan 1989). Furthermore, 111 patients were required, as part of an experimental study, to listen to an audiotaped presentation on the eve of surgery (Ziemer 1983). Group 1 listened to procedural information, group 2 to sensory information and group 3 to procedural and sensory information plus cognitive coping strategies (advice on calming self-talk). However, no significant differences were established among the three groups, although the first two listened to a 5-minute audiotape whereas the third listened to a 22-minute audiotape containing a great deal of information. Such attention bias may have the potential to distort the results, i.e. 5 minutes for one group and 22 minutes for the other two. In a later day-surgery study, this attention bias was more pronounced: 40 day-surgery patients were divided into two groups and provided with both procedural and behavioural information (Beddows 1997). Group 1 were provided with the information on admission whereas group 2 received the information before admission (home visit by the researcher to provide the information). Although anxiety was significantly lower in group 2 (home visit), the extra time spent with this group and the experience of being treated differently were not considered, i.e. Hawthorne effect (Parahoo 1997). In a further review of the literature (Johnston and Vogele 1993), it was highlighted that the most favourable outcomes were gained when both procedural and behavioural information strategies were employed simultaneously.

In an experimental study, 82 patients undergoing orthopaedic surgery were observed (Gammon and Mulholland 1996). Group 1 received a mixture of procedural, sensory and cognitive coping strategies whereas the control group 2 received routine care. Using self-reported measures, the experimental group, i.e. group 1, were significantly less anxious and less depressed. It was therefore concluded that preparatory information was a behavioural guide, an aid to self-efficacy, and a point of convergence for emotional and problem-solving strategies or a necessary part of the 'work of worry'. However, the lack of an 'attention-control group' may render such evidence as bias, e.g. group 1 received 'special attention' whereas group 2 merely received the usual care. Again, this has the potential to lead to considerable attention bias.

In a more recent study (Cooil and Bithell 1997), 42 orthopaedic patients were divided into two groups, where one group received an instructional list of 'dos' and 'don'ts', but the experimental group received the same list although with some personally communicated instruction (procedural and behavioural information) on how to mobilize correctly during the postoperative period. Recall of information was greater in the experimental group, although the issue of attention bias is still prominent. Moreover, patients were obliged to recall the information on the first postoperative day, i.e. while still in pain and discomfort from the previous day's surgery. This may have led to inadequate recall of information by some patients. Finally, 131 cardiac surgery patients who received additional procedural and behavioural information via the telephone on six occasions postoperatively were surveyed (Hartford et al. 2002). The experimental group who had received the extra telephone information were significantly less anxious than the control group who had received normal care, i.e. no telephone contact. However, the experimental group received much more than mere information because during the telephone interviews patients asked many additional psychosocial questions. To assume that just the additional information lowered anxiety may therefore be erroneous.

Behavioural or role information

In an early study of recovery from surgery (Lindeman and Van Aernam 1971), 261 patients were surveyed to explore the positive effects of preoperative teaching. All patients had their lung capacity measured and were then divided into two groups. The experimental group received a programme of helpful breathing exercises whereas the control group received no further intervention. The experimental group were observed to experience a significant reduction in their length of hospital stay. However, this study did not explore any psychological intervention, but merely the behaviour required by the patient to improve physical recovery. Indeed, such is the focus of many studies concerning recovery from surgery, i.e. enhancing physical recovery and not necessarily psychological recovery. Such a focus may raise the moral question about the true purpose of preoperative information provision. Does it concern the gaining of an obliging compliant patient or the true education and empowerment of an anxious patient (Webber 1990, Fleming 1992, Leino-Kilpi et al. 1993, Redman 1993, Pellino et al. 1998, van Weert et al. 2003)? Patient empowerment has been defined as (1) an act of granting autonomy, (2) a process of gaining influence over events and outcomes and (3) a psychological state (feeling of being enabled) (Menon 2002). Unfortunately, few studies concerning preoperative information strongly emphasize patient empowerment.

In a replication by King and Tarsitano (1982) of the above study by Lindeman and van Aernam (1971), 49 patients undergoing surgery were instructed on how to cough and breathe effectively in the postoperative period. Again, using entirely physiological measures, the patients who had undergone the extra instruction had significantly better behavioural outcomes. In a study that considered the benefits of a behavioural information booklet (Young and Humphrey 1985), patients undergoing hysterectomy were contacted 2 weeks before their admission to hospital. Participants were randomly divided into two groups. Group 1 received a preadmission teaching brochure containing specific exercise instructions deemed helpful for recovery whereas group 2 received no teaching brochure. No significant differences with regard to satisfaction or anxiety were established on the morning of surgery. However, the results may have been distorted because some patients had a premedicant, some were to undergo general anaesthesia and others local anaesthesia, and some patients underwent surgery for a malignancy. Such a diverse population sample may have contributed to the inconclusive results.

In a study undertaken to uncover the views of nurses and effective information provision, 159 were asked to complete a questionnaire (Yount and Schoessler 1991). The data gained were compared with the responses of 116 patients on a postoperative questionnaire about preference for information (Schoessler 1989). The nurses rated the behavioural skills training required for a speedier recovery as the most important aspect to teach patients on the day of surgery. However, this was not the most important aspect for the patients on the day of surgery, because they believed psychological support to be of greater benefit. In a similar study of 294 day-surgery patients (Oberle et al. 1994), it was also concluded that nurses emphasized behavioural and sensory information provision on the day of surgery. Conversely, in a day-case survey about information provision (Brumfield et al. 1996), 30 patients and 29 nurses were asked to complete and return a postal questionnaire. Patients ranked situational (behavioural) information as the most important on the day of surgery whereas nurses rated psychosocial support as a priority. It may be that day-case patients made problem-focused coping information (behavioural information) their priority because their stay in hospital was to be so brief, i.e. problem-focused coping information was deemed a high priority because the patients would be caring for themselves at home in a few short hours. In a further study concerning day surgery (Kain et al. 1997), 97 patients undergoing a variety of surgical procedures were surveyed to determine what information they required from their anaesthetist. The questionnaire was administered preoperatively on the day of surgery. The most wanted information concerned pain management, postoperative mobility and the opportunity to meet the anaesthetist, i.e. mainly problem-focused coping information.

Finally, in a review of the literature, both procedural information and behavioural instructions demonstrated the most universal effects in improving measures of postoperative recovery (Johnston and Vogele 1993). However, such information tends to dominate modern surgery and again could therefore be more concerned with compliance on the day of surgery (Andrew 1970, Hill 1982, Young and Humphrey 1985, Wallace 1986a, Suls and Wan 1989, Butler et al. 1996, Linden and Engberg 1996, Fellowes et al. 1999). In addition, although such information is beneficial on the day of surgery, its sole use may be of little benefit in the days and weeks spent at home before and after modern elective surgery.

Sensory information

In an early review of the literature (Miller et al. 1989), it was concluded that the most effective form of information for patients undergoing surgery or a stressful medical procedure was sensory information alone or in combination with procedural information. In a further early review, it was concluded that procedural, psychological (very brief measures to reduce anxiety) and sensory information were noted to have the most effect (Rothrock 1989). A number of studies have therefore employed sensory information in order to gauge its impact on psychological recovery. In an early study (Hill 1982), 40 patients undergoing eye surgery were randomly divided into four groups. A 7-minute audiotape of slightly different information was provided for each group: (1) basic eye anatomy plus behavioural instructions; (2) basic eye anatomy plus sensory information; (3) both behavioural instructions and sensory information plus basic eye anatomy; and (4) general information. The group who received basic eye anatomy plus information about the likely sensations remained hospitalized for a shorter period and reported mobilizing at home significantly more quickly. However, as stated, behavioural measures, e.g. length of time in hospital, now have little or no value in modern inpatient and day-case surgery, and can no longer be regarded as an effective measure of recovery from modern surgery (Karanci and Dirik 2003, Mitchell 2004).

In a study of 20 patients undergoing an unpleasant medical procedure (barium enema where a radio-opaque dye is inserted into the large bowel), significantly less anxiety about the likely sensations was reported by the group who received sensory information as opposed to the group who received procedural information only (Hartfield et al. 1982). However, no anaesthesia was employed with this medical test, which may have rendered the procedure somewhat less threatening because anaesthesia has been viewed as a very anxiety-provoking medical event (Egbert et al. 1964, Ramsay 1972, Male 1981, McCleane and Cooper 1990, Shevde and Panagopoulos 1991, McGaw and Hanna 1998, Mitchell 2000). In a similar study, a teaching film was presented to 50 patients before an unpleasant medical event – nasogastric intubation for gastric content analysis (tube inserted through the nasal cavity, down the oesophagus and into the stomach) (Padilla et al. 1981). Patients were divided into four groups and slightly different information provided, e.g. procedural only, procedural with common distressful sensations, procedural with coping behaviours, and procedural with coping behaviours to relieve the common distressful sensations. Patients reported the sensory and coping behaviour information to be the most effective in helping to decrease discomfort, pain and anxiety. However, again the procedure was only brief and involved no anaesthesia.

In an inpatient study (Schwartz-Barcott et al. 1994), 91 patients undergoing cholecystectomy were studied by dividing patients into three groups: audiotape information, information from a nurse and routine care. The audiotaped information and the nurse both conveyed a mixture of sensory and behavioural information. Both these groups reported significantly less anxiety although only when compared with the routine care group, i.e. normal care received in that particular clinical environment. It is unknown what 'routine care' actually entails because it may differ from ward to ward (Auerbach 1989). Although used in numerous studies, therefore, routine care can frequently be a poor control.

Finally, in a large American postoperative telephone survey (Krupat et al. 2000), 3602 patients were contacted to uncover the most appropriate information after discharge from hospital. It was discovered that, when information provision was good, satisfaction with care was also good. Having some control and being provided with sensory information were both significantly related to satisfaction – although only weakly. Similar results were also obtained in a recent day-surgery survey about sensory information (Bernier et al. 2003). Following the survey of 116 day-surgery patients, a teaching guide with reference to the areas of most concern was produced covering five dimensions of preoperative information provision: situational/procedural information, sensation/discomfort information, patient role information, psychosocial support and skills training. The information judged to be required within the sensation/discomfort dimension was associated with postoperative pain management.

In summary, problem-solving information is a form of teaching used extensively throughout the education and instruction of surgical patients. It is therefore the most common form of patient education and teaching. However, its true purpose has sometimes been questioned because instructional information has frequently been used to gain a compliant patient and not necessarily to provide information to educate and empower patients. Certainly problem-focused coping information has the most universal appeal because both patient and hospital personnel benefit from its application, i.e. patients are provided with essential, practical information required for a quick physical recovery and hospital staff are able to meet the demands of the operating schedule with little delay or complication. It could therefore be argued as most appropriate for use in day-case surgery. However, because of its implicit practical contents, e.g. ability to help patients find practical solutions to meet their individual requirements, such information must be provided before the day of surgery (see 'Timing of information provision' p. 131). Finally, many recent studies have tended not to examine information provision as vigorously as in previous decades. The reasons are twofold: (1) all problem-solving information provision has demonstrated some success in the past and (2) modern day surgery has now rendered such information provision-focused research as somewhat obsolete, as a range of information is now required because considerable self-preparation and self-recovery takes place at home after day surgery. Merely to focus information provision on the few days once spent in hospital is no longer appropriate. Patients need to be informed about home recovery where professional help is not as easily available.

Emotionally focused coping information

Although many studies suggest that problem-focused coping information is the most effective, numerous other studies have recommended emotionally focused coping information as of even greater value. Such evidence may have resulted from patients' perceptions of a health-care situation in which stressors are deemed less susceptible to change, i.e. the situation cannot be circumvented by planned problem-focused coping action. In addition, emotionally focused coping strategies could be the preferred choice for participants using avoidant coping strategies, i.e. when the provision of too much information causes an increase in anxiety (see Chapter 4). Some day-surgery studies have revealed avoidant coping behaviour to be the most common form of coping prevailing in almost a third of all patients (Kerrigan et al. 1993, Garden et al. 1996, Mitchell 2000). The three categories of emotionally focused coping information discussed are cognitive strategies, relaxation and modelling (Table 5.3).

Cognitive strategies

Cognitive coping strategies can be described as a purposeful emotional attempt to have fewer negative thoughts about a given situation, i.e. a mental strategy for avoiding catastrophizing (believing that something will go seriously wrong) (Litt et al. 1999). This can be largely viewed as an active method of cognitive coping. These encouraged thoughts can help a patient to gain assurance that they will be safe, wake up from their

Table 5.3 Emotionally focused coping information categories	
Category	Description
Cognitive strategies	The purposeful emotional attempt to experience less negative thoughts concerning a given situation, i.e. a mental strategy for avoiding catastrophizing (believing something will go seriously wrong) (active). Alternatively, this can involve mentally rehearsing the anxiety-provoking event (work of worry) (passive)
Relaxation	Individual strategies of relaxation or planned programme of relaxation techniques, e.g. music therapy, simple methods of distraction, hypnosis and guided imagery
Modelling	Actively imitating the required or desired behaviour, e.g. via a real-life event, demonstration, teaching, reading hospital leaflets, websites, videotaped programmes and other aspects of the media (direct). Passively imitating the required or desired behaviour, e.g. watching other patients (indirect)

operation, be unharmed and have full recovery, or act as a method of self-calming, i.e. engender a mood of optimism (Fareed 1996) (see Chapter 4). Alternatively, mentally rehearsing an anxiety-provoking event has demonstrated positive results, e.g. work of worry (Janis 1958) (see Chapter 4). In the 'work of worry', no active emotional attempts are made to experience fewer negative thoughts but the stress scenario is merely replayed in the person's thoughts.

First, a number of studies have employed active methods to encourage cognitive coping strategies. In a review of the literature on alleviating the stress experienced by patients in hospital, positive reappraisals and information about possible sensations were viewed as the most beneficial forms of information provision (Wilson-Barnett 1984). In a further review of the literature, problem-focused and emotionally focused coping strategies were considered to be the most effective approaches (Breemhaar and van den Borne 1991). It was suggested that teaching patients mental strategies to aid coping, such as being educated in methods of distraction or emphasizing any or all of the positive aspects of the surgery, could increase cognitive control. This is in contrast to the 'work of worry', which can be viewed as a passive cognitive coping strategy compared with a taught method of distraction which can be viewed as an active cognitive coping strategy (see Chapter 3). In a review of hospital anxiety, 'cognitive re-framing' was a highly recommended approach (Teasdale 1995b, p. 81). Cognitive re-framing is a term used to describe cognitive coping: 'patients who use cognitive re-framing adjust themselves psychologically in such a way that events formerly perceived as threatening are now seen in a more positive light'. Teasdale's (1995b) cognitive re-framing could therefore be considered very similar to the employment of an active cognitive coping strategy, i.e. an individual's emotional attempt to deal with a stressor judged not to be susceptible to change (Lazarus 1966, Folkman and Lazarus 1980, Folkman et al. 1986). Once within a given clinical situation, e.g. hospital ward before surgery, little problem-focused coping can be undertaken so emotionally focused coping may be the only option, i.e. endeavouring to make a more positive cognitive appraisal of the situation.

A comparative study of relaxation strategies and cognitive coping strategies was undertaken (Pickett and Clum 1982) using 59 cholecystectomy patients to investigate their ability to influence postoperative anxiety. Cognitive distraction resulted in the lowest level of self-reported anxiety, although the cognitive distraction involved being provided with more information about the intended surgery. Supplementary information does not necessarily meet with the above definition of cognitive coping strategy, i.e. using a taught method of cognitive re-framing or viewing the situation in a more positive manner. Additional information within the bounds of a research study may not therefore be a valid cognitive distractor.

A number of studies have suggested that patients who employ an avoidant coping style might have a greater preference for this form of preparation, e.g. distraction or positive suggestions, because they generally choose to ignore cues in aversive situations and desire less information than vigilant copers (Miller et al. 1989, Breemhaar and van den Borne 1991, Krohne et al. 1996). Breemhaar and van den Borne (1991) postulated that avoidant copers assume a wait-and-see attitude from the start and are therefore not too concerned about unexpected happenings or sensations. To examine the effect of cognitive strategies (Young and Humphrey 1985), 30 women, about to undergo hysterectomy, were divided into three equal groups: groups 1 and 2 were taught methods of cognitive coping either via a detailed information booklet or by the researcher; group 3 served as attention-control group. The two experimental groups reported lower anxiety than the control group and spent less time in hospital. However, other studies have had mixed results concerning such preparatory methods: 111 patients were required, as part of an experimental study (Ziemer 1983), to listen to an audiotaped presentation on the eve of surgery. Group 1 received procedural information, group 2 sensory information and group 3 procedural and sensory information plus cognitive coping strategies (advice on calming self-talk). No significant differences were established between the three groups, although this was an older study and may be considered too simplistic, i.e. no account taken of people wanting little information.

Conversely, a number of studies have examined cognitive coping strategies by using the 'work of worry' (see Chapter 4). In an early study (Ray and Fitzgibbon 1981), emotional and behavioural outcomes were measured before and after surgery in 36 patients undergoing cholecystectomy. Patients with higher levels of preoperative arousal took fewer drugs, reported less pain and were discharged more quickly. It was therefore concluded that the mental rehearsal of the anxiety-provoking situation had been of benefit. However, as with a number of the studies in this section, the measures of recovery employed are clearly now obsolete in the day-surgery arena (Mitchell 2004). Similar studies have also suggested that preparation in the mere form of information provision may not always be in the patients' best interest (Salmon 1993). Preparation should therefore focus on providing patients with the opportunity to disclose their fears, receive assurance, social support and relaxation. However, data here (Salmon 1993) are drawn from purely objective, physiological measures without enquiring about the patients' emotional responses, e.g. monitoring blood pressure, heart beat, urinary cortisol. In a further study (Vogele and Steptoe 1986), 15 patients undergoing surgery were observed and over a 2-day period both emotional and physiological data were collected. Patients who thought about their operation more preoperatively had reduced levels of stress when measured by a skin conductance monitor. Again, this indicates that the work of worry may have a beneficial impact. The objective data from a further two studies concerning preoperative preparation for surgery were compared to examine the relationship between anxiety and recovery (Wallace 1986b). Participants with increased preoperative anxiety were more likely to have higher postoperative anxiety, although again this did not automatically result in a poorer recovery. Increased stress levels may not, therefore, automatically result in poor postoperative outcomes as postulated by Janis (1958) in the 'work of worry' theory.

Finally, a number of more recent studies have increasingly employed spiritual aspects of coping within preoperative preparation (Wallston et al. 1999, Williams and Clark 2000). Religious coping has been previously associated with social support (Krohne et al. 2000), although it is mentioned here only because other studies have viewed such coping as a form of cognitive or emotional coping. In a study to validate a questionnaire about religious coping, Wallston et al. (1999) describe three types of religious coping strategies: (1) 'God's will', which is described as the self being 'passive' and God 'active'; (2) self 'active' and God 'passive'; and (3) a combination of the two. However, the 'God's will' approach was associated with poorer adjustment in the postoperative period. In a similar study (Tix and Frazier 1998), the religious coping strategies of 58 patients and their partners after urological surgery was investigated, e.g. prayer, church attendance and importance of religion. Such behaviour was associated with better adjustment, although it was moderated by different spiritual beliefs, i.e. appraised differently depending on the individuals' religious orientation.

Relaxation information

A number of studies have advocated relaxation programmes to be a more beneficial form of anxiety management (Goldmann et al. 1988, Caunt 1992, Salmon 1992a, 1993, Markland and Hardy 1993, Schwartz-Barcott et al. 1994). The form of relaxation provided can vary from relaxation exercises, music therapy or hypnosis to distraction (Mitchell 2003b). In a relaxation study, 24 patients undergoing surgery were divided into two groups (Wells et al. 1986). One group was provided with routine ward preparation whereas the experimental group was taught relaxation techniques. The experimental group spent fewer days in hospital and required less analgesia. However, as mentioned previously, routine care may be a poor research control because the relaxation group may experience a greater level of attention and experience a more positive recovery merely because of the additional attention. This issue can also be viewed in a further study where 24 patients undergoing surgery were randomly allocated to two groups (Holden-Lund 1988). One group received an audiotaped series of relaxation techniques whereas the control group were merely advised to have 'quiet periods'. The audiotapes were 20 minutes in duration and were administered once in the afternoon before surgery and again once a day for 3 days in the postoperative period. Using subjective and objective measures the experimental group had lower levels of anxiety and their surgical wounds presented with less erythema (reduced inflammation and quicker healing).

More recently, 92 patients undergoing general anaesthesia for hysterectomy were studied (Miro and Raich 1999b). Participants were randomly divided into two groups: an attention-control group and a relaxation group. The experimental group received 30 minutes of relaxation, 1 week before surgery and were also provided with detailed instructions on how to practise the techniques at home. All participants were tested for preferred coping style, i.e. vigilant or avoidant coping behaviour. The assumption was that avoidant copers would experience less pain when relaxation techniques were used preoperatively. However, all participants in the relaxation group, irrespective of coping style, reported less pain and were more active in the postoperative period. The reasons for this were stated as extremes of vigilant and avoidant coping behaviour not being exclusively employed and patients finding information from other sources. Put simply, a positive result from such a study may be possible only when extreme vigilant and avoidant coping patients are used and information provision is more strictly controlled.

In a review of the literature on the impact of guided imagery (visual or auditory method of distraction/relaxation) (Eller 1999), it was concluded that state anxiety (immediate anxiety arising from stressful experience) may be modified by the use of such guided techniques. In a similar study to demonstrate the effects of guided imagery (Tusek et al. 1997), 130 patients undergoing elective surgery were divided into two groups: group 1 received routine preoperative care whereas group 2 listened to guided imagery tapes for 3 days before their surgical procedures, during induction of anaesthesia, intraoperatively and in the recovery area, and for 6 days after surgery. No difference was established between the two groups with regard to the level of anxiety, although in the experimental group 50% required less opioid analgesia to control their pain.

In a brief review of the literature concerning the physical and psychological preparation of patients for surgery (Walker 2002), one of the main themes to emerge was the use of hypnosis. For some patients, such strategies are beneficial although their practical employment in modern day surgery may be somewhat restricted. In an early day-surgery study (Goldmann et al. 1988), 52 patients undergoing surgery received either a short preoperative hypnotic induction or brief information provision. It was revealed that the hypnotized group required significantly less of the anaesthetic agents during induction of anaesthesia. This group was also significantly more relaxed as judged by a self-rated anxiety measure. In a further study, 60 day-surgery patients undergoing local anaesthesia for plastic surgery were observed to determine the benefits of hypnosis (Faymonville et al. 1997). Patients were divided into two groups: a hypnosis group and an emotional support group (deep breathing, relaxation, encouragement of focus on pleasant memory). It was concluded that the hypnosis group required significantly less sedation than the emotional support group. However, the hypnosis group was significantly more anxious in the preoperative phase and may have opted for the hypnosis to help manage their anxiety more effectively.

Other studies have employed music therapy as a form of relaxation before surgery (Domar et al. 1987, Augustin and Hains 1996, Cruise et al. 1997). Domar et al. (1987) studied 42 patients undergoing skin surgery and provided a 20-minute audiotape of relaxation for half of the group whereas the other half were asked to read a book of their choice for 20 minutes each day. Although the programme of relaxation commenced 3–4 weeks before the day of surgery, no significant subjective differences were established. However, a significant positive result was gained in a similar study of 41 day-surgery patients (Augustin and Hains 1996). Although the experimental group only listened to the music for 15–30 minutes, objective data collection revealed a reduction in anxiety. However, some patients refused to listen to music, which may have reduced the validity of the study as a result of selection bias, i.e. patients able to choose to which experimental group they were allocated for the purposes of the study. Moreover, some patients may refuse to be part of such a study because of the possibility of being assigned to the control or placebo group (Schultz et al. 2003). In a further study (Lepage et al. 2001), the influence of music on sedative requirement was examined in 50 patients undergoing spinal anaesthesia. One group received music via a headset during the surgical procedure plus a patient-controlled administration device containing midazolam (sedative). A second group merely received the same patient-controlled administration device. It was uncovered that midazolam requirements during surgery were significantly less for the group listening to music, i.e. distracted from the environmental impact of their clinical surroundings. A similar study was also undertaken on patients undergoing minor surgery under local anaesthesia (Mok and Wong 2003). Again, the music group experienced significantly lower self-reported anxiety. However, a nurse stood with all the patients during the surgery, which could have influenced the results as patients have been known to experience less anxiety when close to a nurse (Mitchell 2000) (Figure 5.1).

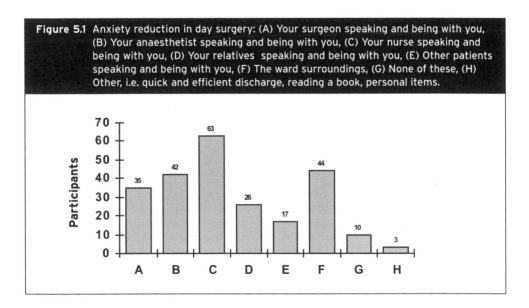

Figure 5.1 Anxiety reduction in day surgery: (A) Your surgeon speaking and being with you, (B) Your anaesthetist speaking and being with you, (C) Your nurse speaking and being with you, (D) Your relatives speaking and being with you, (E) Other patients speaking and being with you, (F) The ward surroundings, (G) None of these, (H) Other, i.e. quick and efficient discharge, reading a book, personal items.

A number of studies have recently examined the 'awake' patient within the operating theatre environment. Operating theatres were not originally constructed for the conscious patient although modern surgery has witnessed many changes, resulting in more conscious patients in theatre, e.g. many more conscious patients, although sedated, now come into the operating theatre. Cruise et al. (1997) studied 121 patients undergoing sedation for eye surgery and assigned patients to one of four conditions: audiotape of relaxing suggestions, normal quiet environmental noise, audiotape of previous operating room noise (during the same surgical procedure) or relaxing music. Using a visual analogue scale to gauge satisfaction, patients were more satisfied when listening to music although they were not less anxious. In a similar study, patients undergoing urological procedures and spinal anaesthesia were randomly divided into two groups: music via headsets or headsets with no music (Koch et al. 1998). The music group was found to require significantly less sedation although the study may have lacked validity because the no-music group did not always wear the headsets throughout the intraoperative period. In a survey of intraoperative care and the conscious patient (Leinonen et al. 1996), the most effective aspect of anxiety management was the mere presence of the nurse. A number of patients who were receiving no music via their headsets removed them. In a final study of the conscious patient in theatre when undergoing a caesarean section, supportive relatives and staff helped in the reduction of anxiety (Kennedy et al. 1992) (see Chapter 3).

Modelling information

Modelling can be described as the direct imitation of the required or desired behaviour in order to help achieve the goal of a quick and successful recovery from surgery. Knowledge about the desired behaviour can be gained via a real-life event, demonstration, teaching sessions, reading hospital leaflets, websites, videotaped programme and other aspects of the media. Such knowledge can also be gained indirectly by passively imitating the required or desired behaviour, e.g. watching other patients within the clinical environment and imitating.

Indirect teaching can occur via videotaped or audiotaped presentations and has therefore been used in many research studies. In a review of 25 research papers about the use of videotaped presentations (Gagliano 1988), it was concluded that such programmes were of great benefit because patients often viewed a good role model or a patient with positive outcomes. Seeing positive comparisons during stressful situations might help some patients cope more effectively, e.g. demonstration of positive methods of managing personal recovery (Taylor and Lobel 1989). A number of studies have all concluded that viewing a videotaped presentation before an unpleasant medical event is of benefit (Shipley et al. 1978, 1979, Tongue and Stanley 1991, Leino-Kilpi and Vuorenheimo 1993). Such presentations helped to reduce the fear associated with the unknown elements, were cheap to run and did not require the patient to have a certain level of literacy skill, as with written information (mode of information presentation is expanded on in Chapter 6).

In a study of 91 patients undergoing surgery (Wicklin and Forster 1994), the effects of two different videotaped presentations were compared. Patients were divided into three groups 1 week before orthopaedic surgery: a factual video for two groups and a factual and sensory-based video, seen through the eyes of a patient, for the third group. Although no significant differences were established, the more anxious patients within each group were identified. In a similar study (Mahler et al. 1993), a 40-minute videotaped programme explaining recovery from cardiac surgery was shown to 127 participants. Participants were divided into four groups: (1) videotape where a nurse provided all the information; (2) a mastery videotape where patients portrayed recovery essentially as a steady upward progression with little mention of any problems; (3) a coping videotape where patients portrayed recovery as having more ups and downs, mentioning some concerns and problems with which they are coping; and (4) no videotape.

> Although all subjects who viewed one of the three preparatory videos indicated significantly less anxiety than no-tape controls, those in the mastery-tape condition had significantly lower anxiety scores than those in either the coping-tape or the nurse-tape conditions.
>
> Mahler et al. (1993 p. 447)

Therefore, the patients who had received the tape demonstrating an optimistic and positive role model experienced the lowest level of anxiety. Conversely, in a study involving both patients and relatives, a videotaped presentation was shown shortly before discharge after cardiac surgery (Mahler and Kulik 2002). The spouses of 226 male and 70 female patients were randomly assigned to view: an opportunistically slanted information videotape, a videotape that featured more ups and downs of recovery, or no videotape. However, no significant differences were established.

In summary, reviews of the literature about emotionally focused coping information have demonstrated some significant advantages in the use of information provision, hypnosis, relaxation, specialist support workers, modelling and close supportive relationship with a nurse who stays with the patient (Rogers and Reich 1986, Johnston and Vogele 1993). Rogers and Reich (1986) concluded further that, because all such aspects have worked at some stage, the answer must lie with individual, specific methods of preparation. The work of worry, although an older psychological concept, may still be used by many patients. Cognitive distraction has demonstrated many advantages and, indeed, may be the sole aspect of anxiety management intervention currently employed in modern elective surgery (see Chapter 3). Relaxation interventions have demonstrated some success although such approaches may lack credible clinical application. Modelling or the imitating of desired/required behaviour might have greater clinical application, e.g. a vast amount of coverage of health-care situations now appears in the media, providing patients with greater insight.

Conclusion

As alluded to throughout this book, information provision before surgery is crucial for effective psychoeducational management in modern day surgery. Both problem-focused and emotionally focused information provision have their part to play. However, a move away from the mechanistic model of problem-focused information, which is primarily aimed at the immediate events surrounding the day of surgery, is required. Modern elective surgical patients must prepare themselves for surgery and attend to their recovery once discharged in a way that previous surgical populations have never experienced. A balance of problem-focused and emotionally focused coping information is therefore necessary because this is a new era of surgery and patients no longer have the benefit of immediate professional attention that was enjoyed by previous generations. Information provision in modern surgery must therefore move towards an effective and efficient balance between information selection and information delivery.

Summary

* Problem-focused coping information includes procedural, behavioural and sensory information. Emotionally focused coping information includes cognitive coping strategies, relaxation and modelling.
* Procedural and behavioural information provision are the most widely employed methods mainly because they serve two central purposes, i.e. they inform the patient of the approaching event and also the behaviour appropriate for necessary medical and nursing intervention. However, many of the measures used to determine the effectiveness of such information derive from objective measurement, e.g. days spent in hospital, blood pressure, painkillers consumed, etc. Such measures could be viewed as obsolete in modern surgery and, more crucially, limited in their 'true' measurement of psychological recovery.
* Sensory information provision, although effective, is frequently presented in a formal manner. Consequently, patients frequently have unrealistic expectations

about postoperative pain after day surgery, e.g. either patients have not been told about the degree and duration of pain or they believe that day surgery is minor surgery and hence not very painful (Bain et al. 1999, McHugh and Thoms 2002, Dewar et al. 2003, Mitchell 2003a).

- Cognitive coping strategies have been viewed as having both an active and a passive focus. Active cognitive coping strategies are associated with cognitively re-framing threatening perceptions and viewing events in a more positive light, e.g. less catastrophizing. Passive cognitive coping strategies can be associated with the 'work of worry', i.e. the time that some people want to spend in repeatedly considering the anxiety-provoking event.
- Relaxation and modelling have demonstrated their effectiveness, although they may have limited application in modern day surgery. However, increasing media coverage of health-care issues and the expansion of information technology may in future facilitate even greater patient insights, e.g. some American day-surgery units use webcams for patients to preview the clinical environment.

Further reading

Audit Commission (1993) What Seems to be the Matter: Communication between hospitals and patients. London: HMSO.

Dixon-Woods, M. (2001) Writing wrongs? An analysis of published discourses about the use of patient information leaflets. Social Science and Medicine 52: 1417-1432.

Fellowes, H., Abbott, D., Barton, K., Burgess, L., Clare, A. and Lucas, B. (1999) Orthopaedic Pre-admission Assessment Clinics. London: Royal College of Nursing.

Health Service Commissioner for England for Scotland and for Wales (1997) Annual Report for 1996-1997. London: HMSO.

Mitchell, M.J. (2001) Constructing information booklets for day-case patients. Journal of Ambulatory Surgery 9: 37-45.

Walsh, D. and Shaw, D.G. (2000) The design of written information for cardiac patients: A review of the literature. Journal of Clinical Nursing 9: 658-667.

Websites

Bandolier – a newssheet concerning clinical information: www.jr2.ox.ac.uk/Bandolier

BMJ Publishing on common clinical topics: www.evidence.org

Information on clinical guidelines from National Service Framework: www.nelh.nhs.uk

Amalgamation of internet evidence-based healthcare resources: www.tripdatabase.com

Chapter 6

Information delivery

Information provision and elective surgery

As discussed in Chapter 5 a number of contentious issues have arisen regarding information provision especially in modern surgery, e.g. measurement of psychological recovery, clinical application of suggested interventions, lack of formal delivery, etc. One major issue concerns the classification of information provision, i.e. information provision to assist problem-focused and emotionally focused coping (see Tables 5.2 and 5.3 in Chapter 5). Problem-focused coping information is the main form of preoperative information provision, although there is currently no distinction between the two forms of information in practice and little choice over the form in which information is received is provided within the UK (Bruster et al. 1994, Scriven and Tucker 1997, Bradshaw et al. 1999, Dixon-Woods 2001, Mitchell 2001, Berry et al. 2003).

In this chapter the contentious issues relating specifically to the delivery of all information in both information categories are discussed, i.e. problem-focused and emotionally focused information provision. The issues to be examined are the indicators for information provision, mode of provision, timing of provision and indicators against provision. These issues are more pronounced when providing preoperative information aimed more at problem-focused coping, e.g. leaflets, educational material, verbal explanations, videotaped presentations and websites, although they are still of concern for information provision aimed more at the emotionally focused aspects of coping with surgery, e.g. relaxation and modelling.

Indicators for information provision

Over many years a plethora of studies has highlighted the lack of information as a source of considerable anxiety during hospitalization. In an early study concerning anxiety on admission to hospital lack of adequate communication was a source of increased anxiety (Volicer 1973). Volicer and Bohannon (1975, p. 358) produced a Hospital Stress Rating Scale, which incorporated the most stressful aspects of hospitalization: 'some

LIVERPOOL
JOHN MOORES UNIVERSITY
AVRIL ROBARTS LRC
TEL. 0151 231 4022

aspects of the experience of hospitalisation which are perceived as very stressful by patients are related to a lack of communication of information or lack of communication in a meaningful way'. Wilson-Barnett (1976) noted that 25% of hospital patients mentioned 'feelings of unease' over the lack of information about their medical condition. A list of the most positive aspects of hospitalization was subsequently produced with four relating directly to communication: talking to the staff nurse, student nurses, the charge nurse and visitors (Wilson-Barnett 1976).

In an early comprehensive survey of preoperative fear (Ramsay 1972), it was revealed that a calm patient who had been given some explanation was easier and safer to anaesthetize: 73% of the patients included in the study had preoperative fears relating to the anaesthesia, e.g. not waking up, induction of anaesthesia with a mask, waking during surgery; 62% were concerned with pain during the operation, 15% with surgical fears and 23% with miscellaneous fears, e.g. a diagnosis of cancer or being naked on the operating table. In a later survey of 150 patients about preoperative fears (Ryan 1975), 84% reported increased feelings of anxiety, 30% were fearful of a diagnosis of cancer (even when a benign diagnosis had been given), 25% had anaesthetic fears (42% death under anaesthesia, 31% lack of anaesthesia, 13% waking up during the operation, 13% postoperative nausea), 17% feared the operation itself and 9% feared the possible postoperative pain. Ryan (1975) concluded that the value of information about surgery before general anaesthesia should not be underestimated. In a survey by Breemhaar et al. (1996) of the inadequacies of patient information provision both patients and health-care providers were interviewed: 50% of participants experienced fear of anaesthesia, pain and discomfort, and 50% wanted more information. Patients wanted more information on the appropriate recovery behaviour once discharged because 'patients received too much information on the day of admission, while they received little information at discharge' (Breemhaar et al. 1996, p. 42).

In an outpatient study employing 210 patients (Strull et al. 1984), 41% would have preferred more information whereas 58% said that they had received the correct amount. Clinicians underestimated the patients' desire for information and debate, although they overestimated the patients' desire to be involved in the decisions. It was concluded that, although much information was required, it was merely to be kept informed and not necessarily an indication of the desire to be more involved in the decision-making process. In a meta-analysis of 68 studies about information provision before a surgical intervention (Hathaway 1986), it was revealed not only that patients who received preoperative instructions had more favourable outcomes but also that the effects were 20% better than in those not receiving preoperative instruction. After a survey of 301 patients admitted to hospital with an acute medical/surgical condition (Bubela et al. 1990), it was concluded that information enhanced the quality of life and encouraged positive feelings of recovery. These sentiments were repeated in a study by Meredith (1993), who conducted a comprehensive survey in which 30 patients and 57 doctors and nurses were interviewed. Patients were first surveyed in an outpatient department and then, postoperatively, in the ward. Time constraints in the outpatient department, the inappropriateness of the doctor's ward rounds for intimate or serious discussion, and the lack of involvement of the relatives in communication and other patients being in constant earshot were all highlighted as serious barriers to effective communication. Moreover: 'In the face of the threat of a public airing of often acutely personal details, some patients will resort to the defence of saying as little as possible to anyone. Not to ask questions of staff becomes a means of avoiding public disclosure of personal information' (Meredith 1993, p. 598).

In a literature review of the need for patient information provision (Leino-Kilpi et al. 1993), two main educational approaches were highlighted: (1) ideological – patients' fundamental right to know about their care and treatment, and (2) practical – the need for patient compliance with the prescribed treatment, e.g. in a study using 42 orthopaedic patients (Cooil and Bithell 1997), two groups of patients were randomly assigned either to read an instructional sheet only or to be provided with an identical instruction sheet plus personal explanations and a demonstration of the required exercises. No differences were established between the two groups in this study. However, the information sheet was merely a brief procedural account containing numerous behavioural 'dos' and 'don'ts'. Therefore, a possibly greater emphasis could have been placed on compliance rather than the patients' fundamental right to know and be informed. In a study by Avis (1994), 22 surgical patients undergoing both general and local anaesthesia were interviewed. It was evident from the study that current educational ideology may lie more within the practical compliance domain than in the patients' fundamental right to know.

> Although patients criticised the lack of information, and expressed a desire for more, they made surprisingly few attempts to question hospital staff. They expected to be told what to do and adopted the role of recipient rather than partner in care.
>
> Avis (1994, p. 294)

In an analysis of nursing textbooks about patient education (Redman 1993), it was stated that the delivery of health education might not always be to an acceptable standard. This may result from patients' impressions of the nurses being too busy or the emphasis resting more with the medical information at the expense of nursing information (Fleming 1992, Cortis and Lacey 1996). In the study by Cortis and Lacey (1996), 1544 recently discharged patients were sent a questionnaire relating to satisfaction with hospital information. One of the conclusions related to patients viewing the nursing staff as too busy to help: 'This resulted in patients not asking as many questions as they would have liked, and not expecting staff to have time to talk things over in any detail' (Cortis and Lacey 1996, p. 680). This, again, may be a reflection of the practical ideology towards information provision by both staff and patients, i.e. the perceived desire for patient compliance (Leino-Kilpi et al. 1993).

The Health Service Commissioner for England, for Scotland and for Wales (1997) highlighted five main areas of complaint against the NHS, three of which related to problems of communication. The Commissioner stated:

> The importance of communication has been emphasised repeatedly in previous Annual Reports and I make no apology for returning to it this year.
>
> Health Service Commissioner for England for Scotland and for Wales (1997, p. 5)

This was reiterated 4 years later in a further report, i.e. complaints about communication with relatives (Health Service Commissioner for England for Scotland and for Wales 2001). In a survey of 150 day-surgery patients (Mitchell 1997) it was discovered that, even on the day of their surgery, many patients were not completely satisfied with the written information received (Figure 6.1). Similarly, Bruster et al. (1994) undertook an extensive survey of 5150 randomly chosen NHS patients recently discharged from acute hospitals in England. The provision of information to this broad group of NHS patients was widely deemed to be insufficient. It was therefore stated that communication was a considerable problem for both medical and surgical patients:

> Patients were often not given important information about the hospital and its routine, their condition or treatment, and particularly about tests and operations they had had. Often when patients were given this information it was given in an upsetting way or with little respect for privacy.
>
> Bruster et al. (1994, p. 1544).

Fourteen per cent of relatives and friends thought that their families were given too little information and 28% thought that they had not received enough information to help in their relative's recovery.

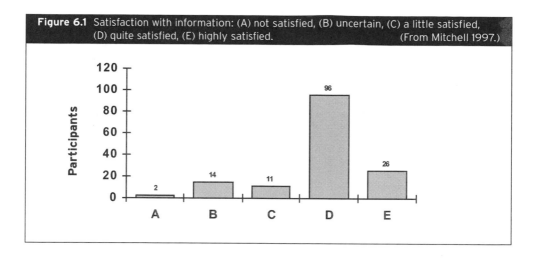

Figure 6.1 Satisfaction with information: (A) not satisfied, (B) uncertain, (C) a little satisfied, (D) quite satisfied, (E) highly satisfied. (From Mitchell 1997.)

In a recent literature review (Lithner and Zilling 1998), it was revealed that preoperative information increased the well-being of adult patients after surgery, with the potential to save both time and money. A further literature review (Mitchell 1999a, 1999b) revealed information provision to be a great challenge for modern day surgery – in the UK, Europe and the USA. In a survey by Lithner and Zilling (2000, p. 34) of 50 patients admitted for cholecystectomy, it was revealed that a great deal of information was required both at admission and at discharge: 'At admission, 94% of the patients wanted to receive information about complications after surgery'. The most valued information to be received related to the anxiety-creating factors of pain and postoperative complications. In a similar study, a telephone survey was conducted with 315 women within 2 days of discharge from day surgery (Markovic et al. 2002): 93% of the women preferred day surgery for both family reasons and increased control.

> Many valued the opportunity to be in control of recovery at their own pace, rather than submitting to a hospital regime.
>
> Markovic et al. (2002, p. 56)

However, some patients were private patients and were significantly less satisfied with the information provided. Such patients may possibly have expected to be provided with more extensive information because they were paying directly for their treatment.

Discharge information was viewed by many studies to be of particular benefit. In a study undertaken in an acute hospital setting, 76 inpatients and 89 recently discharged patients were surveyed (Bostrom et al. 1994). The results demonstrated that patients consistently required similar information, i.e. advice on activities of daily living, skin care and feelings about their condition. The first 2 weeks after discharge were seen as the most important time because patients were frequently striving to regain greater health-care autonomy. Recommendations were made to establish a telephone helpline for patients to contact the hospital at any time, an automatic follow-up telephone service, written discharge information, an unbroken system of communication between the hospital and community teams, and a database for the nurses to help inform patients. In a further medical survey it was revealed that during a 16-month period 939 telephone calls were made to the day-surgery unit (Mukumba et al. 1996): 40% of these callers requested more information. Therefore, many patients were obviously leaving hospital unprepared for the events that lay ahead during their recovery period. Such evidence has led to the utilization of numerous telephone discharge services.

Further support for this view was also provided during an extensive telephone follow-up study using 1400 recently discharged patients (Bostrom et al. 1996). For each patient it was documented in the medical records that he or she had received a great deal of information before discharge. Participants were divided into three research groups: no intervention or encouragement, encouraged to use a nurse-run telephone service and a nurse-initiated telephone call service. Only nine calls were received from patients in the group encouraged to use the nurse-run telephone service, whereas 445 calls were made to patients on two or three occasions in the nurse-initiated group. It was revealed that the information received by patients while in hospital had either been forgotten or not understood because more than 90% of the patients contacted by telephone during the nurse-initiated calls ($n = 445$) had questions relating to their recovery. Recommendations were therefore made to establish an automatic follow-up telephone service and a database for the nurses to help inform patients because clearly patients required more information but were reluctant to make contact themselves.

In an experimental study involving 87 day-surgery patients (Mitchell 2000), in which patients were telephoned 2–4 days after discharge, complete satisfaction with information was not experienced by all patients (Figure 6.2). About 50% were very satisfied, leaving a further 50% experiencing gaps in information provision. In an extensive day-surgery study (Bain et al. 1999), 5069 patients were asked to complete a questionnaire within 2 weeks of discharge from hospital. Patients who received information before admission were significantly more satisfied, as were patients who received an explanation. Moreover, the recovery period after surgery was significantly shorter in the more satisfied patients, i.e. 4.4 days as opposed to 5.5 days. The study therefore recommended improved information, and realistic expectations about pain and recovery experience. In a similar study, Barthelsson et al. (2003b) interviewed 12 patients after day-case laparoscopic cholecystectomy. Pain management was a problematic issue because patients were provided with insufficient information and as a result of their pain and anxiety many forgot some of the information given to them at discharge.

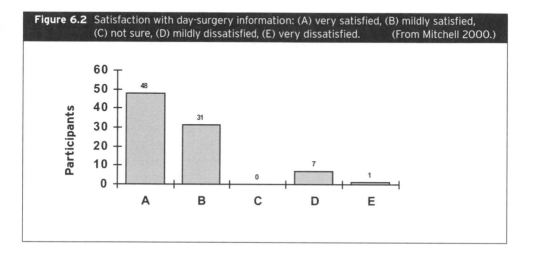

Figure 6.2 Satisfaction with day-surgery information: (A) very satisfied, (B) mildly satisfied, (C) not sure, (D) mildly dissatisfied, (E) very dissatisfied. (From Mitchell 2000.)

Moore et al. (2002) interviewed 20 women about their experiences of diagnostic laparoscopy in day surgery. All the women stated that they were aware of some risk to their life although they viewed this as minimal. One-third of patients did not want to know about any complications, although two-thirds wanted to know about the risks (determined by the researcher as death, major complications and risk of an inconclusive result):

> Women in this study had gathered their information about risk from a number of different sources, such as the hospital, personal and family experiences, work colleagues and the media.
>
> Moore et al. (2002, p. 307)

The study recommended that the risk of major complications should be explained to patients, although the latter should dictate whether or not this information was required. In a similar day-surgery study undertaken to examine the views of 80 female patients undergoing day surgery (Cox and O'Connell 2003), most patients were satisfied with the information provided, although 50% accessed other health-care professionals for further advice. In a new day-surgery procedure for gastro-oesophageal reflux, Barthelsson et al. (2003a) interviewed seven patients 1 week after surgery about their experiences. Forgetting postoperative instructions and the lack of information were all stated as the most negative aspects of undergoing modern surgery, although all would be happy to have such surgery again. A survey by Hazelgrove and Robins (2002) was concerned with the experiences of relatives who cared for the day-surgery patients once home. The provision of limited postoperative written instructions about pain management and the lack of a postoperative contact telephone number were an issue for many carers.

More recently, many studies have focused on the needs of patients who may display vigilant and avoidant coping behaviours as a way of determining information requirements (see Table 4.1 in Chapter 4). Some patients need different levels of information in order to aid effective problem-focused and emotionally focused coping strategies (see Chapter 5). If a mismatch between information provision and individual coping style occurs, anxiety may increase (Krohne et al. 1996, 2000, Royal College of Surgeons of England and Royal College of Psychiatrists 1997, De Bruin et al. 2001). As day-surgery patients have indeed been identified as a group requiring different levels of information (Avis 1994, Mitchell 2000, 2001, Hazelgrove and Robins 2002, Moore et al. 2002, Barthelsson et al. 2003a, 2003b), the development of different levels of information within day surgery may be of considerable benefit.

In an early study about vigilant and avoidant coping behaviour or a sensitizing or repressing coping style, 60 patients were divided into three groups: group 1 viewed an 18-minute videotape of the surgical procedure once, group 2 viewed the same videotape three times and group 3 just talked to the doctor. It is concluded that fear may be reduced with the increase in viewings for some patients termed 'sensitizers' (avoidant copers) whereas repressors (vigilant copers) may benefit from different preparation strategies, e.g. sensitizers prepared extensively and repressors left alone. In a similar study that separated sensitizers and repressors (Shipley et al. 1979), 36 patients undergoing endoscopy were prepared by viewing an explicit videotaped endoscopy programme no, one or three times. The more the sensitizers viewed the videotape the lower their anxiety and heart rate. The opposite occurred for the repressors, e.g. anxiety increased with the number of viewings. In the study by Avis (1994), 12 day-surgery patients were observed throughout their visit to the pre-assessment clinic followed by in-depth interviews. Some patients clearly did not wish to gain much information and were therefore quite prepared to hand over their care to the 'professionals'. Macario et al. (1999) surveyed 101 day-surgery patients to determine the most undesirable aspects of postoperative recovery. Patients rated vomiting, followed by gagging on the endotracheal tube and incision pain, as the most undesirable aspects. However, some patients refused to take part in the study, because they did not want to discuss any unpleasant aspects of their treatment: 'some patients did decline to participate in the study because of their concerns about making adverse outcomes more explicit' (Macario et al. 1999, p. 657). Finally, in an experimental study involving 87 day-surgery patients by Mitchell (2000), almost 33% of the patients rated themselves as avoidant copers (requiring a small amount of information) and about 25% rated themselves as vigilant copers (requiring a larger amount of information) (Figure 6.3).

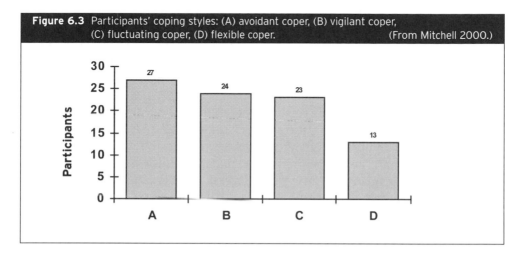

Figure 6.3 Participants' coping styles: (A) avoidant coper, (B) vigilant coper, (C) fluctuating coper, (D) flexible coper. (From Mitchell 2000.)

In summary, information has been consistently highlighted as a problematic issue for surgical patients. The lack of adequate information provision has persisted over many decades. Relatives have also stated that information provision is limiting when attempting to care for relatives at home while they recover from surgery. Numerous studies have suggested that patients require different levels of information provision in accordance with their coping style, i.e. vigilant or avoidant coping. If the success of day surgery is to continue, different levels of information developed to meet such personal requirements must be assembled and used.

Mode of information provision

Several studies have highlighted the conflicting views about the mode of information delivery, e.g. written communication, verbal communication, videotaped presentations and, to a lesser extent, audiotaped presentations. Each of these modes is therefore briefly examined because an extensive number of studies have implicitly used these modes of delivery without examining the method of information provision directly. Therefore, embedded throughout this book are numerous studies that employ these modes of information presentation (Schoessler 1989, Webber 1990, Yount and Schoessler 1991, Lisko 1995, Bostrom et al. 1996, Cooil and Bithell 1997).

First, the provision of written educational material is discussed: 80 patients undergoing minor gynaecological surgery were studied and randomly assigned to one of three groups – routine care only, minimally informative preparatory booklet and maximally informative preparatory booklet (experimental group) (Wallace 1984). Anxiety immediately before surgery, immediately after surgery and 1 week after surgery were lower in the maximal booklet group, i.e. patient anxiety was increased when only routine care or the minimally informative preparatory booklet was provided. Although recommending an increase in the level of information provided, Wallace (1984) states that this may not be suitable for all patients. In a similar study (Wallace 1986a), 63 women undergoing minor gynaecological surgery were randomly assigned to three groups: routine care, minimal information booklet and maximal information booklet. When questioned 2 hours before surgery about knowledge of the procedure and misconceptions, the maximal information group were more knowledgeable. However, the level of anxiety among the groups did not differ. Again, such results question the true purpose of information provision, i.e. education versus compliance.

In a similar experimental study (Gammon and Mulholland 1996), 82 patients undergoing surgery were randomly assigned to two groups. The first group received a mixture of procedural, sensory and cognitive coping strategies whereas the control group received routine care. The patients in the experimental group, i.e. provided with written information, were significantly less anxious and less depressed although, as previously stated, additional intervention or being treated differently may always produce more positive results. In a further study to examine patient education requirements (Bostrom et al. 1994), 76 inpatients completed a questionnaire and 89 patients were interviewed by telephone after discharge. It was established that hospitalized patients were consistent in identifying their learning needs, e.g. written information about medication, treatment, complications and enhancing the quality of life was highly valued. A further survey of 38 day-surgery patients (Law 1997), 2 days after surgery, revealed that 34% of patients could not remember what the doctor had said and 31% could remember only basic information. A leaflet for reference purposes was therefore viewed as invaluable to aid the management of a forgotten or unforeseen event occurring at home. Similar results were also obtained in a study examining brief inpatient surgical stay, e.g. 1–3 days for open cholecystectomy (Lithner and Zilling 2000).

Nevertheless, written material can present many problems and a number of studies have examined the readability of leaflets because patients must obviously be able to understand the information for it to be of any benefit (Ley and Florio 1996, Mumford 1997, Coulter et al. 1998, Walsh and Shaw 2000). Some leaflets have been deemed to be either too simplistic or containing too much jargon. In addition, educational leaflets must be presented in a legible manner. In an evaluation of 184 hospital leaflets collected from 97 hospitals, concerning hysterectomy, Scriven and Tucker (1997, p. 110) discovered that 71% of the leaflets were hospital-produced photocopies, 15% hospital-produced printed booklets and 14% photocopies of commercially produced booklets: 'Leaflets from 27 hospitals were found to be illegible due to blurred printing or faint ink'. The study concludes that hospital educational material should be evaluated by patients and debated by patient discussion groups to determine the content, as opposed to hospital personnel merely determining what is required.

In a critical scrutiny of the publications about patient information leaflets, the biomedical agenda can be clearly distinguished in most leaflets (Dixon-Woods 2001). Two themes emerged: the largest reflects the traditional biomedical model. This is a mechanistic model of interaction in which patients are characterized as passive and open to manipulation in the interests of a biomedical agenda. This agenda has three main motives: medicolegal implications, patient compliance and paternalism (dealing with an irrational, passive, forgetful incompetent patient). The second and smaller theme concerns patient empowerment. However, there is now a political need to reduce inpatient stay and promote modern surgery, i.e. day surgery, for greater efficiency within the NHS and improved cost-effectiveness. So, for patients increasingly to care for themselves at home, they must be more informed and any British government must therefore promote greater patient information if day surgery is to be successful and more patients are to be treated in modern day-surgery facilities.

Some studies have suggested that patients require both written and verbal information. Fifty patients undergoing brief surgical inpatient stay were surveyed (Lithner and Zilling 2000) and it was revealed that much written and verbal information was required both on admission and at discharge. In addition, in an experimental study relating to 87 day-surgery patients by Mitchell (2000), the vast majority of patients required both written and verbal information whereas only very few required a videotaped presentation (Figure 6.4). In a study concerning information about medication by Berry et al. (2003), it is stated that the 'use of more personalised style of presentation ["you" and "your"] resulted in significantly increased satisfaction with a written explanation and significantly reduced perception of risk to health from taking the medication' (Berry et al. 2003, p. 135). A more personalized written and verbal approach may therefore aid compliance. In an experimental study by Fagermoen and Hamilton (2003, p. 289), it was again concluded that patients required both written and verbal information: 'Patients valued the nurses' interaction and approach and rated this higher than informational needs'. However, the information provided within this study may lack some validity for modern elective surgery because some of the patients underwent surgery for a malignancy. The requirements of such patients may be increased as a result of the nature of their condition.

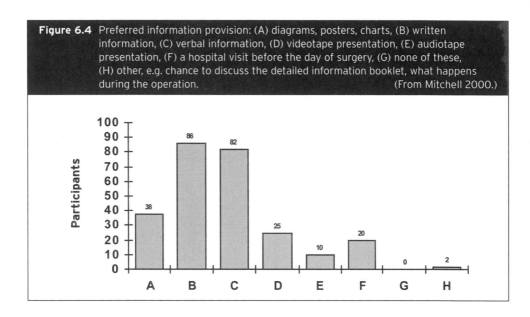

Figure 6.4 Preferred information provision: (A) diagrams, posters, charts, (B) written information, (C) verbal information, (D) videotape presentation, (E) audiotape presentation, (F) a hospital visit before the day of surgery, (G) none of these, (H) other, e.g. chance to discuss the detailed information booklet, what happens during the operation.   (From Mitchell 2000.)

Conversely, some studies have suggested that written information has little impact and recommended increased verbal information. In a study of 30 female patients undergoing hysterectomy (Young and Humphrey 1985), patients were assigned to three groups. The first two groups were taught methods of cognitive control over anxiety, either via a detailed booklet (group 1) or verbally (group 2). The final group was employed as an attention-control group, i.e. time spent discussing hospital routines only. Little difference was established between the two experimental groups so it was concluded that the provision of mere verbal information was more cost-effective than the production of leaflets. In a similar study (Young et al. 1994), 38 female patients admitted on the day of surgery were randomly assigned to two groups. Patients were either sent an information leaflet by post before admission or received no information.

Objective measures of physical recovery in hospital were recorded and participants were asked to complete satisfaction, stress and social recovery questionnaires. Again, no significant differences were established between the two groups. Therefore, routine verbal information was viewed to be just as effective as written information. In an ambulatory surgery study to determine opinions about information provided (Linden and Engberg 1996), 110 patients completed a questionnaire. Patients did not find the written information as adequate or as satisfactory as the oral information. Patients therefore desired written information to be supported by verbal information. In addition, one-third of patients found both the written and the verbal information to be unsatisfactory. A lack of the required information was significantly associated with more pain during their stay and immediately before discharge.

The final mode of presentation concerns videotaped programmes. Again, a considerable number of studies have examined this aspect and so other studies employing videotaped programmes are implicit throughout the book (Shipley et al. 1978, Mahler et al. 1993, Wicklin and Forster 1994, Brumfield et al. 1996, Mahler and Kulik 2002). In a literature review of the strengths and weaknesses of videotaped programmes about patient education (Gagliano 1988), 25 studies were reviewed. It was concluded that videotapes were economical, easy to stop and rewind for repeated viewing, capable of reaching a wider audience and did not depend on the literacy skills of the listener. In a further brief review (Lisko 1995), videotaped programmes were viewed as a positive adjunct to modern day surgery because of the minimal preparation time, increased client throughput and patient anxiety. In a survey of 30 patients undergoing orthopaedic surgery (Leino-Kilpi and Vuorenheimo 1993), over 50% required information a few days before surgery and 50% stated that they would have preferred to view a videotape of the procedure before admission. In an experimental study to demonstrate that an instructional videotape viewed preoperatively could improved patient knowledge (Zvara et al. 1996), 178 patients were randomly assigned into two groups: group 1 received a 10-minute videotape about anaesthesia and surgery whereas group 2 received no videotape. Only one significant aspect emerged from a knowledge test given at the end of the preassessment visit and after the routine visit from the anaesthetist. Group 1 knew the correct procedure if they felt unwell on the day of surgery. Almost 85% of the patients who viewed the videotape thought that it was beneficial whereas 41% who did not see the videotape said that it would have helped.

In a further day-surgery study to examine the effects of a videotaped presentation (Done and Lee 1998), 127 patients were divided into two groups on the day of surgery. The experimental group was shown a 7-minute videotape about their general anaesthetic whereas the control group had no videotape. Although the knowledge of general anaesthesia was significantly increased in the experimental group, no difference between anxiety levels was established. The study concludes that a video-taped educational programme should be used in a designated area although the day of surgery may not be the most effective time for viewing information because almost half the patients (44%) preferred to have information earlier. In a similar study (Doering et al. 2000), 100 patients undergoing hip replacement surgery were surveyed. A videotape programme was designed that was 12 minutes in length and featured a patient (who had undergone the surgical procedure) explaining events. The presentation was broadly aimed at the anticipation of events with some additional procedural information. The participants were randomly divided into two: a control and an experimental group. The experimental group viewed the videotape on the eve of surgery whereas the control group received no viewing. Using behavioural, emotional and physiological measures, the experimental group had lower anxiety, although only when using physiological measures, so the videotape may have had some, albeit limited, impact.

In recent reviews of the literature specifically about videotaped educational presentations (Krouse 2001), it was concluded that such programmes were beneficial to patient knowledge, anxiety management and self-efficacy enhancement.

> The main benefit from video and written information was an increased level of patient knowledge about risks and the process of anaesthesia and pain management.
>
> Lee et al. (2003, p. 1427)

However, no increase in patient satisfaction was uncovered within the reviews. Finally, a convenience sample of 96 adult patients viewed an educational videotaped presentation in the preassessment clinic before surgery (Krenzischek et al. 2001). The length of videotape varied, e.g. general anaesthesia patients 14 minutes, regional anaesthesia 16 minutes and local anaesthesia 9.5 minutes. Ratings of the most preferred method for receiving information were conducted. The videotape was preferred by 50%, instruction by staff 47%, written information by 9% and internet by 3%. Most patients therefore required a videotape presentation plus instruction from staff before surgery.

Some studies have also employed audiotape programmes (Baskerville et al. 1985). In the study by Baskerville et al. (1985), 119 day-surgery patients scheduled for hernia repair were provided with a 20-minute audiocassette tape explaining the condition, its repair and the postoperative care: 90% of patients found the information adequate, 6% requested more information and the number of times the audiotapes were used ranged from 1 to 20 (56% listened to the tape more than twice). Bondy et al. (1999) undertook a study to evaluate the effects of educational materials posted to patients before day surgery. Patients were recruited by telephone before their surgery and asked about their access to an audio-cassette recorder/player and their limitations regarding hearing or vision. Patients were then randomly divided into two groups: two pamphlets and an audiocassette describing general and regional anesthesia posted to their home or no additional information or audiocassette presentation. The audiocassette presentation lasted 10 minutes and highlighted the sequence of events before, during and after surgery, i.e. procedural information. A significant difference in anxiety was observed between the two groups because the control group was more anxious. However, 49% of the control group participants expressed an interest in having additional information before their surgery, so almost half of the control group required more information although they received none. Such an occurrence could lead to bias in the results because so many participants who wanted extra information received nothing.

In summary, all modes of information delivery have experienced some success. Nevertheless, written information with the opportunity to discuss issues further with professional staff remains the most effective approach. Studies suggesting verbal information to be as effective as written information were largely conducted before the increase in modern elective day surgery. Written information to be used by the patients and their relatives for reference purposes throughout the days after discharge is now highly desirable and essential for the eradication of postoperative 'trial-and-error' learning.

Timing of information provision

Although the number of patients undergoing intermediate elective inpatient surgery is diminishing, such patients have an increased amount of time (relative to day-surgery patients) in which to gain information and glean answers to questions to allay fears (Lepczyk et al. 1990, Pellino et al. 1998). Before a decrease in this amount of time that patients spend in hospital, timing of information provision did not therefore necessarily present as a problematic issue, e.g. the day(s) spent in hospital during the preoperative phase were frequently used to educate the patient and establish a nurse–patient relationship (Vogelsang 1990). However, as the length of hospital stay has fallen and the amount of elective day surgery risen, the issue of the timing of information provision has gained momentum (Donoghue et al. 1995).

In one of the early studies by Johnston (1980) to examine the issue of timing of information provision, 136 patients undergoing various types of surgery were surveyed. It was concluded that an increase in anxiety was experienced many days and/or weeks before surgery and for at least 5–6 days after surgery. On an individual basis the exact time when anxiety begins and when it eventually falls were not clearly established. Preoperative anxiety is therefore not a minor, short-term emotional disturbance; it results from the rational fear of a serious life-threatening event, which can last for many days/weeks before and after surgery (Johnston 1980). In a comprehensive study of 1420 patients undergoing various surgical procedures (O'Hara et al. 1989), it was concluded that anxiety was greatest on the day of surgery and had no sudden end postoperatively. Some patients experienced increased anxiety 6–8 weeks before surgery. In addition, 14% of participants reported high levels of psychological distress up to 3 months after surgery. However, not all surgery was discrete, i.e. simple singular event, because some patients underwent surgery for suspected malignancy.

In a study of 41 patients undergoing cardiac surgery (Christopherson and Pfeiffer 1980), an information booklet was sent by post before surgery at different times. Patients were randomly divided into three groups and sent no information (group 1), an informational booklet 1–2 days before surgery (group 2) or an informational booklet 3–35 days before surgery (group 3). The level of patient anxiety and knowledge about surgery were measured using a self-rated questionnaire. Group 3 experienced the lowest anxiety preoperatively and group 2 the lowest anxiety postoperatively. Therefore, patients in receipt of early information experienced the lowest anxiety preoperatively. Being more informed well in advance must therefore have made a difference. However, the paradox, which arises between the two groups, may have arisen as a result of two research design issues. First, the exact time each member of the two groups read the information can only be assumed: many participants in group 3 could have received the information 3, 4 or 5 days before surgery or read it immediately; many in group 2 who received the information booklet 2 days before surgery could also have read it immediately. The difference between receiving and reading information 3, 4 or 5 days before surgery and receiving and reading information 2 days before surgery may be indistinguishable. Second, the information booklet sent to participants in groups 2 and 3 was 16 pages long. From a practical viewpoint, patients in group 2 may not have had sufficient time to read and comprehend the entire 16-page booklet 2 days before surgery.

In a similar experimental study about patients undergoing cardiac surgery (Cupples 1991), one group were provided with information 5–14 days before admission (experimental group), whereas a second group (control group) received routine teaching on admission. In the postoperative period the experimental group had a greater level of knowledge, more positive self-reported mood states and increased physiological recovery. However, no differences were observed in anxiety levels even though, in comparison, the experimental group spent a far greater amount of time with the nursing staff. In a similar study by Levesque et al. (1984), 125 cholecystectomy patients were randomly assigned to one of three groups: group 1 received specific detailed information 2 weeks before surgery, group 2 received specific detailed information on the eve of surgery and group 3 were the control group and therefore received usual care, i.e. no extra information. No significant differences were uncovered using psychological and physiological measures, so no difference was determined in the most effective time to receive information. However, the experiment could also have been flawed as a result of the behaviour of the nursing staff: 'staff members reported that the additional teaching was not seen as a priority for the experimental patients and little reinforcement was given for the appropriate pre and post-operative behaviours' (Levesque et al. 1984, p. 234). The nursing staff realized to which research group the patients were assigned and adjusted their teaching responsibilities accordingly.

In a study using a detailed audiotaped educational presentation lasting 40 minutes (Mavrias et al. 1990), 37 cholecystectomy patients were tested for desired timing of information. Patients were randomly divided into three groups: group 1 prepared 2 weeks before surgery, group 2 prepared the day before surgery and group 3 not prepared. Again, no significant differences were established using anxiety, pain ratings, mood, physical recovery, length of hospitalization and analgesia usage. In a parallel study examining the effects of preoperative instruction on 72 patients undergoing cardiac surgery, Lepczyk et al. (1990) randomly divided the group into two. One group received instruction as inpatients the day before surgery whereas the second group received instruction as outpatients 4–8 days before surgery. No significant differences were found using the measures employed, although there was a significant relationship between knowledge about the operation and personal knowledge of someone who had previously undergone cardiac surgery. However, this had no influence on the level of anxiety experienced.

In an evaluation of a pre-hospital educational booklet for total hip replacement surgery (Butler et al. 1996), patients were randomly assigned to receive either an education booklet by post 4–6 weeks before surgery or no booklet. Although there was no significant difference between the anxiety levels of the group, patients who had received the booklet were on average less anxious during admission to hospital. In addition, these patients were, on average, more likely to have practised the physical exercises before admission and so required significantly less physiotherapy while in hospital.

Schoessler (1989) conducted one of the earliest studies on preference for timing of information provision with regard to modern surgical practices, e.g. patients admitted to hospital on the morning of surgery. Data were collected from 116 patients undergoing various surgical procedures and general anaesthesia. It was discovered that 50% of participants required information on admission, 41% wanted the information before admission and some merely wanted the information immediately before surgery. It was concluded that 'healthcare providers must now focus on exploring methods to deliver effective pre-operative education in a dramatically altered environment' (Schoessler 1989, p. 136). In a similar survey of women admitted on the morning of surgery for hysterectomy, the utility of a preadmission teaching brochure sent by post was examined (Young et al. 1994). Patients were randomly assigned to receive either the educational brochure or no additional information. However, the information brochure was very behaviourally oriented, containing such advice as postoperative exercises, length of hospital stay, etc. No significant differences were established about anxiety.

A number of day-surgery studies have recommended that information should be mailed to the patient during the preoperative phase because receipt on the day of surgery had been demonstrated as being too late (Oberle et al. 1994, Brumfield et al. 1996, Mitchell 1997). In a survey by Brumfield et al. (1996), 30 patients undergoing general anaesthesia for laparoscopic day surgery were interviewed. Most patients wanted teaching to occur before admission, i.e. patient information received by post during the preoperative phase. In a similar day-surgery study by Oberle et al. (1994), 294 patients undergoing various surgical procedures were surveyed and a large number of patients were dissatisfied with the timing of information provision because the bulk of it occurred on the ward immediately before surgery. It was concluded that most patients would have preferred to receive information before admission either by post or during the preassessment visit. In a comparable qualitative study by Donoghue et al. (1995, p. 173), 31 day-surgery patients were interviewed between 1 and 3 weeks after day surgery: 'Many of the participants reported that there were experiences they had not anticipated, surprises that they did not welcome and things that they would have liked to have known before the operation'. The study therefore recommended improved education and a review of the timing of educational programmes. In a further survey by Mitchell (1997) of 150 patients undergoing minor gynaecological day surgery and general anaesthesia, 6% stated that they would have preferred to receive the information a few months before surgery, 24% a few weeks before surgery, 48% a few days before surgery and 20% a few hours before surgery (Figure 6.5).

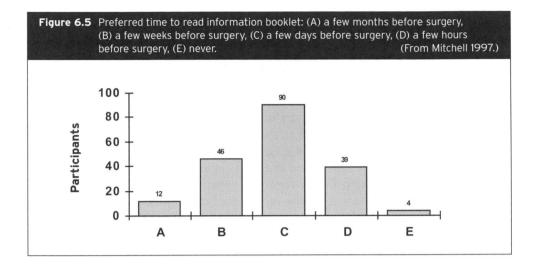

Figure 6.5 Preferred time to read information booklet: (A) a few months before surgery, (B) a few weeks before surgery, (C) a few days before surgery, (D) a few hours before surgery, (E) never. (From Mitchell 1997.)

In an experimental day-surgery study to examine the effects of timing of information provision (Coslow and Eddy 1998), 30 patients undergoing general anaesthesia for laparoscopic sterilization were divided into two groups: the control group received information 1 hour before surgery whereas the experimental group received a structured individual tutorial lasting 20 minutes, 1–2 weeks before surgery. This included a tape–slide presentation and a six-page booklet to take home. The only significant difference emerging between the two groups, however, concerned pain management, e.g. requests for and consumption of analgesia significantly increased in the control group, indicating possibly that a more informed patient experiences less pain. Unfortunately, no self-reported measures of

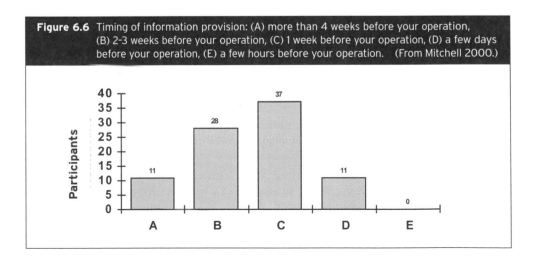

Figure 6.6 Timing of information provision: (A) more than 4 weeks before your operation, (B) 2-3 weeks before your operation, (C) 1 week before your operation, (D) a few days before your operation, (E) a few hours before your operation. (From Mitchell 2000.)

anxiety were used. However, the attention bias between the two groups was considerable. Finally, in a comprehensive study to evaluate patients' views of day surgery in Scotland (Bain et al. 1999), 5069 day-case patients from 13 hospitals were asked to complete a questionnaire within 2 weeks of surgery. Patients who received information before admission were significantly more satisfied as were patients who received an explanation. The study therefore recommended improved information about pain and recovery before hospital admission. In a similar study by Mitchell (2000), female patients undergoing gynaecological surgery were surveyed about the preferred time to receive information: 1–3 weeks before surgery was viewed as the most appropriate time. Crucially, no one wanted the information on the day of surgery (Figure 6.6).

In summary, timing of information provision has gained greater importance with the advent of modern day surgery because contact with hospital personnel is frequently brief and hospitalization minimal. Indeed, the British government has a target of no waiting lists by 2008, thereby allowing for a greater focus to fall on patient choice (Cook et al. 2004). The continued expansion in day surgery is central to this target. Many studies have reported that patients prefer information before the day of surgery. However, this can differ between 1 and 3 weeks before surgery. Nevertheless, it is clear that with this new era of surgery patients desire written information to be provided in advance of their surgery in conjunction with the opportunity to discuss aspects with a member of staff.

Indicators against information provision

For many years the utility of information provision has been debated and frequently determined not to be required or at least not as a panacea for all preoperative psychological preparation. In a study by Christopherson and Pfeiffer (1980), 41 patients were asked to read an information booklet before cardiac surgery. As many patients completely refused to read any such pre-surgery material, the control group was self-selecting, e.g. some patients, possibly avoidant copers, did not want any additional information. In an earlier experimental study (Ziemer 1983), 111 patients were presented with differing audiotaped information programmes on the eve of surgery. Participants were divided into three groups: procedural information only, procedural and sensory information, sensory and coping information. No significant differences were established using physiological and emotional measures. Therefore, the provision of extra information was not observed to be beneficial. However, the study may have been somewhat biased because the first two groups had a 5-minute audiotape whereas the third group received a 22-minute tape.

A number of early studies demonstrated that information provision is insufficient when it is the sole means of preoperative psychological preparation (Anderson 1987, Elsass et al. 1987a, Martelli et al. 1987). In a study of 74 patients admitted for elective general surgery by Elsass et al. (1987a), 84% stated that the emotional support provided by the nurses preoperatively was more effective than the written information. Moreover, detailed medical information provided by the anaesthetist served only to increase anxiety for some patients. Similarly, Martelli et al. (1987) studied 46 patients undergoing local anaesthesia for oral surgery and concluded that emotionally focused coping strategies were the most effective methods for patients who were very anxious and in a situation where there was little possibility for personal choice. Furthermore, using emotional and behavioural measures to survey patients before cardiac surgery, Anderson (1987) concluded that information alone did not reduce anxiety although it did help to increase feelings of control.

Teasdale (1993) in a critical appraisal of the relationship between information provision and anxiety reduction emphasized that to assume that one automatically follows the other may be an oversimplification of a very complex issue, i.e.

Patient + Information = Reduced anxiety.

Teasdale suggests that all information is partial because it is impossible to tell the patient everything and extremely difficult to be truly objective. In addition, it is very difficult to remain truly confident that the information is required or indeed that it has been properly understood. Unless it is requested, it is unclear whether the patient wishes to receive the information being provided. Moreover, factual information given to the patient, however neutral and objective, may not be interpreted in the way in which it was originally intended: 'Therefore, to ask whether information relieves anxiety is conceptually flawed' (Teasdale 1993, p. 1128). It can be assumed when using this mechanistic model only that the information provided has had the desired effect, e.g. reduced the patients' anxiety or improved their ability to cope. Such answers are very difficult to establish although they do reflect the psychological theory of vigilant and avoidant coping, e.g. some people may not benefit from the acquisition of information in the preoperative phase.

A number of studies have demonstrated that, when patients undergoing surgery and general anaesthesia are forced to comply with a preoperative educational programme, i.e. receive preoperative information, their level of anxiety can actually increase (Salmon et al. 1986, Salmon 1992b, Kerrigan et al. 1993). Salmon et al. (1986) and Salmon (1992b), following a study of 17 patients, discovered significantly higher

LIVERPOOL JOHN MOORES UNIVERSITY
LEARNING SERVICES

levels of cortisol in the urine of patients on a ward where they were requested to comply with preoperative procedural information giving. Therefore, patients experienced an increased stress response as a result of hearing the information. In one of the first day-surgery studies by Goldmann et al. (1988) focusing on relaxation before surgery, 52 female patients undergoing general anaesthesia for gynaecological surgery were studied. Participants were divided into two groups before anaesthesia and one group received extra information and the second group received 3 minutes of hypnosis. The main conclusions were associated with information provision.

> The provision of information does not have a uniformly positive effect. Patients may either wish to be informed about the details of their operation, remain uninformed, or a mixture of both.
>
> Goldmann et al. (1988, p. 468)

In a comparable experimental study by Bondy et al. (1999), using patients admitted on the same day as surgery, information pamphlets and a 10-minute videotaped presentation were sent to each patient in a randomly allocated experimental group, whereas the control group received routine care, i.e. no additional written information. Using a self-administered anxiety questionnaire (Spielberger et al. 1983), the experimental group were significantly less anxious immediately before surgery. However, of the 65 participants in the experimental group, 10% preferred no information and in the control group 24% preferred (and received) no information. Therefore, an element of self-selection by the control group may have occurred. Patients who did not want much information may have given their permission to be involved in a study in which they would receive little information. In a further experimental study (Lamarche et al. 1998), 54 inpatients were randomly assigned to two groups: 28 patients in the experimental group were telephoned before cardiac surgery in order to provide information and the opportunity to pose questions; 26 participants in the control group received no telephone call – merely routine care. Using a visual analogue scale on the day of admission to gauge anxiety, a significantly higher level of anxiety was established in the experimental group, i.e. the extra information had increased anxiety.

Kerrigan et al. (1993) surveyed 96 men undergoing general anaesthesia for elective inguinal hernia repair. The aim of the study was to observe the possible changes in anxiety after receiving detailed information about potential complications. Although the detailed information did not increase patients' self-ratings of anxiety, 25% of those who randomly received the detailed information stated that they had received too much, i.e. one in four patients who received detailed information did not want it. In a similar study by Hawkshaw (1994) expressly concerned with day surgery, 1008 patients were telephoned at home on their first postoperative day. Patients were judged to require differing levels of information concerning their surgical experience:

> This is reflected in the 729 (72.3%) patients who reported that they were happy with the information they had acquired. This includes 274 (27.2%) who received no information but were satisfied.
>
> Hawkshaw (1994, p. 349)

Lepczyk et al. (1990) studied 72 patients after cardiac surgery and discovered that 81% of patients, once told of their need for surgery, sought details about their operation themselves. Therefore, they may not have required additional information once admitted to hospital because adequate information had already been gained.

Guadagnoli and Ward (1998, p. 336) also suggest that there are problems in the balance between the doctor and patient interactions: 'there will always be some imbalance in the patient–physician relationship since the patient is sick and vulnerable and the physician has the expert knowledge.' Patients in this situation may feel it unwise, even foolish (rightly or wrongly), to question the 'specialist', i.e. they trust the doctor and may not wish to challenge his or her wisdom. However, if they do not ask, the doctor will have no knowledge of their questions. Avis (1994), in a study of 22 surgical patients, also alluded to this issue. Patients wanted to be informed although they expected to be told what to do and assumed a passive role. Furthermore, after a judicial decision involving informed consent a number of medical practitioners in Australia undertook a review of consent (Stanley et al. 1998). The aim of the study was to determine the degree to which patients understood the risks associated with a surgical procedure. In the study 32 patients were surveyed and randomly allocated to two groups: routine consent and additional detailed verbal and/or written information. Using emotional measures on two separate occasions, i.e. before surgery and 6 weeks after discharge, the study was unable to establish a difference in anxiety or knowledge level between the two groups. Therefore, the additional information group was no more informed or any less anxious than the routine care group.

Many recent studies have demonstrated the need for psychosocial interventions and not merely information as such. In a meta-analysis 2024 patients receiving psychosocial treatment preoperatively were evaluated against 1156 control individuals (Linden et al. 1996). Here the vital role of the psychosocial aspects of care was emphasized, i.e. patients receiving psychosocial treatment preoperatively had more positive outcomes, mobilized more quickly, experienced less pain and were more satisfied. In addition, it is suggested that more psychosocial interventions are urgently required in this modern surgical era. In a further meta-analysis of 37 studies examining recovery from surgery, Dusseldorp et al. (1999, p. 516) also strongly recommended the need for psychoeducational programmes and stated that future studies must consider the type of care required: 'Program components explicitly focusing on the reduction of anxiety and depression are rarely elaborated on in the studies. For example, some stress management programs were described only in general terms as counselling for stress or anxiety, or as group discussion of ideas, thoughts, and feelings about the heart attack and its effects'.

More recently, the lack of psychological interventions available to help patients in the postoperative period has been repeatedly identified (Hartford et al. 2002). Hartford et al. (2002) state that the inpatients' stay for cardiac surgery has been cut by 50% over the last decade, making adequate information provision an essential aspect of care: 131 patients undergoing cardiac surgery were randomly assigned to two groups. Group 1 patients and partners received six post-discharge telephone calls over a 7-week period whereas group 2 received no telephone calls. The anxiety level of patients in the telephone group was significantly lower than in the experimental group but only on one occasion, i.e. 2 days after discharge. Moreover, the pre-discharge information was all procedural and behavioural information, i.e. no psychological elements. All the psychosocial concerns during the telephone calls came from the patients in the form of questions – none from the hospital staff. Therefore, no psychosocial aspects of care were provided on a formal basis – just procedural and behavioural information.

Finally, in a study by van Weert et al. (2003, p. 109) the videotaped interactions between doctor and patient, nurse and patient, and health educator and patient on the day of admission for cardiac surgery were analysed:

> The communication between the physicians and the patients appeared to be primarily about medical topics. However, in the nurses' encounters, almost one-third of the time (29.8%) was spent on medical topics as well.

The study goes on to state that 75% of all patients were not informed pre-operatively about the psychosocial consequences of cardiac surgery. Although such evidence comes from the vast amount of studies undertaken concerning cardiac surgery (Dusseldorp et al. 1999, Walsh and Shaw 2000, Koivula et al. 2002a, Mahler and Kulik 2002, van der Zee et al. 2002), no evidence is available to suggest that this is any different from any other type of surgery. Indeed, cardiac surgery has received the most psychosocial attention because of (1) the vast number of patients under-going treatment, (2) the vast resources subsequently made available and (3) the huge psychological implications to the patients undergoing such surgery. Therefore, if psychosocial aspects of care were being adequately provided, this would be the group most likely to have been receiving it. However, tangible psychological interventions recommended by the vast number of studies involving patients undergoing cardiac surgery remain minimal (Dusseldorp et al. 1999, Parent and Fortin 2000, Hartford et al. 2002, Koivula et al. 2002b, van der Zee et al. 2002, van Weert et al. 2003, Tromp et al. 2004).

In summary, not all patients require an exhaustive amount of information. Indeed, many may find the provision of detailed information anxiety provoking, as highlighted in the vigilant and avoidant coping styles (see Chapter 4). Information is therefore not a panacea for the treatment of preoperative anxiety. Many patients require not only information but additional tangible psychological interventions (outlined in Chapters 3 and 4) to aid preoperative anxiety management. First, however, such interventions require formal construction and presentation in a clinically acceptable manner for use in modern elective day surgery.

Conclusion

For many years the provision of information to patients undergoing surgery has been problematic. All too frequently patients have received too little information. However, the length of inpatient stay could, to some extent, compensate for this shortfall once patients were in hospital awaiting surgery. Time was available for patients to ask questions and gain additional information with previous traditional surgical episodes. However, the growth in the amount and complexity of day surgery has exacerbated this longstanding issue. Day-surgery patients and their carers need to be informed in order to care for themselves adequately once home. In addition, it has been well established that some patients (vigilant copers) want to be more fully informed. As highlighted earlier, and in the previous chapters, little or no account for coping style appears in many studies of this type, e.g. vigilant and avoidant coping. The future success of day surgery may depend, in part, on the availability of improved modes of information provision and the availability of differing levels of information.

The mode of information provision must include, for the vast majority of patients, written material with the opportunity to discuss the material with a professional member of staff. Some patients may also benefit from the use of a videotaped or audiotaped presentation. However, given the rapid rate of recovery from elective day surgery, a number of patients may find such a mode of provision unnecessary. But, for day-surgery patients who do not undergo discrete elective surgery, i.e. not a single surgical event, such additional educational material may be most welcome.

Timing of information provision has become a considerable issue with the increase in day-surgery activity. Previous early studies focusing on inpatient surgery did not always establish preadmission information as essential. However, this is not the case with modern elective day surgery. Day-surgery studies have repeatedly recommended that written information must be provided before the day of surgery. Unfortunately, this is not always achieved and in one day-surgery study it was established that 60% of patients had not received any written information before the day of surgery (Mitchell 2000). Finally, not all patients wish to receive a full account of surgery and anaesthesia. It is therefore, again, essential that different levels of information provision are made available, together with tangible aspects of psychological care. The provision of different levels of information is a crucial element in the effective delivery of preoperative psychoeducational care. However, effective preoperative psychoeducational care will be incomplete and far less effective without the additional components described in Chapter 4.

Summary

- A plethora of studies have revealed information provision to be a challenge to modern surgery. Almost all studies on the subject have determined information provision to be inadequate for many patients. With adequate information, anxiety was widely viewed to be lower and the whole recovery process quicker. The challenge remains for modern surgery to develop an information provision strategy that enables patients to extract the type and level of information most suitable for their needs.
- Patients prefer to have written information about their surgery supported by a discussion with the doctor or nurse. However, media-based products, e.g. videotaped programmes and websites, are growing in popularity alongside minimal hospital stay and reduced hospital staff contact. Many studies demonstrate the need for psychoeducational nursing interventions. The goal for numerous studies was to have a more informed patient, although this did not necessarily equate with a less anxious patient.
- Videotaped educational preparations have demonstrated considerable benefit for patients, e.g. improved information, less anxiety and improved pain management. However, many of the studies failed, first, to identify patients who

required the extra information before its provision, e.g. vigilant and avoidant copers. A number of recent studies based in modern day surgery have identified videotaped presentations as a useful adjunct during a period when time is limited and patient numbers substantial.

- Many of the original studies about timing of educational provision established little difference between educational materials provided before admission and those provided after admission. However, many of these studies employed procedural and behavioural educational material and did not focus solely on psychological welfare, e.g. compliance versus patient empowerment. This is particularly the case with cardiac surgery patients. More recent studies, especially associated with modern elective day surgery, have established that patients require information provision before hospital admission.

- A number of studies have demonstrated information provision alone to be of little psychological benefit to patients both before and after surgery. This has been verified by its lack of ability to reduce anxiety for some patients and its inadequate educational level for others. More recently, modern surgery has made it possible for patients to be in hospital for minimal periods of time. However, the information provided in such circumstances has had a principally medical emphasis and is not linked with other psychosocial aspects of care and advice. A psychoeducational plan of care suitable for use in modern elective day surgery is therefore urgently required.

Further reading

Bruster, S., Jarman, B., Bosanquet, N., Weston, D., Erens, R. and Delbanco, T.L. (1994) National survey of hospital patients. British Medical Journal 309: 1542-1546.

Edmondson, M. (1996) Patient Information. In: Penn, S., Davenport, H.T., Carrington, S. and Edmondson, M. (eds), Principles of Day Surgery. London: Blackwell Science.

Mumford, M.E. (1997) A descriptive study of the readability of patient information leaflets designed by nurses. Journal of Advanced Nursing. 26: 985-991.

Scriven, A. and Tucker, C. (1997) The quality and management of written information presented to women undergoing hysterectomy. Journal of Clinical Nursing. 6: 107-113.

Websites

Guild of Health Writers: www.healthwriters.com
Media Medics: www.media-medics.co.uk
Medical Journalists' Association: www.mja-uk.org
Society of Medical Writers: www.lepress.demon.co.uk
Toolkit for Producing Patient Information: www.doh.gov.uk/nhsidentity
Virtual day surgery tour: www.carlesurgicenter.com

Chapter 7

Anxiety management in day surgery

Preoperative psychoeducational care

Modern surgical practices are inexorably leading to considerably shorter episodes in hospital (Charalambous et al. 2003). Medical practices have advanced greatly to ensure that such developments occur. However, such elective surgical health care is dominated by minimal access surgery (key-hole surgery), rapid anaesthesia and recovery, reduced nurse–patient contact, and considerable patient self-preparation and self-recovery (see Chapter 2). Consequently, psychoeducational aspects of care have become almost completely submerged in the wake of medical fervour associated with such surgical and anaesthetic advances.

Numerous advances are likewise now required for the psychoeducational management of the adult elective day-surgery patient in order to keep pace with this new surgical era. Historically, preoperative anxiety management has relied almost exclusively on information provision, and interpersonal and communication skills (see Chapters 2 and 3). However, it has been suggested that simply teaching nurses interpersonal, interviewing or counselling skills does little to tackle the entrenched subculture of technical medicine (Nichols 1985). Ad hoc psychological aspects of care to aid preoperative management have been used although these have been largely on an informal basis, e.g. no psychological plan of care developed, implemented and documented in the nursing notes. In this new era of speedy surgical intervention and minimal hospital stay, considerably more attention must be given to patient information provision and other wider psychological considerations because much recovery now takes place away from immediate professional help and attention. A more structured plan of psychological care and information delivery is required to prevent this difficult situation from continuing. In addition, improved information provision may soon have to become an integral aspect of modern day surgery because the Audit Commission for Local Authorities and the NHS in England and Wales (1998b, p. 3) states: 'The overriding finding is that day surgery rates have increased very significantly for all 20 basket procedures.' This is an indication of the continuing rise in the amount of day surgery being undertaken and thereby an increase in the surgical population experiencing day surgery. The Audit Commission (1998b) also urged those health-care trusts that currently undertake very little day surgery to increase their capacity. More recently, a further report by the Audit Commission surveyed over 300 day-surgery units as part of an ongoing assessment (Audit Commission for Local Authorities and the NHS in England and Wales 2001). Six of the ten measures or indicators employed to determine 'good practice' were concerned with the provision of information. This has been demonstrated throughout this book to be a central theme for good psychological care provision.

Moreover, psychoeducational interventions will become a more prominent issue as the number and complexity of day-surgical procedures increase (Rawal et al. 1997). Day-surgery facilities are set to expand to become known as treatment centres. 'A further twenty-three NHS-run Treatment Centres and a further 32 independent sector Treatment Centres are in development and expect to be operational by the end of December 2005. In all we expect there will be 80 Treatment Centres by the end of 2005 providing up to 250,000 additional operations per year' (Department of Health 2003, p. 7).

It is recognized that completely eliminating anxiety for all patients undergoing day surgery may be an unrealistic goal. However, helping all patients to manage the psychological experience of, and recovery from, day surgery more effectively in the twenty-first century is a very realistic and achievable goal. The provision of a more formal psychoeducational plan of care is central in the achievement of this goal. A plan of care is therefore put forward that draws on the evidence from the previous chapters. The features of the formal psychoeducational plan are first described followed by the issues about implementation.

Intervention

Psychoeducational framework

A combination of the psychodynamic and transactional approaches to coping is required in order to provide an effective psychoeducational framework of care in this new era of surgical intervention (Figure 7.1). In this way consideration of individual traits alongside the dynamic experience of the day-surgery environment will occur (see Chapter 4). From a psychodynamic viewpoint, individuals clearly focus on different aspects when experiencing the adversity of day surgery as a result of personality differences and past experiences, e.g. vigilant and avoidant coping styles, health locus of control, self-efficacy appraisal. As the average length of stay in day surgery has been stated as 6.5 hours (Pfisterer et al. 2001) and individual requests for care are restricted as a result of the vital medical agenda implicit within day-surgery practice, a wholly psychodynamic approach to coping will be restrictive (little room for individual wishes or semblance of control available).

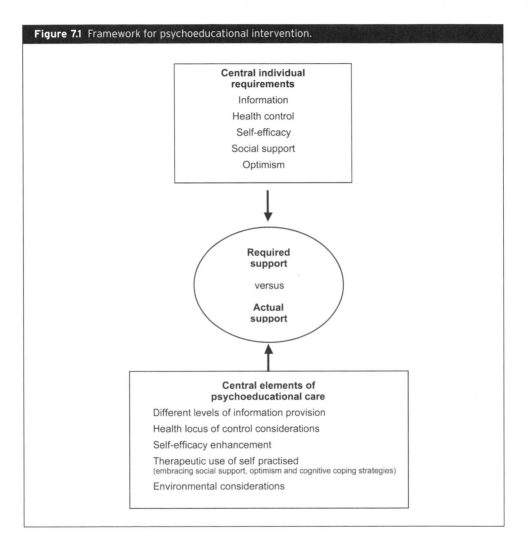

Figure 7.1 Framework for psychoeducational intervention.

From a transactional viewpoint, a number of issues may also prevent the adoption of a wholly transactional approach to coping. Patients remain in day surgery for a very brief period, the environment is completely unfamiliar and the hospital staff, although professionals, are almost always complete strangers. Therefore, a considerable amount of primary and secondary appraisal will be prevented, e.g. problem-focused coping strategies will be largely curtailed leaving only emotionally focused coping strategies on the day of surgery. Indeed, emotionally focused coping strategies have been identified as the main focus for anxiety management in modern day surgery (Mitchell 2003b) (see Chapter 3).

Using a combination of the specific psychological approaches (which all stem from the two broad approaches to coping), the basis for psychoeducational support required by the modern surgical patient can be established. The main components of an effective psychoeducational plan identified in Chapters 4 and 5 are information provision, health locus of control, self-efficacy and therapeutic use of self (embracing social support, optimism and cognitive coping strategies). The acceptance within modern surgery of patients with different informational requirements plus the need to focus on health locus of control, self-efficacy and therapeutic use of self (social support, optimism and cognitive coping strategies) is of paramount importance. Therefore, each aspect is described in detail together with its potential application. Of equal importance is the ability of the modern elective surgical environment to meet such psychoeducational requirements (see Figure 4.3, Chapter 4). However, it is largely unknown what features of the day-surgery environment contribute to an increase in patient anxiety. Therefore, a study is currently under way to help determine such influences. Others have also suggested a similar framework for psychological health care (Ridner 2004) and a balance between modern surgical service demands and individual desires (Menon 2002).

Information provision

The desired level of information provision is the most important element for effective psychoeducational intervention before day surgery. This is principally because it is essential in (1) establishing a coping style/information provision match (vigilant copers receive full information disclosure whereas avoidant copers receive standard disclosure), and (2) promoting the positive influence that the desired level of information can have on health locus of control experience and self-efficacy enhancement. From the plethora of studies about information provision in modern surgery it is evident that many patients are dissatisfied with the information provided (see Chapters 2, 3 and 6). In addition, many day-surgery units recognize that information provision may be less than adequate. In a survey by Thoms et al. (2002) only 66% of UK anaesthetic departments contacted returned a questionnaire about patient information provision. Of the departments who did return the questionnaire, 85% stated that information provision required improving. However, the study goes on to state: 'If, as is likely, responders gave more attention to this topic than non-responders, then our results may overstate the extent of information provision' (Thoms et al. 2002, p. 919). Such a situation of reduced information provision has been exacerbated in modern day surgery as a result of the rapid treatment and discharge of patients, e.g. limited time for psychological aspects of care because of the busy surgical schedule (Cox and O'Connell 2003).

Not all patients, however, want a large amount of information. A number of studies have strongly suggested that forcing a full level of information disclosure on patients can prove detrimental (Janis 1958, Salmon et al. 1986, Salmon 1992b, Kerrigan et al. 1993, Hawkshaw 1994, Lamarche et al. 1998) (see Chapter 2). However, essential preoperative information, e.g. fasting times, 24-hour carer, pain management, etc., can all too frequently be overlooked by patients who do not wish to read too much information about their surgery. If provided with brief highly relevant information, which does not detail treatment, such an issue could be avoided. To promote such individual responses to information provision a different outlook must be adopted. In a modern surgical health-care environment, the provision of information that recognizes vigilant and avoidant coping styles has been strongly recommended (Moerman et al. 1996, Kain et al. 2000, Mitchell 2000, Moore et al. 2002) Moreover, vigilant and avoidant coping behaviours have been identified in day-surgery patients (Mitchell 2000) (see Figure 4.4 in Chapter 4). In the study by Mitchell (2000), almost 33% of all day-surgery patients were deemed to be avoidant copers, i.e. wanted only a standard level of information disclosure because too much might increase anxiety. Conversely, just over 25% of patients were deemed to be vigilant copers, i.e. wanted a full level of information disclosure because too little might increase anxiety. A minimum of two levels of information provision is therefore highly recommended, i.e. standard and full disclosure of information. In this way vigilant copers will receive an abundance of information to read whereas the avoidant coper will receive brief, direct information more suited to their needs. Once such a system is established, crucial patient instructions, important to avoid the cancellation of surgery, may not be overlooked by the patient.

As can be seen in Figure 4.4 not all people fall neatly into the extremes of vigilant and avoidant coping behaviour. Four types of coping behaviour have been identified: vigilant, avoidant, fluctuating and flexible coping (Krohne 1978, 1989). Vigilant coping is characterized by the desire for maximum levels of information, avoidant coping by the desire for minimum levels of information, fluctuating coping by the desire for a variable level of information and flexible coping by adaptable informational requirements (Table 7.1). It is for this reason that a third level of information will be necessary, e.g. standard, intermediate or full disclosure.

The correct level of information provision is of crucial importance for the effective psychoeducational management of adult patients before day surgery. The third level can consist of a balance between the two extremes, e.g. some patients may prefer to know many details in a certain area of their care. This has given rise to the term 'fluctuating coper'. Patients with a mixed desire for information provision have been viewed as the most difficult to care for in respect of anxiety management (Rosenbaum and Piamenta 1998).

Table 7.1 Coping style definitions

Term	Definition
Vigilant coping	Coping style for dealing with a stressful situation characterized by the desire for maximum levels of information. The provision of too little information may give rise to an increase in anxiety
Avoidant coping	Coping style for dealing with a stressful situation characterized by the desire for minimum levels of information. The provision of too much information may give rise to an increase in anxiety
Fluctuating coping	Coping style for dealing with a stressful situation characterized by the desire for variable levels of information. The information desired may be highly specific. Incorrect communication of the desired amount or selected areas of information may give rise to an increase in anxiety
Flexible coping	Coping style for dealing with a stressful situation characterized by assuming an adaptable stance regarding information provision. Generally, whatever information is provided will be acceptable

As the ability to gain the desired level of information before day surgery is extremely limited (reduced opportunity and contact with hospital personnel), a deliberately planned effort on the part of the medical and nursing staff is required. It cannot be assumed that the desired level of information will be automatically provided by other formal mechanisms within the outpatient or preassessment visit or on the day of surgery because studies have demonstrated that this does not occur informally (van Weert et al. 2003). Apart from the day of surgery being too late for such information delivery, psychoeducational considerations are frequently overlooked on the day of surgery as a result of other vital medical issues. To compensate for this, formal mechanisms for receiving information before the day of surgery must be established and the provision of different levels of information made a necessity, not a desirable option. It must be accepted in modern surgical practices that patients have different information requirements and that one level of information provision is no longer appropriate or acceptable, especially when so much recovery takes place at home (Table 7.2).

Table 7.2 Psychoeducational management plan

Intervention	Rationale
Provision of different levels of information	Some patients (vigilant copers) may require more information than is generally available in the modern day-surgery environment. Too little information for such patients may increase anxiety. Therefore, in such a health-care environment where the opportunity to gain the desired level of information is often minimal, direct action by the medical and nursing staff is essential
Health locus of control considerations	Some patients do not feel in control of events in the health-care situation. Therefore, in an acute modern surgical environment where the opportunity for such personal inclusion is often minimal, a planned programme of health-care control considerations by the medical and nursing staff is essential
Self-efficacy enhancement	Some patients perceive their ability to cope in a modern surgical environment as limited. Therefore, in such a health-care situation where much recovery occurs at home, a planned programme of self-efficacy enhancement by the medical and nursing staff is essential
Therapeutic use of self	1. Social support: the close physical presence of the nurse is a form of social support and may be one of the most effective methods of preoperative anxiety management. Doctors and nurses are viewed as the experts. Therefore, being physically close to the patient frequently offers the perception of safety
	2. Optimism: constantly dwelling on the negative aspects of the proposed anaesthesia and/or surgical treatment could give a false impression of safety. Therefore, in such an active health-care environment as day surgery, where the opportunity to discuss fears is often minimal, direct action by the medical and nursing staff is essential
	3. Cognitive coping strategies: part of emotionally focused coping information and defined as the purposeful emotional attempts to prompt less negative thoughts about a given situation. In such an active health-care environment as day surgery, where the opportunity to discuss fears is often minimal, the use of phrases and utterances provided to engender a more realistic impression of safety are important, e.g. 'You will be safe because . . .?'
Environmental considerations	Positive implicit and explicit environmental appraisals can have an advantageous effect on patients' perception of safety. Therefore, in such a busy health-care environment as day surgery, where the opportunity to discuss events is minimal, positive appraisals of the environmental are essential

Health locus of control enhancement

Many studies have suggested that an increase in health locus of control can have a positive influence on recovery (see Chapter 4). The health locus of control theory is based on the assumption that 'internals' have a greater belief in their ability to shape their own destiny, whereas 'externals' feel more influenced by luck, fate and powerful others. Locus of control has previously been considered as a 'fixed' aspect of personality (Rotter 1966). However, a number of studies have recommended that health locus of control may not be this rigid. In an early study (Seeman and Seeman 1983), it was suggested that individual control in the health-care situation can be self-determined or, conversely, a product of the situation, i.e. not just reflective of individual desires. Peterson and Stunkard (1989, p. 820) stated: 'Personal control resides in the transaction between the person and the world; it is neither just a disposition nor a characteristic of the environment.' Control was therefore deemed to be context specific and open to manipulation, especially by 'powerful others' (Johnston et al. 1992, Avis 1994, Halfens 1995). When in groups, people may possess a 'collective' appraisal of control, e.g. the group norm for 'control' in that specific situation. If the collective appraisal of control in a particular group is perceived as weak (shared belief of more powerful others), individual perceptions of control may also be influenced in a similar direction (Peterson and Stunkard 1989).

The modern surgical environment provides a strong example of how such a shift in external health locus of control appraisal can occur, e.g. sparse information provision, brief hospital admission for surgery and anaesthesia within an environment dominated by rigid schedules, consent signing, enforced fasting, undressing and administration of powerful drugs, all maintained by uniformed doctors and nurses (powerful others). The influence of powerful others in uniforms in such a situation could considerably enhance the belief in powerful others and consequently become a very potent force. In a classic psychological study about the power of authority (Milgram 1974), it was vividly demonstrated how powerful others in uniform could greatly influence perceptions and subsequently dramatically shape behaviour.

The level of control required by day-surgery patients may need to be only minor and 'real or perceived', e.g. in an older study, as mentioned in a previous chapter, an increase in control was demonstrated merely by permitting blood donors a simple choice of which arm to be used during the procedure (Mills and Krantz 1979). Which arm to be used mattered little to the hospital personnel but for the patient it bestowed the perception of choice. If patients were provided with a perception of choice – real or perceived – their experience of health control may therefore greatly increase. As the ability to exercise some control in an acute day-surgery situation is very limited and the perceived ability to retain some aspects of health-care control is reduced in some patients (Mitchell 2000), a deliberately planned attempt on the part of the medical and nursing staff is required. Doctors and nurses must therefore identify simple aspects of intervention, which have the ability to bestow a perception of choice, e.g. choice to remain dressed if their surgery is later in the operating schedule, relatives to remain with the patient if desired, staggered admission times, etc. These need only be minor aspects of care, although if each member of the team were to behave in such a manner, the overall perception of health control would be considerable.

Self-efficacy enhancement

Many studies have suggested that an increase in self-efficacy can have a positive influence on recovery (see Chapter 4). Self-efficacy or the confidence in one's ability to behave in such a way as to produce a desirable outcome can give rise to considerable distress if these abilities are reduced. As patient stay in day surgery is so brief and preparation and recovery at home the greater part of the surgical experience, patients require superior self-efficacy beliefs in order to encourage a positive recovery. Dental surgery studies (a similar experience to day surgery) have demonstrated that recovery is enhanced when patients experience an increase in self-efficacy appraisals (Litt et al. 1995, 1999). Again, the modern surgical environment may negate personal attempts to establish an increased level of self-efficacy, e.g. brief hospital admission, strange environment, rigid schedules and powerful uniformed others determining complex medical events. As the perceived ability to cope with day surgery is reduced in some patients (Mitchell 2000) and much recovery occurs at home, a deliberately planned effort on the part of the medical and nursing staff to enhance self-efficacy appraisal is needed. Doctors and nurses must therefore identify simple aspects of intervention that can aid the enhancement of self-efficacy, e.g. explaining all events and providing the desired degree of information, guarantee of a nurse-initiated telephone call during the postoperative period, degree of information provision confirmed at discharge. If each member of the team were to behave in such a manner and such care became standard, the overall perception of self-efficacy enhancement/encouragement would be considerable (see Table 7.2).

Therapeutic use of self (social support, optimism and cognitive coping strategies)

In Chapter 4, social support was highlighted as an important factor in the psychological recovery of patients from surgery. However, the modern surgical environment precludes, to a large extent, the presence of relatives or other supportive members. In such circumstances the presence of a doctor or nurse as an agent of social support has been viewed as highly beneficial, i.e. therapeutic use of self (Elsass et al. 1987a, 1987b, Leino-Kilpi and Vuorenheimo 1993). Their presence has been compared with the assuring attendance that a parent or guardian bestows on an infant, e.g. the infant feels safer when the parent is in sight (Teasdale 1995a). Therefore, merely being close to and communicating with the patient provides a considerable element of safety (see Figure 5.1 in Chapter 5). Such a reassuring presence has also been demonstrated in the ambulatory surgery setting. A study was conducted using 19 day-surgery patients to ascertain which behaviours were deemed to be caring ones (Parsons et al. 1993). Various categories emerged but the three most effective caring behaviours identified were the nurses' reassuring presence, verbal reassurance and attention to physical comfort. Therefore, the mere presence of the nurse in close proximity to the patient while he or she was in the day-surgery facility and expressing concern was viewed as very helpful during periods of increased anxiety. In addition, in a study undertaken in an acute hospital setting, eight patients were interviewed to examine the experience of 'being reassured'. Two main themes emerged: internal experience (perception of an unthreatening and caring environment, receiving information, feeling of control, optimistic outlook provided by staff) and external experience (nurse being near the patient, well cared for or nurses demonstrating that they cared) (Fareed 1996).

In a number of recent studies therapeutic use of self has even been viewed as more important than information provision (see Chapter 6). In a study by van der Zee et al. (2002, p. 131) increased information did not have an overall beneficial effect on anxiety: 'the social and communication qualities of the anaesthesiologist seem to have an important impact on patient's faith in the medical staff and thereby on their pre-operative anxiety levels.' Therefore, the perception of being cared for by well-trained professionals with good interpersonal skills helped patients to manage their anxiety more effectively. In a comprehensive study by Koivula et al. (2002a), almost all the patients awaiting cardiac surgery had some anxiety. However, the presence of the nurses helped to ease this: 'ample overall support from the nurses involving both emotional, informational and tangible support [time spent talking with and being close to the patient] had a significant association with milder anxiety than if the amount of support was low' (Koivula et al. 2002a, p. 442). Such an approach to preoperative nursing intervention was also reiterated in a study in which 10 patients were interviewed after their operation together with 10 nurses who provided their care (Lindwall and von Post 2003). Listening to the patients' experiences, and acting on the patients' verbal and non-verbal cues to engender feelings of safety were stated as important features of perioperative nursing.

The use of social support, self-efficacy enhancement and encouragement of a more optimistic outlook can collectively be considered as therapeutic use of self techniques. When nurses are in close proximity to the patient it is not just their presence but also the spoken word. Communicating empathy, encouragement and support have clearly demonstrated superior benefit than presence alone (Spector and Sistrunk 1979), such as during intensely anxious moments in the nurse–patient or doctor–patient interaction, e.g. immediately before induction of anaesthesia, distraction of the patient is a common ploy used to help the patient endure the experience (Mitchell 2003b). Therapeutic use of self techniques are frequently employed during such stages by the use of a combination of social support (close physical presence, touch, comforting words of assurance), self-efficacy enhancement (physical presence and supportive statements) and encouragement of a more optimistic outlook (dispelling myths associated with surgery and anaesthesia).

Finally, cognitive coping strategies are used as part of emotionally focused coping information and defined as the purposeful emotional attempts to prompt less negative thoughts about a given situation, e.g. a mental strategy for avoiding catastrophizing (see Chapter 4). The application of such care will inevitably overlap with self-efficacy enhancement and the encouragement of a more optimistic stance. However, the central importance of such intervention has been established in many studies (see Chapters 2, 3 and 4). Nevertheless, no studies have uncovered the most appropriate words of assurance during such interactions. Doctors and nurses merely employ phrases and utterances that they personally deem to be most appropriate. Such information about the most effective and appropriate phrases and utterances is vital for a comprehensive preoperative psychoeducational plan of care. Research is ongoing to uncover the most effective cognitive coping strategies, e.g. most helpful phrases and encouraging statements, for use in such situations (see Table 7.2).

Environmental perceptions

The final part of this proposed formal psychoeducational plan of care directly concerns the environment. When on board an aircraft waiting to take holiday-makers to a place in the sun, many people may look around the aircraft in order to gain assurance (or not as the case may be) that the aircraft is flightworthy, the aircrew competent and the aircraft able to land safely at their destination. Patients may scrutinize the day-surgery environment in a very similar manner because they are also experiencing a stressful and potentially life-threatening situation, with little control over events and totally in the hands of strangers. Again, no studies have been undertaken of the impact of the day-surgery environment on patients as they assess the doctors'/nurses' competence and aspects of the environment, which may increase or decrease the stress response.

Some evidence suggests that patients undertake similar evaluations in the health-care environment because they have been observed to choose with which nurses to interact during their hospital stay (Teasdale 1995b). In an analysis of the concept of reassurance in health care by Teasdale (1995b), patients watched the nurses to see how they interacted with other patients and then chose them (or not) to communicate with on the strength of these observations. In a study by Fareed (1996), the external aspects of 'feeling assured' emanated from an unthreatening, friendly, kind and pleasant atmosphere where patients were encouraged to express their feelings. However, what is considered an unthreatening, friendly, kind and pleasant atmosphere within the day-case surgery arena is unclear.

A number of studies have examined the theatre environment and the conscious patient (Kennedy et al. 1992, Gnanalingham and Budhoo 1998), but very few have surveyed patients about the ward day-surgery environment (see Chapter 3). In a dental surgery study by Cohen et al. (2000, p. 387), the negative aspects of the environment were highlighted: 'In general, people disliked the sight and sound of dental equipment, the smell of the dental environment and the vibration of the drill.' In a further survey of 87 day-surgery patients about satisfaction with information provision and anxiety (Mitchell 2000), the aspect of care that helped to reduce anxiety the most was the presence of the nurse, closely followed by the ward environment (see Figure 5.1 in Chapter 5). In this study the ward surroundings were described as quiet, calm and professional, with music playing quietly in the background. However, the precise elements that contributed to this assessment of safety by the patients is unknown. The implicit and explicit messages of safety present within the day-surgery environment require further examination so that future action can be taken to enhance the positive influences and diminish the negative experiences (see Table 7.2).

Implementation

Administrative and legal issues

The implementation of such a psychoeducational plan of care would require spearheading by a dedicated team, ideally with the help of a nurse specialist (psychoeducational intervention in modern surgery). Extensive reports about the psychological care of surgical patients (Royal College of Surgeons of England and Royal College of Psychiatrists 1997, Audit Commission for Local Authorities and the NHS in England and Wales 1998b) suggest that nurses should be the coordinators of information provision within modern day surgery in order to alleviate some of the many associated problems (see Chapters 5 and 6). Such a nurse could be based in the preassessment clinic and help coordinate and implement the complete psychoeducational programme of care throughout modern elective surgery, e.g. preassessment visit, care on the day of surgery, discharge information and post-discharge contact. In a recent day-surgery survey by Mitra et al. (2003, p. 12), named nurses were given the specific task of spending extra time with their patients to ensure that they had sufficient information to care for themselves once discharged: 'They [the patients] had access to a telephone helpline and selected patients were visited on the first post-operative by the day surgery community nurse from the day care unit.' In a large study by Thompson et al. (2003, p. 908) to determine information requirements of patients undergoing gastroscopy, the nurse was viewed as a central figure in its provision: 'Nurses are thus in a unique position to provide essential information and reduce initial anxiety to patients and their families.' If the proposals put forward in *The NHS Plan* (Department of Health 2000) are to be realized, i.e. 75% of all elective surgery undertaken on a day-case basis, such changes outlined here may no longer be viewed as optional.

Little in the way of extra resources would be required to implement the formal psychoeducational plan of care because it could be established alongside existing practices. The formulation of the different information booklets, a degree of staff training and a staged period of introduction would be the main requirements, but the financial cost of such a plan may not be prohibitive, e.g. booklet production and resource costs, because it may be possible to use work already undertaken and available via numerous internet websites. Different levels of information could be established centrally and downloaded by individual day-surgery units or, indeed, by the patients themselves whenever required. Such innovative methods of communicating with patients are supported in a recent NHS report (Department of Health 2001) which is just one of numerous reports emerging that recommend the wider use of technological advances to augment patient communication.

Educational material must be presented in a structured and easily understood manner, e.g. in a questions answered format (Kent 1996). This format has been viewed as a very direct and concise method of conveying information. Indeed, a vast number of internet websites employ a very similar method, e.g. frequently asked questions (FAQs). This format could be used together with a logical sequence for day-surgery leaflet construction, e.g. phase 1 before admission, phase 2 on admission and phase 3 on discharge (Audit Commission for Local Authorities and the NHS in England and Wales 1990, pp. 43–44) (Tables 7.3–7.5). However, any blueprint for a patient information pack will need rigorous patient and multidisciplinary evaluation before its use. In addition, local variations in practice may necessitate some adaptations. Moreover, the implementation of such a system would possibly require a slow introduction to one surgical speciality or even one surgical procedure at a time. This may be necessary, because it would involve devising different levels of information for each surgical procedure and a degree of staff training. Also, such changes may benefit from a stable and sustained partnership between nurse clinicians and nurse educators, because the introduction of innovative clinical research can be a very challenging endeavour for all concerned (Hunt 1987). Indeed, medical education must now consider ambulatory surgery as a substantial part of its curriculum (Dent 2003).

Table 7.3 Framework for preassessment information construction (not exhaustive)

Phase 1: preassessment clinic

What is day surgery?
Explain modern surgical and anaesthetic practice, minimal access surgery, intermediate surgery, reduced waiting list time, one morning or afternoon in hospital, recovery at home, etc.

What do I need to know about the day-surgery unit?
Explain location, parking, telephone number, arrival and approximate discharge times, where to go on arrival, arrangements for relative/friend, identification of staff, brief definition of staff roles in the day-surgery unit, etc.

What operation will I have?
Provide avoidant coper with a standard account, written information, emphasis on relaxation, etc. Provide a fluctuating coper with an intermediate account of procedural, behavioural and sensory information, written information with requested additional elements. Provide a vigilant coper with a full account of procedural, behavioural and sensory information with diagrams, a chance to visit the unit, full written information, take-home video, etc.

Table 7.3 continued

Phase 1: preassessment clinic (continued)

What type of anaesthetic will I have?
Provide avoidant coper with a standard account, emphasis on relaxation, etc. Provide a fluctuating coper with an intermediate account with requested additional elements. Provide a vigilant coper with a full account of procedural, behavioural and sensory information with diagrams, etc.

What are the benefits of having this surgical procedure?
Explain avoidance of future complications, improved health status, reduced waiting time, minimal hospital stay, surgery at patient convenience, avoidance of hospital-acquired infections, issues specific to type of surgery, etc.

Why is a preassessment visit needed?
Explain medical suitability ensured, social circumstances, information provision, recovery advice, psychoeducational management, etc.

What arrangements should I make before the day of surgery?
Explain transport, relative/carer to accompany, 24-hour postoperative care by adult, plan adequate convalescence period, social and employment arrangements, pain management provision, wound management advice, issues specific to type of surgery, etc.

What do I need to do before I arrive at the hospital on the day of surgery?
Explain nil by mouth, suitable clothing, what to bring and what not to bring, medication, relative/carer, arrival and approximate discharge times, special instructions, etc.

Table 7.4 Framework for day-surgery information construction (not exhaustive)

Phase 2: day of surgery

What will happen to me once I arrive at the hospital on the day of surgery?
Briefly reiterate procedural, behavioural and sensory information, although concentrating mainly on emotional coping information provision, e.g. cognitive coping strategies, relaxation, modelling, etc.

If I am anxious how will I be helped?
Explain implementation of psychoeducational plan of care

Who are the people caring for me and when will I meet them to discuss my care?
Introduce self, other staff, surgeons and anaesthetist, time for brief discussions, etc.

How will my carer be kept informed of my progress and eventual discharge?
Explain to carer to remain with patient for as long as possible, telephone contact, prearranged telephone call, special arrangements, etc.

What will my anaesthetic be like?
Explain local, regional or general anaesthesia briefly, answer questions, explain length of anaesthesia, method of induction, etc.

Table 7.4 continued

Phase 2: day of surgery (continued)

What will happen after my operation before my discharge home?
Explain recovery room, ward recovery, warning of possible use of medical equipment
(intravenous infusion, cannula, etc.), analgesia, antiemetics, medications, wound
management advice, medical certificate, issues specific to type of surgery, etc.

Table 7.5 Framework for discharge information construction (not exhaustive)

Phase 3: discharge

On discharge home from the hospital what should I do?
Explain immediately return home, rest, take the recommended medications at the times
specified, e.g. analgesia, antibiotics, allow time for convalescence, manage wound as
advised, issues specific to type of surgery, etc.

If I experience any pain how will I manage it?
Explain that a little pain and discomfort are expected, rest completely for the first 24–48
hours, avoid sudden or excessive movement for the first 24–48 hours, take the
recommended analgesia exactly as advised for at least the first 24–48 hours, etc.

What side effects may occur at home and how can I recognize them?
Explain excessive pain, tiredness, nausea, wound problems, sore throat, fatigue, specific
issues, etc.

What support will I have at home?
Explain adult carer main support for a minimum of 24 hours, telephone helpline number,
24-hour nurse-initiated telephone call, GP, district nurse, hospital follow-up appointment if
required, issues specific to type of surgery, etc.

How will the operation affect my normal lifestyle?
Provide brief advice on returning to normal, e.g. sleeping, eating and drinking, bathing,
mobility level, returning to work, stretching, advice on sexual matters, bowel and bladder
function, housework, lifting, driving, exercise and sport, weight loss/gain, issues specific to
type of surgery, etc.

Whom can I contact for more advice or the early results of my surgery?
Provide day-surgery telephone number, GP, district nurse, early hospital appointment,
issues specific to type of surgery, etc.

Where can I obtain more information about my surgery?
Discuss day-surgery unit contact, consultant surgeon, GP, district nurse, British Association
of Day Surgery website, etc.

What are the possible complications of this type of surgery?
Discuss degree, duration and possible sites of pain, nausea and vomiting, wound infection,
usual and unusual events plus how to recognize them as such, possible sensations, issues
specific to type of surgery, etc.

For legal and surgical consent purposes all patients must receive a certain level of information before surgery (Kaufmann 1983, Redman 1993, Kent 1996). The legal minimum requirements could become the starting point for both full and standard information booklet construction because there are currently no criteria defining full and standard information booklet construction. The Clinical Negligence Scheme for Trusts (CNST) (Sanderson 1998) has 11 standards, which must be adhered to in order for health-care trusts to gain insurance against medical negligence claims. Only one standard (standard 7) relates to information provision (Table 7.6).

Table 7.6 Standard 7: Clinical Negligence Scheme for Trusts

Information on the risks and benefits of proposed treatment or investigation

There is patient information available showing the risks/benefits of 10 common elective treatments (minimal cover)

All consent forms used comply with NHS Executive Guidelines for design and use (maximal cover):

1. There is patient information available showing the risk/benefits of 20 common elective treatments
2. There is a policy/guideline stating that consent for elective procedures is to be obtained by a person capable of performing the procedure

There is a clear mechanism for patients to obtain additional information about their condition

From Sanderson (1998).

All information provided must contain between 10 and 20 risks–benefits common to elective surgical treatment, depending on the level of legal cover required. In addition, patients must be given instructions on how to obtain additional information, if desired. Increasingly, discharge information provision will be required to help patients recognize the possible development of complications. Patients need to be made aware of the signs and symptoms of complications at an early stage to ensure that they seek help swiftly (Smith 2000). In a recent day-surgery review of laparoscopic bowel injuries resulting from minimal assess surgery, delayed recognition was a major factor in the assessment of liability (Carroll et al. 1998, Vilos 2002). This is a view supported by the British government as a result of the extent of medical negligence claims (Towse and Danzon 1999). In addition it has been stated: 'as the proportion of surgery which is done as a day case increases so the proportion of cases [negligence claims] resulting from day case surgery will increase correspondingly'

(Leigh 1995, p. 410). Day-surgery management teams have therefore been advised to implement cost-effective risk-management policies such as the provision of sufficient discharge information.

Preassessment clinic

A proposed psychoeducational management plan such as the one outlined above will help systematically to coordinate tangible nursing activities and aid anxiety management. Effective psychoeducational nursing care based on contemporary research evidence can then be delivered in the way suggested to aid, for the first time in a formal manner, patients undergoing modern surgery. No such preoperative psychoeducational management plan currently exists, although such formalized interventions are manifestly required for the future of modern day-case surgery. However, such a plan of care will be ineffective unless a competent method of delivery is proposed.

When day-surgery patients attend the preassessment clinic in the days and weeks before surgery, the process of delivering the psychoeducational plan of care can begin. First, and most importantly, alongside the essential medical preassessment checks, patients must be able to decide which level of information they require. Time consuming questionnaires will not be needed for this, merely an overview of the information or the 'information options' available. A chart could be displayed on a wall in the preassessment clinic, highlighting the information options, e.g. option 1 avoidant coper requiring a standard level of information, option 2 possibly a fluctuating coper requiring an intermediate level of information and option 3 vigilant coper requiring a full level of information (Table 7.7) (the name of the coping style will not be required for the patient versions and is merely employed here for explanation purposes). Once an information provision/coping style match has been established the information package containing the correct level of problem-focused information (procedural, behavioural and sensory information) and emotionally focused information (cognitive coping strategies, relaxation and modelling) could be provided (see Tables 7.3–7.5). All written material could then be discussed with the patient either in the preassessment clinic or by telephone before surgery. The identified level of information should continue through to discharge and the patient be sent home with the appropriate level (see Table 7.5).

Although standard and full information provision options are required, an intermediate information provision option is also important, because not all patients will want the extremes of information, e.g. not all patients will be vigilant or avoidant copers. However, the degree

Table 7.7 Proposed information option chart

Information options	Avoidant coper (standard disclosure)	Fluctuating coper (intermediate disclosure)	Vigilant coper (full disclosure)
Preassessment clinic visit	Standard verbal/written, problem-focused and emotionally focused information about treatment, care and recovery	Intermediate, verbal/written, problem-focused and emotionally focused information about treatment, care and recovery	Full verbal/written, problem-focused and emotionally focused information about treatment, care and recovery
Day of surgery	Brief verbal reiteration, standard problem-focused and emotionally focused information	Brief verbal reiteration, intermediate problem-focused and emotionally focused information	Brief verbal reiteration, full problem-focused and emotionally focused information
Following discharge	Standard verbal/written problem-focused and emotionally focused information for home use	Intermediate verbal/written problem-focused and emotionally focused information for home use	Full verbal/written problem-focused and emotionally focused information for home use

of provision of information for fluctuating copers (intermediate information provision) has proved very difficult to ascertain because they themselves are unsure what information they need and what will help reduce their anxiety. In a study, by Rosenbaum and Piamenta (1998), of patients scheduled for hernia repair, fluctuating copers were viewed as the group experiencing 'dispositional conflict', i.e. a tendency to attend to and ignore threatening cues at the same time (unsure of what information to listen to and what to ignore). These participants were 'rated by the nurses on the ward as the worst copers in comparison to all other groups of subjects' (Rosenbaum and Piamenta 1998, p. 841). Therefore, because of their uncertainty about information provision, anxiety of such patients has been viewed as the most difficult to manage. Flexible copers are not included in the 'information options' because, for them, information provision is not viewed as an anxiety-provoking issue. Such patients can therefore make their choice from the options already available.

This type of visual display will elicit a speedy reply because most patients are fully aware of their information requirements (coping style) and have previously been able quickly to identify the level of information appropriate for them (Mitchell 1997). Once chosen, the corresponding level of information could be provided in commercially produced booklets, videotaped programmes, database systems or via specific internet sites. An internet site or hospital database may possibly be the most effective method because the desired level of information could be viewed and printed for the patient immediately or, as in the case of an internet site, the website address provided for home use.

To ensure that the correct information option is followed on the day of surgery, a simple identification system could be established in the pre-assessment clinic and used on the day of surgery, e.g. a simple traffic light colour-coding system could be used, e.g.

Red	Avoidant coper	→	Stop	→	Provide standard information.
Amber	Fluctuating coper	→	Caution	→	Provide intermediate information.
Green	Vigilant coper	→	Go	→	Provide full information.

Red would indicate a patient requiring a standard level of information (avoidant coper), amber a patient requiring an intermediate level of information (fluctuating coper) and green a patient requiring a full level of information (vigilant coper). This system could take the form of an inexpensive, appropriately coloured wrist tag or marker for the back of the hand, bed or trolley. The whole process would take only a matter of minutes to execute, its simplicity would ensure that little staff training is required, it would benefit patients enormously and provide a greater sense of satisfaction for the medical and nursing staff, and save a considerable amount of time spent explaining unwanted or unnecessary information to highly anxious patients on the day of surgery.

Such a system may require an increase in time spent in the preassessment clinic. However, this extra time may not be a considerable issue because only those patients who require full disclosure may need a slightly longer visit. In a study of 74 patients undergoing preassessment, Pellino et al. (1998) randomly assigned patients into one of two groups: group 1 received routine education in the preassessment clinic whereas group 2 received routine education plus additional time within an educational centre. The patients in group 2 had significantly increased self-efficacy appraisals in comparison to group 1. However, the study may have been somewhat flawed because many patients refused to take part in the control group (group 1 – routine education) and to a lesser extent the experimental group. Patients would therefore not take part in a study that did not correctly identify their educational requirements. The study also demonstrated the additional time needed to discuss issues adequately with patients because the impact of the medical agenda prohibited adequate information provision.

Although the orthopaedic clinic nursing staff are very knowledgeable about pre-operative preparation, the time and environment to

> adequately provide pre-operative teaching is severely hampered by additional patient obligations.
>
> Pellino et al. (1998, p. 57)

A visit and planned programme to discuss surgery in this way, and later re-establishing contact with a familiar nurse on the day of surgery, have helped to reduce anxiety in day-case surgery (Vogelsang 1990). Unfortunately, where preassessment interviews are conducted via the telephone, this potentially beneficial relationship is far less achievable, e.g. in one study telephone preassessment took an average of 14 minutes to complete (Ellis 2002). Such methods of preassessment, which deal almost exclusively with the medical agenda, are gaining in popularity because they are quick and effective (Healy and McWhinne 2003). Although clinically efficient, they are less than ideal from a psychological viewpoint. Such an approach also seeks to perpetuate the medical domination of the preassessment visit (Keenan et al. 1998) and again marginalizes essential psychological aspects of care.

Day of surgery

During phase 2 (admission), information provision should be provided as part of the formal psychoeducational management plan outlined earlier (see Table 7.2). All aspects of the plan **must** be fully used at this most stressful phase. The type of information required here might be brief procedural, behavioural and sensory information (see Table 7.3). However, in a study of 116 inpatients admitted on the morning of surgery (Yount and Schoessler 1991), it was concluded that psychosocial support should be the main emphasis on the day of surgery. The long wait on the day of surgery has been viewed as a source of considerable anxiety (Menon 1998, Mitchell 2000) (see Figure 3.2 in Chapter 3). Patients scheduled for surgery late on the operating list may therefore require full exposure to the psychoeducational plan of care. A number of studies have also identified the lack of knowledge about the role and qualifications of the anaesthetist as a problematic issue (Lonsdale and Hutchison 1991, Farnill and Inglis 1993, McGaw and Hanna 1998), e.g. patients did not know who the anaesthetists were or their role in caring for them. Meeting the anaesthetist has been viewed to help aid anxiety management and provide the opportunity to gain answers to FAQs, e.g. 'Does induction of anaesthesia involve a mask or needle and how long will the anaesthetic last?' (Goldmann et al. 1988).

On the day of surgery, ways in which the chosen information pathway, e.g. how standard, intermediate or full information disclosure can be maintained, must be established. This is crucial because some patients, possibly vigilant copers, may experience greater anxiety when not fully aware of all events. An instant means of identifying the selected pathway of desired information will make such a task far easier, e.g. appropriately coloured wrist tag, coloured skin marker on back of the hand, bedside identification note. In this way all staff involved in day surgery, e.g. nurses, surgeons, anaesthetists, theatre staff, medical and nursing students, will be able immediately to identify the patients' educational requirements.

Help for the relatives, if present, in the management of their anxiety during this phase is also required. In a study of the coping strategies employed by 40 patients' spouses while waiting during a loved one's surgery (Trimm 1997), tangible aspects of problem-focused and emotionally focused coping were identified (Jalowiec et al. 1984). Overall, relatives employed mainly problem-focused coping methods whereas at an emotional level they preferred to remain optimistic. Relatives therefore need the nurses to keep them informed of progress on the day of surgery, to be available to answer any questions, and again provide optimistic phrases and utterances.

Discharge and home recovery

During phase 3 (discharge) the emphasis moves to recovery at home. Again, information provision should be made as part of the formal anxiety management plan outlined earlier and all aspects of the plan **must** be fully used, especially the enhancement of self-efficacy (see Table 7.2). Patients will be at home in a few hours managing their own care. They should therefore be provided with the desired level of verbal and written information, e.g. standard, intermediate or full information disclosure. Again, this should be in the form of problem-focused and emotionally focused coping information (see Table 7.5).

In a comprehensive study by Bostrom et al. (1996), it was discovered that many patients although requiring more information were reluctant to ask for it. Patients were randomly allocated to three experimental groups: group 1 received a nurse-initiated telephone call, group 2 were expressly advised to telephone the day-surgery unit for advice when required (patient-initiated telephone call) and group 3 were the control group, i.e. no telephone call or encouragement to telephone the day-surgery unit. Over a 4-month period only 9 patient-initiated telephone calls were received whereas the nurses initiated 445 calls. However, every patient called had several questions for the nurses when contacted. 'Telephone follow-up with discharged patients revealed that several areas of self-care were not fully understood' (Bostrom et al. 1996, p. 50). The nurses stated that much information had been given before discharge but this had either been forgotten or not understood once home. A hospital database of information, which the nurses could use to inform the patients and thereby deliver an unbroken line of communication between the hospital and community services, was therefore recommended. The provision of the identified level of information is necessary throughout the whole day-surgery experience, i.e. pre- and postoperatively. For the patient who initially requests a standard level of disclosure but subsequently requires more information in the postoperative period (and indeed for all patients in the postoperative period), a nurse-initiated telephone call 24–48 hours after surgery should also be established. Many studies have vigorously supported such a move because pockets of undisclosed or forgotten information can quickly be provided (Lewin and Razis 1995, De Jesus et al. 1996, Wedderburn et al. 1996, Willis et al. 1997, Heseltine and Edlington 1998, MacAndie and Bingham 1998).

This aspect of 'returning to normal' is a considerable theme within the literature on recovery at home after day surgery, together with pain management, sleep disturbance, nausea and the desire for information (Ruuth-Setala et al. 2000, Robaux et al. 2002, Mitchell 2003a). Many studies have also uncovered the patients' desire to be informed of the possible complications in the postoperative period and also how such complications can be recognized (Bubela et al. 1990, Farnill and Inglis 1993, Bostrom et al. 1994, 1996, De Jesus et al. 1996, Ruuth-Setala et al. 2000). Donoghue et al. (1995, p. 173) interviewed 31 day-surgery patients and 'Many of the participants reported that there were experiences they had not anticipated, surprises that they did not welcome and things that they would have liked to have known before the operation'. The provision of information about 'returning to normal', may therefore help to prevent issues of 'trial-and-error' recovery (Kleinbeck and Hoffart 1994). Some patients wanted information about the safe time to resume activities, warning of the possible problems, and again what to regard as 'normal or unusual' in the postoperative period (Linden and Engberg 1995, 1996). In an Australian survey, 40 patients were asked on the eve of surgery to rank 13 categories of information into the most preferred order (Farnill and Inglis 1993). When they were able to eat after surgery, when they were able to get out of bed and the common complications were all rated as the most desirable.

In a study of 165 inpatients after surgery it was revealed that patients were fairly consistent in prioritizing their learning needs (Bostrom et al. 1994). Information about medication, treatment and complications, and enhancing the quality of life were more valued than information about activities of daily living, community follow-up, skin care and feelings about the condition. In a wide-ranging postal questionnaire sent to 550 day-surgery patients concerning their experiences, a number of post-discharge problems were identified (Royal College of Surgeons of England and East Anglia Regional Health Authority 1995). The main problems were sleep disturbance, asking for help, wound care, mobility, returning to work and nausea. In a further two day-surgery studies (Linden and Engberg 1995, 1996) the most common problems at home were pain management (42%), sleep (15%) and nausea (11%). In a literature review of day surgery and information provision a leaflet construction guide highlighted the main patient requirements (Bradshaw et al. 1999). The guide recommended inclusion of information about postoperative pain management, common wound problems, aspects of bathing, stretching, heavy exercise, returning to work, driving and advice on sexual matters.

Community health-care support has also featured in a number of studies (see Chapter 2). In a survey of 70 patients after day surgery it was uncovered that only 7% contacted the hospital within the first 3 days of discharge and only 7% their GP (Kennedy 1995). In a postal survey of 205 patients 12 months after gynaecological day surgery (Bhattacharya et al. 1998), day-case surgery patients and inpatients were compared. It was revealed that there had been no significant effect on GP consultations between the two groups. Moreover, hospital costs for day surgery were significantly less than inpatient surgery for the same gynaecological procedure. An audit of 268 patients who had undergone a variety of day-surgery procedures was also undertaken to evaluate the level of community health-care involvement (Woodhouse et al. 1998). The common reasons for visiting the GP were found to be for medical certificates, discussion on return to work and wound care. The study therefore recommended encouraging patients to use the day-surgery telephone helpline, the provision of clear instructions on discharge about returning to work plus the provision of medical certificates in order to combat any increased use of community health-care resources. A similar study also examined the impact of day surgery on GP workload and recommended improving information provision, analgesia provision and the distribution of medical certificates (MacAndie and Bingham 1998).

However, as a result of the rapid rise in day surgery and the increase in more complex day-surgery procedures, community service input after day surgery may be rising (Marshall and Chung 1997). In a comprehensive study by Kong et al. (1997, p. 292) undertaken to establish the demands of day surgery on GPs, 1798 questionnaires were sent to day-surgery patients: 'Of the 1478 completed questionnaires, 247 (16.7%) patients consulted their general practitioner after day surgery.' The most common reason for visiting was pain management (34.3%). Therefore, almost one-third of the patients consulted their GP for pain or a surgical procedure related infection: 'An increase in workload for general practitioners is inevitable when more ambitious procedures are performed on less fit patients on a day case basis' (Kong et al. 1997, p. 294). In addition, the continuing increase in day surgery has led to a corresponding rise in patient and lay-carer involvement throughout the pre- and postoperative period (Mitchell 2003a). The impact that day-surgery expansion is having on patients and their carers' contribution to care is a challenging issue for modern day-case surgery. During interviews with 252 carers of day-surgery patients, 90% were concerned about the patients' pain, wound care, sleep disturbance and nausea (Knudsen 1996). A leaflet especially constructed for carers was therefore highly recommended. Day-case surgery and its future expansion are extremely reliant on a willing and able layperson to provide essential care for relatives/friends.

Finally, the provision of the desired level of information is a crucial factor in the swift and uneventful recovery of day-surgery patients. Lay carers are willing to provide the care for their relative or friend although they require adequate information to help them undertake this role. Patients frequently encounter experiences in the postoperative period about which they have little or no knowledge. The provision of a nurse-initiated telephone call and a helpline are therefore essential prerequisites for an effective dedicated day-surgery unit fit for the twenty-first century. Overall, greater emphasis on psychoeducational aspects of care is required in this new era of increasing ambulatory surgery (Table 7.8).

Table 7.8 Overview of complete psychoeducational care

Preassessment clinic visit

- Medical assessment for day surgery, e.g. physical ability to undergo surgery and anaesthesia
- Nursing assessment for day surgery, e.g. correct level of information gained in order to (1) satisfy individual coping style, (2) ensure effective home preparation for surgery and (3) ensure effective home recovery
- Psychoeducational plan of care commenced, e.g. information provision/coping style match, health locus of control considerations, self-efficacy enhancement, therapeutic use of self practised and attention to environmental considerations
- Choice of information selected and provided, e.g. standard, intermediate or full disclosure
- Colour-coding scheme relevant to information requirements initiated
- Information provision and psychoeducational plan coordinated by identified nurse specialist and implemented by all staff
- Relative/carer involvement where possible

Day of surgery

- Psychoeducational plan of care continued, e.g. information provision/coping style match, health locus of control considerations, self-efficacy enhancement, therapeutic use of self practised and attention to environmental perceptions

Table 7.8 continued

Day of surgery (continued)

- Colour-coding scheme relevant to information requirements continued
- Full psychoeducational plan of care implemented especially for patients appearing late on the operating schedule
- Relative/carer kept informed where possible

Discharge planning

- Psychoeducational plan of care continued, e.g. information provision, health locus of control, self-efficacy considerations, therapeutic use of self practised and attention to environmental considerations
- Nurse-initiated telephone call to patients 24–48 hours after surgery
- Telephone helpline number provided for all patients
- Discharge planning, information provision and psychoeducational plan coordinated by identified nurse specialist and implemented by all staff
- Relative/carer involvement where possible

Conclusion

Day-case surgery has become the most common form of elective adult surgery. Increasingly, more elective surgical procedures will move from the inpatient arena into the day-surgery arena. Likewise, surgical procedures once performed as day surgery are moving into the outpatient arena. Quite simply, the length of hospital stay for an elective surgical procedure is rapidly diminishing, e.g. reduced from weeks to hours. As a result of such revolutionary changes in the delivery of surgical health care the need for effective psychoeducational management has grown rapidly. There is currently no formal psychoeducational plan of care, although there is a desperate need for such intervention. A detailed psychoeducational plan of care has therefore been suggested based on research evidence. The plan has five major elements: three levels of information provision, health locus of control considerations, self-efficacy enhancement, therapeutic use of self practised and environmental considerations.

First, three levels of information are required, e.g. full, intermediate or standard disclosure. Full disclosure may be required for vigilant copers because too little information will give rise to an increase in anxiety in such patients. Standard disclosure may be required for avoidant copers because too much information will give rise to an increase in anxiety. Fluctuating copers or patients who have high information requirements in a specific area and lower requirements in other areas may need to have a balance between the two extremes of standard and full disclosure.

The second major element concerns health locus of control. It has been demonstrated that some patients appreciate a little more control than is readily available in the health-care situation in order to enhance their recovery prospects. Such health-care control need only be minor (real or perceived). In a health-care situation such as day surgery where the opportunity for such personal inclusion is often minimal, a planned programme of health-care control enhancement by the medical and nursing staff is essential. The third major element concerns self-efficacy enhancement. It has been demonstrated that some patients do not feel as able to cope with the events of day surgery, e.g. minimal professional care, maximum self-care. Therefore, in the short time available in the preassessment clinic and on the day of surgery it is essential to have a planned programme of self-efficacy enhancement by the medical and nursing staff. The fourth major element concerns the therapeutic use of self. This aspect combines social support, optimism and the doctors' and nurses' utterances in the promotion of the perception of safety, e.g. helps to diminish catastrophizing thoughts and enhance more realistic positive perceptions. The fifth and final major element concerns the perception of the environment. Although little research has been undertaken about this aspect, the impact of the health-care environment should not be underestimated. The positive implicit and explicit messages of safety, once identified in greater detail, must be employed in full.

Such a psychoeducational plan of care will require adequate preparation. The appointment of a nurse specialist role may be a vital first step. Such a role will help to coordinate the entire psychoeducational experience of day surgery, e.g. preassessment clinic visit, day of surgery, discharge planning and home recovery. However, all staff within the day-surgery unit will be involved in the implementation of the psychoeducational plan. Construction and agreement of the information to be provided at each level, e.g. standard, intermediate or full disclosure, will be required. In addition, such educational material will need to be presented in a clear and logical order with due care and attention given to the legal requirements.

The preassessment visit can no longer remain dominated by formal medical issues. Although medical assessment within day surgery is vital for safety purposes, the opportunity for a formal nursing assessment with regard to psychoeducational issues is gaining greater importance. This is especially the case when more ambitious surgical procedures are being undertaken on less fit patients (Cook et al. 2004). Patients need to be provided with a choice of information during the preassessment visit and this choice noted in order for the patients to be colour coded for the day of surgery. In this way the agreed information, wanted by the patients, can be provided on the day of surgery with little need for further evaluation.

On the day of surgery the information provision/coping style match must continue together with the implementation of the full psychoeducational plan of care. This is especially the case for patients appearing later on the operating schedule because they are likely to become most anxious. Finally, on discharge the information provision/coping style match must continue together with the implementation of the full psychoeducational plan of care. Patients will be endeavouring to return to 'normal' once discharged home and may therefore require some additional nursing assistance, e.g. nurse-initiated telephone call, district nurse visit, GP visit. In this way information about the recognition and management of possible unforeseen events can be provided.

Summary

- No formal psychoeducational plan of care exists in any aspect of surgical nursing intervention.
- A psychoeducational plan of care is desperately needed in modern elective day-case surgery especially as more ambitious surgical procedures are being undertaken on less fit patients.
- The psychoeducational plan of care outlined here has five major components: three levels of information provision, health locus of control considerations, self-efficacy enhancement, therapeutic use of self practised and environmental considerations.
- The implementation of such a care plan may need coordinating by a nurse in a nurse specialist role although implementation will be the responsibility of all nurses.
- Information provision is central to the psychoeducational plan and therefore the correct identification of the patients' coping style during the preassessment visit is of paramount importance.
- The provision of an information provision/coping style match throughout all stages of the day-surgery experience is essential.
- All five major components of the psychoeducational plan are required during the whole day-surgery experience in order to embrace effective preoperative psychoeducational intervention fully.

Further reading

Allen, D. (2004) The Changing Shape of Nursing Practice: The role of nurses in the hospital division of labour. London: Routledge.

Burden, N., DeFazio-Quinn, D.M., O'Brien, D. and Gregory-Dawes, B.S. (2000) Ambulatory Surgical Nursing, 2nd edn. London: W.B. Saunders.

Chester, G.A. (ed.) (2004) Modern Medical Assisting. New York: Saunders.
Clifford, C. and Clark, J. (2004) Getting Research into Practice. London: Churchill Livingstone.

Websites

National Electronic Library for Health: www.nelh.nhs.uk
Patient information sites:

    www.nhs.uk/nhsmagazine
    www.youranaesthetic.info
    www.ich.ucl.ac.uk/factsheet
    www.users.bigpond.net.uk
    www.wcvh.com.au

Chapter 8

Twenty-first century elective surgical nursing

Day-surgery innovation

Modern elective day surgery has ensured many permanent changes to the future of surgical nursing intervention. The extensive inpatient surgical procedures once performed in the past have reduced considerably and day surgery is now the norm for most patients undergoing elective surgery. Day-surgery procedures frequently employ both minimal access techniques and individually tailored anaesthesia to ensure a rapid recovery. Such practices consequently demand little second phase postoperative physical nursing intervention. It is now commonplace for patients to be admitted to a day-surgery facility and to be treated and discharged within a matter of hours with 'greet 'em, treat 'em and street 'em' being the new maxim. Moreover, this modern surgical trend is irreversible and expanding constantly both in the number of surgical procedures that can be undertaken and in the number of patients able to undergo day surgery.

Correspondingly, the need for physical nursing intervention has reduced considerably, because patients experience less physical trauma and are therefore able to be discharged home within a few short hours of surgery. The escalation of this new surgical era is of crucial importance to the nursing profession, because the impact of such medical advances on surgical nursing practices has far-reaching implications, e.g. as the amount of day surgery continues to grow and medical advances ensure a more rapid recovery from surgery for an even greater proportion of the surgical population, many traditional surgical nursing skills will increasingly become obsolete. The nursing profession must gain a constant appreciation of the events transforming its future and ensure that it adapts its surgical practices accordingly in order to maintain a valuable contribution to the patient's experience of modern surgery. This will necessitate developing areas of surgical nursing intervention once largely marginalized, e.g. psychoeducational aspects of care. Traditional, more physically based nursing intervention in modern elective surgery is now on the decline and psychoeducational aspects of care in the ascendancy. However, psychoeducational aspects of care are still largely overshadowed by the political forces placed on the nursing profession to embrace more devolved medical tasks rather than to look towards its own body of evidence. The role of the surgical nurse in such a new and stimulating era must endeavour to embrace new nursing challenges, evolve its own body of knowledge fit for twenty-first century elective surgical nursing and, most importantly, use such knowledge in the clinical setting. Therefore, in this final chapter the additional advances that have the potential to influence surgical nursing intervention further are highlighted together with the expansion of day surgery in the form of treatment centres and the future direction for modern surgical nursing.

Surgical and anaesthetic advances

Throughout the next decade treatment in day-service facilities will continue to expand as a result of: (1) government initiatives (see 'Treatment centres' p. 178), (2) economic incentives, (3) advances in surgical and anaesthetic practices (increasing use of regional anaesthesia together with medical equipment for home management), (4) the growing number of patients deemed eligible to undergo day surgery, and (5) additional day-surgery capabilities.

First, many day-surgery studies continue to be undertaken in order to demonstrate the suitability of new and different surgical procedures or the cost savings to be made or to extol the effectiveness of different anaesthetic techniques for the common inclusion into day-surgery practices (Fleming et al. 2000, Klein and Buckenmaier 2002, Cartagena et al. 2003, Charalambous et al. 2003, Guy et al. 2003, Law et al. 2003, Lemos et al. 2003, Nielsen et al. 2003). In a study by Fleming et al. (2000), 45 patients undergoing laparoscopic cholecystectomy were surveyed. An overall success rate of 80% was achieved, which resulted in a cost saving of $Aus984 per patient treated. Each patient received a nurse-initiated telephone call within the first 24 hours of surgery and the study recommended that, when agreed protocols were implemented, e.g. all patients receive ondansetron (anti-emetic) intraoperatively, such a level of success is possible. In a study by Guy et al. (2003), the cost and outcomes after day-surgery haemorrhoidectomy were compared with inpatient haemorrhoidectomy. A $Sing300 saving was made for each patient because the mean hospital inpatient stay was 2.6 days. The procedure was therefore recommended as suitable for day-case surgery, although preferably such operations should take place in the morning and the patient be provided with detailed advice. Surgery during the morning session was recommended because 16% of day-surgery patients require readmission with less time to recovery before the closure of the unit at 5pm.

Second, different anaesthetic techniques are increasing the level of surgical procedures possible in day-surgery facilities. In a study of patients undergoing hernia repair (Gupta et al. 2003), 40 patients were randomly assigned into two groups: one group received spinal anaesthesia with bupivacaine 6.0 mg whereas the second received spinal anaesthesia with bupivacaine 7.5 mg (long-acting local anaesthesia). Although few differences were established between the two groups, group 1 (bupivacaine 6.0 mg) required significantly more intraoperative analgesia. Spinal anaesthesia with bupivacaine 7.5 mg and fentanyl was therefore recommended as an alternative to general or local anaesthesia for ambulatory inguinal herniorrhaphy. However, it is documented that the long discharge times and risk for urinary retention restrict its routine use in all patients. In a further study concerning hernia repair (Weltz et al. 2003), 29 patients underwent a thoracic/lumbar paravertebral procedure, involving an injection of local anaesthetic immediately lateral to the vertebral column where the cord divides into the dorsal and ventral rami. This method was selected because the advantages of regional anaesthesia include prolonged sensory block with minimal postoperative pain and opioid use, reduced nausea and vomiting, avoidance of general anaesthesia and shorter hospitalization. The use of the paravertebral block was effective in 93% of the cases in this study. In a further study of regional anaesthesia (Clough et al. 2003), 42 patients undergoing unilateral orthopaedic foot surgery were randomized into two groups: group 1 received general anaesthesia with supplementary foot block (0.5% bupivicaine) whereas group 2 received general anaesthesia alone. Group 2 received more intraoperative analgesia and antiemetics although no significant differences in pain scores were established during the first 24–48 hours. However, with the supplementary foot block group, the time period before the onset of pain was extended.

In a further regional anaesthesia study (Watson and Allen 2003), the outcomes of 400 patients undergoing surgery and spinal anaesthesia were audited. Patient preference, respiratory disease, obesity and cardiovascular disease were cited as the main reasons for use of spinal anaesthesia. Although access to day surgery was extended to people who may have otherwise have been unsuitable, some patients experienced an increased amount of time in the day-surgery unit after their surgery, e.g. knee arthroscopy. Similarly, in a study of 96 inpatients undergoing hernia repair (Erdem et al. 2003), participants were randomized into two groups: spinal anaesthesia group and local infiltration group. It was revealed that the spinal anaesthesia group remained in hospital significantly longer than the local infiltration group (2–4 days). The use of local infiltration as opposed to spinal anaesthesia was therefore recommended because of the reduced hospital stay, reduced costs and applicability to all patients.

In addition, modern anaesthetic techniques are permitting even faster recovery from anaesthesia. In an extensive study by Apfelbaum et al. (2002, p. 71), 2354 were surveyed in order to demonstrate how the first-stage recovery area or post-anaesthesia care unit (PACU) could be bypassed for a 'fast-track' recovery:

> New anesthetics with improved pharmacokinetic and pharmaco-dynamic properties, specifically a shorter elimination half-life, permit a faster emergence from anesthesia and allow the evaluation of immediate postoperative recovery at an earlier time point.

The criteria put forward to warrant suitability for bypassing the first-stage recovery area are the patient being awake and alert, minimal pain (no parenteral medication), no active bleeding, vital signs stable, nausea minimal and no vomiting; if neuromuscular blocking agent is used additional checks must be made and oxygen saturation must be 94% or higher.

Third, a number of day-surgery studies are increasingly employing the use of supplementary medical equipment to aid pain management during the first few postoperative days (Ganapathy et al. 2000, Boada et al. 2002, Nielsen et al. 2003). A number of additional operations could be performed as day surgery although pain management at home frequently renders some operations restrictive. Patient-controlled regional anaesthesia using elastomeric pumps (Eclips), or similar devices, are therefore increasingly being employed. Local anaesthesia is delivered via a catheter near to the nerve, thereby reducing sensation in the limb. In a study to examine such patient-controlled regional analgesia (Ilfeld et al. 2002), 30 participants were randomly divided into two groups after upper limb orthopaedic surgery. Group 1 received ropivacaine 0.2% (long-acting anaesthesia) whereas group 2 received sterile 0.9% saline; both were delivered via an infraclavicular brachial plexus perineural catheter (armpit) for 3 days (essentially a patient-controlled analgesia pump delivering local anaesthesia into the nerve supplying the arm). Supplementary use of oral opioids and related side effects were significantly decreased in the ropivacaine group. In addition, sleep disturbance was 10 times greater for the saline group and overall satisfaction was significantly greater in the ropivacaine group. The continued use of such a form of anaesthesia during upper limb orthopaedic surgery was therefore recommended.

In a similar study (Rawal et al. 2002), 60 patients scheduled for ambulatory hand surgery underwent the procedure with an axillary plexus blockade. After surgery, a plexus catheter was connected to an elastomeric, disposable 'homepump', containing 100 ml of either 0.125% bupivacaine or 0.125% ropivacaine (both are local anaesthetic for wound infiltration). The aim of the study was to compare the analgesic efficacy of bupivacaine versus ropivacaine brachial plexus analgesia after ambulatory hand surgery, because previous studies have found epidural bupivacaine to be 40% more potent than epidural ropivacaine. However, no significant differences were established between the two groups although both ropivacaine and bupivacaine provided effective analgesia via this method of delivery and patient satisfaction with patient-controlled regional anaesthesia was high.

Fourth, a number of studies have examined the feasibility of increasing day surgery for older adults (Chung et al. 1999, McCallum et al. 2000, Aldwinckle and Montgomery 2004). In a comprehensive study by Chung et al. (1999) 17,638 ambulatory surgery patients were audited during a 3-year period and it was documented that 27% of patients were 65 years or older. Although the older people had a higher incidence of intraoperative cardiovascular events, postoperatively there were no significant differences in comparison to all other patients. The study therefore recommended that the risks to older people undergoing day surgery did not justify their exclusion. However, it was stated that this population might require more careful intraoperative cardiovascular management. McCallum et al. (2000) also reached similar conclusions in a study in which patients were surveyed 12 weeks after day surgery. An increase in age of 70+ did not result in a greater use of community services or the need for extra help during the postoperative period. Day-surgery patients were commonly younger and in good general health, although there was no detrimental evidence about the effects of day surgery for older people. However, improved selection at the preassessment clinic and enhanced information provision were recognized as having the potential to boost outcomes.

Aldwinckle and Montgomery (2004) undertook a retrospective review of 1647 older patients (70+) over a 2-year period to assess postoperative outcomes. Of the 74% (n = 1226) who responded to the questionnaire, 95% were satisfied with the service and 5% were very satisfied. Only 1.4% required any help from the primary health-care team during the first 24 hours and overall readmission rates were 1.6%, which is below the recommended Royal College of Surgeons of England rate of 3%: 'We could find no evidence that age > 70 years should in any way be an exclusion criteria for day surgery' (Aldwinckle and Montgomery 2004, p. 59). Moreover, patients deemed less physically fit are also increasingly admitted to day-surgery facilities. Various methods of assessment are employed to gauge physical ability to undergo general anaesthesia, e.g. American Society of Anesthesiologists' physical status (ASA scale 1–5), body mass index (BMI), etc. (Hilditch et al. 2003a, 2003b, Ansell and Montgomery 2004, Carlisle 2004). Patients with an ASA 3 rating have previously been considered unsuitable for day surgery although this too has now been questioned (Ansell and Montgomery 2004).

Finally, some day-surgery units have begun to operate on minor emergency cases resulting in considerable cost savings (Conaghan et al. 2002, Charalambous et al. 2003). The aim of the study by Conaghan et al. (2002) was to assess the feasibility of treating patients with minor and intermediate general surgery emergency conditions as day cases, e.g. superficial abscesses, acutely painful hernias and thrombosed prolapsed haemorrhoids. Patients were previously frequently admitted via accident and emergency and spent a night in hospital before surgery the next day. In the study patients were randomized to two groups: a day-surgery group (if criteria for physical fitness established) and inpatient surgery group. When comparing the two methods, i.e. sent home to return for day surgery within 48 hours versus admitted as an inpatient for surgery the next day, day-case patients spent significantly less time in hospital than the inpatient group. In addition, the inpatient group were frequently admitted to inpatient wards and placed last on the operating list for the next day. If any case over-ran the emergency surgery was frequently cancelled. This occurred far less with day-surgery operating lists. However, day-surgery emergency follow-up treatment by district nurses led to a rise in their work, e.g. dressing wounds. Nevertheless, a saving of £147 was made per patient although it was recommended that such a service could be successful only in a dedicated day-surgery unit.

In a similar study by Charalambous et al. (2003), 83 patients experiencing minor orthopaedic trauma were audited in the defined period. When the patients were informed that they would have to stay in hospital for the night before surgery the following morning 23% made the decision to go home and return the next morning. The study therefore recommended a protocol for minor orthopaedic surgery patients where patients could go home and return the next morning for surgery to the day-surgery unit. In addition, the opposite is also occurring, i.e. more minor surgery is departing from day-surgery facilities (Kremer et al. 2000). More minor day-surgery procedures are increasingly moving away from the main hospitals to more community practice settings in line with the planned increase in the number of treatment centres (see 'Treatment centres'). In a study of 50 patients undergoing local anaesthesia for hernia repair in the primary care setting (Smith 1998), 98% were very happy with the service and the absence of the problems associated with general anaesthesia.

Treatment centres

The current UK government has launched a number of initiatives to help aid the expansion of day surgery (Cook et al. 2004), although only three central initiatives will be highlighted here. First, there are wide differences in day-surgery activity throughout the UK caused by such issues as reduced capacity in terms of premises, preferred medical practices, staffing, etc. If all the day-surgery units in the UK were as efficient as the best performers 120,000 additional day-case procedures could be undertaken in day-surgery facilities nationally (Audit Commission for Local Authorities and the NHS in England and Wales 2001). Efforts are therefore being made to help day-surgery units enhance their potential and provide a wider range of day-surgery work (Cook et al. 2004, NHS Modernisation Agency 2004).

Second, alongside such encouragement to transform practice, national tariffs or 'payment by results' for surgery undertaken is being planned: 'It will mean that NHS organisations are paid more fairly for the treatment they provide. Money will be linked directly to patients and patient choice so the more productive and efficient an NHS Trust, the more it will benefit from extra resources' (Cook et al. 2004, p. 61). 'In particular, the Department [DoH], with the NHS, will look to develop incentives that help to reduce unnecessary hospitalisation' (Department of Health 2004b, p. 69). The more efficient NHS trusts that undertake more day surgery will thereby be financially rewarded. Trusts that undertake a greater proportion of inpatient surgery will not benefit from such extra resources. Any trust that does not provide a high percentage of the surgical procedures detailed in the 'basket of procedures' or 'trolley of procedures' in day-case facilities (see Chapter 1) may therefore become somewhat disadvantaged. However, the true impact that such a policy will have on the day-surgery rates and expansion of more day-surgery facilities within all UK trusts remains to be seen. Nevertheless, national tariffs will be phased in over the next few years and be fully operational by 2008, so the financial incentives for pursuing a more day-surgery-oriented approach are imminent.

Third, the government is currently in the process of commissioning the building of new day-surgery facilities in the form of treatment centres within both the NHS and the independent sector (Fuller 2003, Department of Health 2004b). About 60–80 treatment centres are planned for England by the end of 2005 and a further 100 by 2006 (Moore 2003). A detailed map of fully operational schemes, centres under development and independent sector schemes is widely available (Fuller 2003, Department of Health 2004a). Treatment centres therefore feature large in the plans to deliver an increased day-surgery service and reform the NHS. It is planned to reduce the NHS waiting time for inpatient surgery to 6 months by December 2005 and remove all waiting time completely by 2008, so that choice of health-care provision becomes the central focus as opposed to the period of waiting (Department of Health

2004a, 2004b). A sum of £2 billion has been assigned for the building and development of new treatment centres (Bostock 2003) and it is envisaged that there will be three types: (1) centres undertaking short-stay inpatient work, frequently focusing on a single specialty such as orthopaedics, (2) centres focusing on day-case or outpatient work and sometimes referred to as 'surgi-centres' and (3) centres based in the community concentrating on diagnostic work (endoscopy, ultrasonography) and minor surgical procedures (excision of cysts or lesions and vasectomies) (Department of Health 2004a).

'Department of Health figures suggest that 68% of elective operations in 2000–2001 were day cases' (Stephenson 2002, p. 9), although this is acknowledged as too high as a result of incorrect reporting and the inclusion of too many outpatient cases. In an audit by Raftery and Stevens (1998, p. 152), it was established that inpatient procedures rose by 22% whereas day-case procedures rose by 102% during the period 1990–1995: 'Success in increasing the proportions treated as day cases appears to have been achieved through large increases in the volume of day surgery rather than through substitution of in-patient treatments by day case work.' It is the government's intention that day surgery will remove from the inpatient surgical lists procedures that can be reliably undertaken on a day-case basis. Day surgery is viewed as a method of relieving some of the burden placed on inpatient surgery, and hence the advent of the 'basket of procedures' and 'trolley of procedures' (Cahill 1999). Transfer of surgery to day-surgery facilities will also help to free up additional capacity in the hospitals and reduce bed shortages. With the use of careful patient selection, it is envisaged that many treatment centres will flourish without the problem of unplanned admissions and delayed discharges (Moore 2003). It is for this reason that some day-surgery treatment centres are being built away from acute hospital services to avoid the potential for other surgery intruding on elective surgery sessions.

The additional 60–80 treatment centres planned for the end of 2005 will be treating an extra 250,000 patients per year (Department of Health 2004b). About 50% of these treatment centres will belong to the independent sector (Ganguli 2003), which has been encouraged to bid for such health-care provision to help relieve some of the pressure on the NHS in certain 'bottleneck' areas.

> The Department of Health is considering Independent Sector involvement where there are real bottlenecks and the NHS does not have the capacity in terms of premises, staff, or management capacity to deliver NHS-run Treatment Centres.
>
> Department of Health (2004a, p. 1)

It is also suggested that the NHS does not make full use of its capacity in day surgery because it is either over-regulated or the medical staff receive no incentives (D. Carlisle 2003). Conversely, it has been put forward that 'The Independent Centres were designed not only to address waiting lists but also to destabilise the NHS and the wider UK health economy by using contestability to challenge the vested interests in the system' (D. Carlisle 2003, p. 12). Broadly speaking 'contestability' equates to opening NHS health care up to 'market forces' so that primary care trusts (main consumers) will have the option of purchasing care for their patients from the most reliable, efficient and cost-effective treatment centres. Primary care trusts in the future will control 80% of the NHS budget (Department of Health 2004b) and will therefore become very powerful consumers of the services offered in such modern elective surgical facilities.

Staffing of independent sector treatment centres, for medical staff in the first instance, will be on a sessional basis whereas nurses may be 'poached' from the NHS (D. Carlisle 2003).

> Plans to allow the new centres to take up to 70% of their staff on secondment from existing NHS facilities have raised the fear that little additional capacity [of staff] may be created in return.
>
> Bostock (2003, p. 6)

Independent sector treatment centres have therefore been subsequently advised to use overseas teams working on a contracted package basis (Department of Health 2004a). However, as day-surgery expansion continues some nursing roles will eventually be offered on a sessional basis, similar to the medical staff, and nurses employed to perform specific tasks to assist in the delivery of an efficient surgical schedule, i.e. largely employed to undertake devolved medical tasks (see 'Nursing roles').

It is clear therefore that the expansion of both NHS and independent sector treatment centres is highly dependent on the employment of surgeons, anaesthetists, nurses and technical staff. It is also evident, from the inclusion of a wider range of patients able to undergo day surgery, that the growing modern surgery population will predictably require a greater degree of formalized psychoeducational intervention. Although such interventions currently remain submerged beneath the torrent of medical and administrative fervour associated with the expansion of this new surgical era, there is considerable evidence confirming that patients will inescapably require additional psychoeducational aspects of care (see Chapters 2 and 3). Treatment centres that deliver a comprehensive service to the consumer by providing an all-inclusive service will doubtless become a considerably more attractive option for surgical intervention (see 'Ambulatory surgery nursing unit' below). Once treatment centres are more commonplace, 'market forces' will drive the inclusion of ambulatory surgery nursing units within a modern surgical service. From the huge amount of evidence (see Chapters 2 and 3) it is abundantly clear that patients will opt for their day surgery to be undertaken within the treatment centres that provide such a comprehensive service. Demands from patients for such a service can only help to promote nursing knowledge and the unique contribution that the profession can offer this new surgical era. The profession therefore needs to petition during the development of treatment centres to ensure that such essential nursing issues are included on the expansion agenda.

Nursing roles

Current UK practices

The vast majority of nurses employed within the day-surgery setting throughout the UK function within a multiskilled role. This largely comprises the nurse initiating many aspects of care throughout the patients' whole surgical experience, i.e. admission, brief preoperative interventions, ensuring that essential medical tasks and tests are undertaken, transfer to theatre, second phase recovery (Audit Commission for Local Authorities and the NHS in England and Wales 1998a) and discharge (Thapar et al. 1994, Cheng et al. 2003, Joshi 2003). Such a role helps to guarantee the steady throughput of patients in the limited time available and also ensures that the surgery scheduled for each day is undertaken. Indeed, such multiskilled roles are central to the expansion of new day-surgery treatment centres.

Although nurses employed within such treatment centres will principally remain in the familiar multiskilled day-surgery role, future employment may be based more on a competency rating, i.e. ability to perform such tasks as venepuncture, cannulation, reading electrocardiographs (ECGs), etc. (Moore 2003). It is suggested that nurses should welcome such changes, because new opportunities will become available, e.g. more convenient working hours, scope for extended roles, improved continuity of patient care, new well-equipped clinical environments and the possible introduction of new 'school term' contracts (Ganguli 2003, Moore 2003). However, the development of such competency-based interventions intrinsically signifies the continued adoption of devolved medical tasks, with seemingly little or no input from nursing knowledge about the most effective nursing intervention for the modern surgical patient.

Many new roles for nurses are being developed within day surgery in this manner, e.g. the nurse anaesthetist (Audit Commission for Local

Authorities and the NHS in England and Wales 1997, NHS Management Executive 2000, Walker et al. 2003), surgeon's assistant (Burns 1993, Royal College of Surgeons of England and Royal College of Nursing 1999), laparoscopic nurse (Caballero and McWhinnie 1999) and pre-assessment nurse (Carroll 2004, Gilmartin 2004, Ormrod and Casey 2004, Walsgrove 2004) all feature widely. Many experienced nurses have embraced such roles because they welcome the added challenge and additional skills that the new roles bring. However, the nursing profession frequently has little control over the development of such positions because they are often initiated by (1) medical staff eager to improve an aspect of their practice or (2) as a direct result of NHS directives (Cameron and Masterson 2000). The reduction in junior doctors' hours is frequently the underlying reason for many such initiatives highlighting that many of these new extended nursing roles are created in an effort to replace the tasks once undertaken by junior doctors (Cameron and Masterson 2000). New nursing roles promoting nursing knowledge and the contribution that the profession can afford to modern surgical practices are largely absent.

In numerous studies and government reports it is stated that many tasks in modern surgery can be undertaken by nurses, after additional training, because they are viewed as a flexible workforce (NHS Management Executive 1996, 2000, Keenan et al. 1998, Clark et al. 1999, Fellowes et al. 1999, Department of Health 2000, 2001, J. Carlisle 2003, 2004, Hilditch et al. 2003a, Rai and Pandit 2003, Carroll 2004, NHS Modernisation Agency 2004). It is therefore clear that the present British government is keen for the nursing profession to develop in this direction. A number of recommendations have been put forward to assist nurses in the medical assessment of patients because it is recognized that many aspects of preoperative assessment, for example, encompass tasks once undertaken by a junior doctor (Clark et al. 1999, Hilditch et al. 2003a, 2003b). Indeed, a distance-learning programme has been developed to help disseminate such knowledge (NHS Modernisation Agency 2002). As day surgery is set to dominate future elective surgery, such skills, once undertaken by junior doctors, will almost certainly become an implicit part of pre-registration nurse education programmes of study at some stage in the future.

Although such preassessment practices are valuable to modern elective surgery they exclude the exposition of nursing knowledge and the potential contribution that it can bring to modern surgery. Some studies have demonstrated the value of nursing skills in the preassessment clinic (Clinch 1997, Gilmartin 2004), although it has been established that it is the interpersonal skills of the nurses that have also contributed to the patients' positive experiences (Macdonald and Bodzak 1999, Malkin 2000). This may highlight a fundamental difference in the medical and nursing focus within modern surgery. The medical staff principally focus on (and rightly so) the safety of the proposed surgery and cure of the health problem. Conversely, the nursing staff essentially focus on a combination of the wider social, psychological and physical aspects of care. However, within the modern surgical setting, enhancement of the impact of the nurses' interpersonal skills, the provision of information and other psychological aspects of care remain marginalized by the principal medical tasks and are thereby commonly delivered in an impromptu manner (Grieve 2002) (see Chapter 3).

The government, medical staff and indeed many nursing staff welcome the increase in the availability of extended roles. For the former, it helps to fill the void largely created by the reduction in junior doctors' hours whereas, for the latter, it brings additional challenges and the gaining of new skills (at least for the minority of nurses who are able to secure such roles). For most nurses employed within the day-surgery setting the multiskilled role predominates. It is within this multiskilled role that the nursing profession can and must develop new and innovative ways of implementing psychoeducational aspects of care. Innovation will come from within the nursing profession only when it presents valid and reliable evidence for change. The present government's focus for nursing is clearly different from the views expressed here, although the weight of evidence demonstrating the need for such changes is palpable within the modern surgical setting (see Chapters 2 and 3).

Fortunately, there is some prospect for change as the need for improved information provision and greater patient choice is recognized (NHS Modernisation Agency 2003). The Modernisation Agency states (2003, p. 1): 'NHS staff have an unprecedented opportunity to develop models of care that embrace the modernisation agenda and genuinely reflect care pathways that are truly patient-centred'. In addition, there are nine core characteristics appertaining to treatment centres, the seventh of which states: 'A Treatment Centre provides a high quality, positive experience for patients' (NHS Modernisation Agency 2003, p. 3). This core characteristic has five subdivisions, one of which states: 'Information for patients will be accessible and comprehensive and will help patients to be active partners in their own care' (NHS Modernisation Agency 2003, p. 3). It is therefore the profession's responsibility to act as the patient's advocate and provide the evidence to initiate change to generate and use nursing-based knowledge to help achieve such goals. A nursing assessment primarily concerning the psychoeducational needs of the patient desperately requires implementation by the profession for the benefit of patient care in all modern elective surgery. This could be placed alongside the medical assessment and add to the growing comprehensive provision of day-surgery intervention.

Currently, the medical assessment predominates and to a large extent this is because the nursing profession has not yet developed its own assessment tools and strategy for effective psychoeducational intervention. However, the psychoeducational plan of care discussed in Chapter 7 could be used and implemented alongside the essential medical interventions if day-surgery nurses were made more aware of the potential nursing knowledge available to aid psychological management. Unfortunately, in a recent survey of 267 staff nurses employed in day surgery throughout the UK, it was revealed that insight into the nursing knowledge of modern surgical practices within their pre-registration programmes of study was almost nil (Mitchell 2005). Almost 80% of staff nurses experienced very little or no theoretical input into modern day-surgery nursing practices, e.g. extended roles, multiskilling, preassessment clinics, pain management. Likewise, little or no relevant political healthcare issues with the potential to impact greatly on future surgical nursing intervention could have been conveyed, e.g. expansion of treatment centres, national tariffs. Most nurses surveyed were exposed only to traditional surgical nursing knowledge. Traditional surgical nursing intervention is defined here as: (1) preoperatively – a patient admitted in advance of the day of surgery and requiring much physical, social and psychological aspects of care; and (2) postoperatively – a patient who remains in hospital for more than 24 hours requiring much physical, social and psychological aspects of care.

On the basis of this study by Mitchell (2005), the priorities within nursing programmes of study must be completely reversed. Changes are required, because the potential contribution that the profession can offer must become an integral part of all pre-registration nurse education programmes. Change will not arise if nurses, new to modern surgery, are not informed of the wider issues and potential nursing contribution. The majority of pre- and postoperative surgical nurse education should now be more concerned with modern surgical practices and patients who experience 24 hours or less in hospital. The minority of pre- and postoperative nurse education should be concerned with inpatient surgical practices and patients who experience 48 hours or more in hospital. Traditional aspects of nursing intervention are on the decline. Modern, elective surgery has rendered many such interventions obsolete. The profession must recognize such changes and embrace an innovative and more formal psychoeducational role. If nurse educators, in collaboration with clinical colleagues, do not expose students new to the nursing profession to the potential contribution that nursing knowledge can offer this new surgical era, from where is the evidence for effective surgical nursing fit for the twenty-first century to arise? If the current trend continues, the profession is destined merely to follow in the wake of day-surgery medical advances, accumulating devolved medical tasks and re-labelling them as surgical nursing intervention with little or no discrimination in between.

A greater emphasis must also be placed on the generation and use of clinical research in modern, surgical, nursing practices to prevent the profession falling even further behind in this day-surgery revolution. Once the profession recognizes the considerable evidence and potential influence that the application of such knowledge can bring to the quality of modern surgical nursing practices, many nurses may become extremely interested in the development of roles that employ a greater degree of nursing-based knowledge. Currently, this is not an option for most nurses with such an interest, because largely roles that seek to develop devolved medical tasks predominate.

Fortunately, in some day-surgery units, different nursing roles have developed that do embrace some nursing issues. Such roles have developed largely as a result of the introduction of new surgical procedures or because of the more rural setting of the day-surgery unit (Hunt et al. 1999, Fleming et al. 2000, Nielsen et al. 2003). Such innovative nursing roles have the potential for further development because there is the likelihood that patients potentially meet the nursing staff on a number of occasions, e.g. during the preassessment visit, on the day of surgery and during home contact (see Chapter 2). Again, alongside the essential medical tasks, a nursing assessment of the patients' psychoeducational care can be undertaken, implemented and continued for a brief period once the patients are discharged home.

Ambulatory surgery nursing units

As the amount and complexity of day surgery increase in the UK new nursing roles could be developed. However, this will involve changes to the current preassessment clinic structure. Day-surgery preassessment has been widely recommended because it helps to increase efficiency by embracing junior doctors' work (Carroll 2004, Walsgrove 2004), ensuring that patients are able to undergo the planned surgery and informing patients of their surgical procedure (NHS Modernisation Agency 2002). Essentially, the work therefore involves the undertaking of many medical tasks because this is its original purpose, i.e. guaranteeing that each patient is suitable for surgery on the day of surgery. However, if the scope of the preassessment clinic were to be widened as the amount of day surgery were to increase, it could also embrace a nursing assessment to aid the implementation of a more comprehensive service.

Such a service could be provided by an 'ambulatory surgery nursing unit' where patients could undergo a psychoeducational nursing assessment, thereby helping to resolve many of the patient issues highlighted earlier (see Chapters 2 and 3). Such intervention would incorporate the information provision framework discussed in Chapter 7 (see Tables 7.3–7.5) and thereby begin to deliver information in a more formal manner. The ambulatory surgery nursing unit would be a resource centre for information provision, disseminating all information to patients by post, telephone or during the patient preassessment visit. Self-directed reading facilities for patients wanting full disclosure of information could also be made available, e.g. internet amenities, viewing of specific digital television channels, posters, tours around the day-surgery facilities, group discussion opportunities and written information to take home. A number of digital television channels currently exist for a wide range of medical health-care issues and a future channel could exist specifically for day-surgery intervention. Indeed, an NHS digital television channel presenting such information has already been recommended (Department of Health 2004b).

Brief nursing notes would ensure that the psychoeducational nursing assessment is a succinct undertaking and communicated in electronic format on a database accessible to both nurses in the ambulatory surgery nursing unit and the day-surgery unit (Figure 8.1). The use of electronic communication has been strongly recommended in day surgery (Fuller 2003) and is in line with other electronic schemes, i.e. e-booking, e-prescribing, HealthSpace (personal records held in secure internet area for patient to view) and NHS Online (Department of Health 2004b). Such a nursing assessment, together with the implementation of the other aspects of the psychoeducational plan (see Table 7.2), would help guarantee a more informed and less anxious patient at all stages of the day-surgery experience. In addition, a more integrated and expansive ambulatory surgery nursing unit would remove from the day-surgery unit the obligation to provide patient information in the brief time period available. Frequently, on the day of surgery, many patients are too anxious before surgery to retain the information provided and, after surgery, in too much discomfort to remember the information (Hutson and Blaha 1991) (see Chapter 2).

The electronic ambulatory surgery nursing unit notes would state what information the patient had received and the level of information wanted, e.g. standard, intermediate or full disclosure (see Table 7.8). In addition, such e-nursing notes could provide brief details of the other aspects of the psychoeducational plan employed, e.g. health locus of control considerations, self-efficacy enhancement, therapeutic use of self considerations and environmental considerations. A nurse-initiated preoperative telephone call 24–48 hours before surgery to (1) check that the patient intends to keep the appointment and (2) reiterate essential medical advice (nil by mouth) could also become part of the unit's role. The ambulatory

Figure 8.1 Prototype electronic nursing notes.

E L E C T R O N I C   N U R S I N G   N O T E S

NAME   ....

ADDRESS   ....

          ....

TELEPHONE   .... MOBILE ....

E-MAIL   .... @ ....

SURGERY DATE ....

CONSULTANT   ....

N U R S I N G   A S S E S S M E N T

P H A S E   I (see Table 7.3)

	YES	NO
MEDICAL ASSESSMENT COMPLETED	[ ]	[ ]

PSYCHO-EDUCATIONAL INTERVENTION (see Table 7.2)

		YES	NO
1) DESIRED INFORMATION OPTION	STANDARD DISCLOSURE	[ ]	[ ]
	INTERMEDIATE DISCLOSURE	[ ]	[ ]
	FULL DISCLOSURE	[ ]	[ ]

BRIEF NOTES - ....

....

	YES	NO
2) HEALTH CONTROL ENHANCEMENT	[ ]	[ ]

BRIEF NOTES - ....

....

3) SELF-EFFICACY ENHANCEMENT	[ ]	[ ]

BRIEF NOTES - ....

....

4) THERAPEUTIC USE OF SELF	[ ]	[ ]

BRIEF NOTES - ....

....

5) ENVIRONMENTAL CONSIDERATIONS	[ ]	[ ]

BRIEF NOTES - ....

....

....NURSE -

P H A S E   I I (see Table 7.4)

	YES	NO
PRE-OPERATIVE NURSE-INITIATED TELEPHONE CONTACT (date)	[ ]	[ ]

BRIEF NOTES - ....

....

....NURSE -

	STANDARD	INTERMEDIATE	FULL
DESIRED INFORMATION CONTINUED	[ ]	[ ]	[ ]

	YES	NO
PSYCHO-EDUCATIONAL PLAN CONTINUED PRE-OPERATIVELY	[ ]	[ ]

1) DESIRED INFORMATION

....

....

2) CONTROL ENHANCEMENT

....

....

3) SELF-EFFICACY ENHANCEMENT

....

....

4) THERAPEUTIC USE OF SELF

....

....

5) ENVIRONMENTAL CONSIDERATIONS

....

....

....NURSE -

Figure 8.1 continued.

PREOPERATIVE INTERVENTIONS, i.e. recovery, pain management, discharge analgesia, etc.
BRIEF NOTES - ....
....
....
....
....
....NURSE -

P H A S E   I I I (see Table 7.5)

	YES	NO
PSYCHO-EDUCATIONAL PLAN CONTINUED POST-OPERATIVELY	[ ]	[ ]

	STANDARD	INTERMEDIATE	FULL
DESIRED INFORMATION CONTINUED	[ ]	[ ]	[ ]

1) DESIRED INFORMATION
....
....

2) CONTROL ENHANCEMENT
....
....

3) SELF-EFFICACY ENHANCEMENT
....
....

4) THERAPEUTIC USE OF SELF
....
....

5) ENVIRONMENTAL CONSIDERATIONS
....
....
....NURSE -

F O L L O W I N G   D I S C H A R G E

	YES	NO
PRIMARY HEALTHCARE TEAM CONTACT (date)	[ ]	[ ]

BRIEF NOTES - ....
....
....
....
....
....NURSE -

	YES	NO
POST-OPERATIVE NURSE-INITIATED TELEPHONE CONTACT (date)	[ ]	[ ]

BRIEF NOTES - ....
....
....
....
....
....
....
....NURSE -

	YES	NO
POST-OPERATIVE HOME VISIT (date)	[ ]	[ ]

BRIEF NOTES - ....
....
....
....
....NURSE -

	YES	NO
DISCHARGE (date)	[ ]	[ ]

BRIEF NOTES - ....
....
....NURSE -

surgery nursing unit would therefore totally coordinate both the medical and psychoeducational nursing assessment, provide the necessary patient information and communicate all aspects of nursing intervention to the day-surgery unit.

Ideally, it would be appropriate for all day-surgery patients to report to the ambulatory surgery nursing unit on the day of surgery. On arrival patients could be escorted by a familiar nurse to the day-surgery unit and be formally transferred to a day-surgery nurse without the need for the patient to repeat previously supplied information. The purpose of this is twofold. It has been demonstrated that patients greeted by a familiar nurse are less anxious on the day of surgery (Vogelsang 1990). As each patient will have previously visited the ambulatory surgery nursing unit for medical and nursing assessment, and met with many of the nursing staff, this may help to alleviate some of the associated anxiety on the day of surgery. Second, when asked constantly to repeat previously supplied demographic details, surgical inpatients have become apprehensive and unsure of the credibility of the service (van Weert et al. 2003). Again, the formal transfer of care from the ambulatory surgery nursing unit to the day-surgery unit and the nursing notes available in electronic format will obviate the need for repetitive patient questioning. Once care is transferred the day-surgery nursing staff would be able to update the e-nursing notes with a brief summary of the important pre- and postoperative events, e.g. anxiety intervention, brief pre- and postoperative interventions.

Once patients have been discharged home the ambulatory surgery nursing unit would re-establish contact with all patients. This could be by either telephone contact or home visit, depending on the complexity of the surgery undertaken. Increasingly, day-case surgical procedures require patients to look after medical equipment (e.g. vacuum pumps, patient controlled analgesia pumps) during the first few postoperative days and thereby frequently require a visit to help them undertake this role (Boada et al. 2002, Ilfeld et al. 2002, Rawal et al. 2002). As the day-surgery population grows together with the complexity of the surgery, issues of increased information provision and post-discharge support will prevail. Coping with unexpected pain and unforeseen events is already a common problem for many day-surgery patients (see Chapter 2). However, with the advent of the ambulatory surgery nursing unit such a challenge may be reduced considerably, because nurse-initiated contact is guaranteed. Furthermore, patients can be encouraged to visit or make telephone contact with the unit whenever necessary. Again, additional contact or intervention can be briefly added to the e-nursing notes.

The ambulatory surgery nursing unit would become a resource centre for all general practitioners and district nurses involved in the postoperative care of day-surgery patients. Many GPs and district nurses frequently have too little information about their patients in order to manage their care effectively (see Chapter 2). Frequently, relevant information arrives many weeks after surgery has occurred when the patient is fully recovered and has resumed normal activities (see Chapter 2). In addition, many primary health-care professionals are unaware of the new developments in day surgery and require information to update their knowledge and practices. The provision of an ambulatory surgery nursing unit would help to resolve these issues and become a pivotal point of contact for patients and health-care professionals in both the acute and the primary setting.

As communication with the day-surgery unit, patients, GPs and district nurses is a central feature of the proposed ambulatory surgery nursing unit, such a unit would be need to be fully computerized (Pollard 2004). All patient information for all surgery undertaken on a day-case basis must be available on a database for the nurses in the ambulatory surgery nursing unit to relay to the appropriate people. In addition, such a database must contain advice on the course of action for the patients to take in the postoperative period should an unforeseen event arise. The growing and diverse nature of day surgery will necessitate such an approach, because the unit nurses cannot be expected to have detailed information immediately available for all surgical procedures. As the nurses in the ambulatory surgery nursing unit coordinate the overall care of each patient, all further intervention can immediately be added to the e-nursing notes. All nurses in the ambulatory surgery nursing unit, irrespective of personal knowledge of an individual patient, will then have a complete overview of any patient to deal with any enquiry, whether it is from a patient or health-care professional.

Conclusion

Day-service delivery of health care will continue to rise as a result of government initiatives and progressive medical advances. An increasing number of surgical procedures will continually be available to day surgery, improved regional anaesthesia will allow a wider and less physically fit surgical population to undergo day surgery, and increasingly day-surgery patients will be discharged home with medical equipment. Such advances will inevitably lead to the need for ambulatory surgery nursing units to coordinate the demands of such an industrious ambulatory surgery health-care structure.

The current British government is in the process of expanding day surgery in the form of new treatment centres. Over the next 4–5 years day surgery will grow to encompass 75% of all elective surgery. The demand for psychoeducational nursing intervention in modern day surgery will become even greater during this period. Primary care trusts (which will be the largest purchasers of health care) will doubtless require an increased level of communication for their staff and patients in order to care more effectively for this growing and largely self-managing surgical population. The nursing profession must embrace this new surgical era, provide the evidence to demonstrate how nursing can make an effective contribution and transform its practices.

Currently, new nursing roles have largely been guided by the reduction in junior doctors' hours. Backed by NHS incentives and medical projects, such roles have gained much attention and nurses who have secured such roles help to deliver a highly effective service, e.g. preassessment clinics primarily ensure, in advance, that patients are physically able to undergo the scheduled surgery and this has helped to reduce the surgical cancellation rate (see Chapter 2). Nevertheless, the multiskilled nursing role still dominates in modern elective surgery and is set to continue with the introduction of new treatment centres. However, all skills frequently promote the transfer of devolved medical tasks with little or no nursing knowledge able to add to the quality of the patients' experience. A more complete assessment and holistic provision of care for the patient are suggested in the form of an ambulatory surgery nursing unit. Such a unit would not only undertake a medical and nursing assessment but also coordinate nursing intervention for the day-case patient. This would encompass the preoperative visit, brief visit on the day of surgery and postoperative communication. To help initiate such change, the nursing profession must undertake more clinical research concerning the role of the nurse in the modern elective surgery setting to help establish new nursing knowledge fit for the twenty-first century.

Summary

- Day-case surgical and anaesthetic capability will continue to advance, ensuring more extensive surgery with faster recovery periods on a growing surgical population.
- Such advances will also guarantee that patients are increasingly discharged home with medical equipment primarily to aid pain management.
- Older, less fit patients and patients requiring acute, minor emergency surgery will increasingly be common additions to dedicated day-surgery operating schedules.
- By the end of 2005, 60–80 new day-surgery treatment centres will be treating an extra 250,000 patients per year. A further 100 treatment centres are planned for the end of 2006.

- The increasing adult, day-surgery population and expanding number of patients deemed eligible to undergo day surgery will ultimately require a greater degree of communication. Essentially this is because a larger proportion of the surgical population will increasingly be required to manage their own care.
- Primary care trusts, the largest purchasers of health care, will ultimately demand a greater degree of communication to enable their patients and staff to manage this ever-expanding patient self-caring role.
- Primary care trusts will be able to purchase care from whom they choose. Treatment centres that provide a more comprehensive package of care will therefore prosper.
- Currently, new nursing roles largely embrace devolved medical tasks and do not espouse nursing issues. The profession must embrace this new surgical era and uncover evidence to demonstrate how it can make an effective contribution.
- Ambulatory surgery nursing units will be able to undertake a medical and nursing assessment. In addition, they will be able to coordinate and implement the formal pre- and postoperative psychoeducational interventions required by all day-surgery patients.
- Nursing professionals involved in the discussions about treatment centres must petition for the greater use of nursing knowledge and the profession as a whole must undertake clinical research to help develop new surgical nursing knowledge fit for the twenty-first century.
- As the number of patients undergoing day surgery expands, the demand from the consumers for the potential care offered by ambulatory surgery nursing units will make them an essential component for all successful treatment centres.

Further reading

Allen, D. (2004) The Changing Shape of Nursing Practice: The role of nurses in the hospital division of labour. London: Routledge.
Chester, G.A. (2004) Modern Medical Assisting. New York: Saunders.
Clifford, C. and Clark, J. (2004) Getting Research into Practice. London: Churchill Livingstone.
Englebardt, S.P. and Nelson, R. (2004) Health Care Informatics: An interdisciplinary approach. New York: Mosby.
Stanton, J. (ed.) (2004) Innovations in Health and Medicine: Diffusion and resistance in the 20th century. London: Routledge.

Websites

Pre-operative Association: www.pre-op.org
National Association of Theatre Nurses (online courses): www.natn.org.uk

Glossary

American Society of Anesthesiologists (physical status grading system)

A grading system to help gauge the physical status of a patient requiring general anaesthesia, e.g.

> Level 1: healthy patient (localized surgical pathology with no systemic disturbance).
> Level 2: mild/moderate systemic disturbance (the surgical pathology or other disease process). No activity limitation.
> Level 3: severe systemic disturbance from any cause. Some activity limitation.
> Level 4: life-threatening systemic disorder. Severe activity limitation.
> Level 5: moribund patient with little chance of survival.

Anxiolytic

Pharmacological preparation employed in the preoperative period to sedate patients in an effort to help control their anxiety.

Attention bias

When conducting an experimental research study where, for example, a group of patients are randomly divided into two groups, it is important that the researcher/nurse spends a similar amount of time with each group. When an increased amount of time is spent with one half of the group in comparison with the other, irrespective of the differing treatment/information provided, the patients within that group may have improved prospects of recovery simply because the health-care professional(s) spent more time with them (see Hawthorne effect).

Avoidant coping

A coping approach in which the individual makes efforts to withdraw from threatening information. A minimal level of simple information is frequently desired because too much will cause an increase in anxiety.

Such individuals may prefer to trust in the doctors and nurses, minimize events and give positive interpretations to events. Also referred to as blunting and repressing coping styles.

Barbiturates

Barbiturates are drugs that act as central nervous system (CNS) depressants. By virtue of this they produce a wide spectrum of effects from mild sedation to anaesthesia.

Basket of procedures

List of 20 intermediate surgical procedures deemed suitable for day-case surgery and put forward by the Audit Commission (1990).

Behavioural or role information

The behaviour(s) or action(s) the patient is required to undertake before, during or after the surgical procedure, e.g. adopting a certain position for the procedure, keeping a limb elevated, gentle movements only, deep breathing exercises, no lifting for 6 weeks, etc.
  Studies in the USA often refer to this as role information.

Benzodiazepines

The benzodiazepines are pharmacological agents with hypnotic, anxiolytic, anticonvulsive and muscle relaxant properties. They are used in the short term for the relief of severe, disabling anxiety although their prolonged use is discouraged because of possible dependency.

β Blockers

Pharmacological preparations that block the effect of adrenaline (epinephrine) on β-receptors found mainly in the heart, lungs and arterioles, e.g. block β-receptors in the heart and reduce the potential rise in heart rate. They can therefore be useful for reducing the heart rate of an anxious patient awaiting general anaesthesia.

Blunters

Coping style (comparable to avoidant coping) where individuals prefer very little information.

Catecholamines

The most common catecholamines are adrenaline and noradrenaline (norepinephrine). Both adrenaline and noradrenaline are neurotransmitters, which act on the sympathetic nervous system, e.g. generally prepare the body for exercise. Catecholamine levels in the blood are largely associated with the physiological response to stress.

Cognitive or emotional coping strategies

A cognitive coping strategy can be described as a purposeful emotional attempt to have less negative thoughts about a given situation, i.e. a mental strategy for avoiding catastrophizing (believing something will go seriously wrong). These positive thoughts can help a patient to gain assurance that they will be safe, awake from their operation, be unharmed and gain a full recovery.

Confounding variables

Variables that the researcher fails to control or cannot control, although they may influence the results of the study.

Convergent or combined approach to coping

Approach to coping that incorporates both the psychodynamic and transactional approaches to coping. Coping is viewed as a process by which personality traits and individual motives must be considered, together with the interplay of human interactions within the environment.

Cortisol

Cortisol is a corticosteroid hormone produced by the adrenal glands. Serum cortisol levels fluctuate in response to a number of other interactions, e.g. stress illness, pyrexia, trauma, surgery, pain, physical exertion or extremes of temperature. It can also be released in response to long-term stress.

Day surgery

A person suitable for day surgery is currently defined in the UK as 'a patient who is admitted for investigation or operation on a planned non-resident basis and who nonetheless requires facilities for recovery' (Royal College of

Surgeons of England 1992). A further definition of a day surgery candidate by Cook et al. (2004, p. 11) states: 'A patient admitted electively during the course of a day with the intention of receiving care who does not require the use of a hospital bed overnight and who returns home as scheduled. If this original intention is not fulfilled and the patient stays overnight, such a patient should be counted as an ordinary admission'.

Emotionally focused coping

Emotionally focused coping refers to an individual's emotional attempts to deal with a stressor, i.e. the conscious thoughts and feelings associated with the prospect of admission to hospital to undergo general anaesthesia and surgery, e.g. a person may gain assurance from knowledge that it is a good hospital with an excellent reputation. Emotionally focused coping strategies are frequently employed when the stressful event cannot be changed or avoided by the individual.

External health locus of control

Strong belief that one's future is influenced more by luck, fate or powerful others, i.e. doctors, nurses, employer. Such individuals may therefore readily assume that decisions will be made on their behalf.

Flexible coping style

A coping approach for dealing with a stressful situation characterized by assuming an adaptable stance about information provision. Generally, whatever information is provided will be acceptable.

Fluctuating coping style

A coping approach in which the individual has a desire for variable levels of information. Some information required may be highly detailed whereas other aspects may be only minimally specific, e.g. details about the operation only. Incorrect communication of the desired amount or selected areas of information may give rise to an increase in anxiety.

Guided imagery

A visual or auditory method of distraction/relaxation where the patient tries to imagine that he or she has been transported elsewhere, e.g. to a beautiful location.

Hawthorn effect

A selected group of patients in a research study being treated differently or in a special manner, which may influence their experience and thereby possibly enhance their evaluations or improve their recovery prospects, i.e. the effect on participants of simply being the focus of study.

Hospital Anxiety and Depression Questionnaire (HADS)

Commonly used questionnaire employed to assess anxiety and depression. However, it was largely designed to be used by patients experiencing mental ill-health.

Intermediate elective surgery

Defined here as the planned uncomplicated surgery under general anaesthesia which can be undertaken in an operating theatre in less than 1 hour.

Internal health locus of control

Strong belief in one's ability to shape the future and therefore a desire to be firmly involved in the decision-making process. Control can be real or perceived, i.e. not necessarily much control granted although a semblance of control perceived.

Modelling

Directly by actively imitating (behaviourally or cognitively) the required or desired behaviour, e.g. via a real-life event, demonstration/teaching, reading hospital leaflets, websites, videotaped programmes and aspects of the media. Indirectly by passively imitating (behaviourally or cognitively) the required or desired behaviour, e.g. watching other patients.

Monitor-blunter-style scale (MBSS)

Commonly used questionnaire, which endeavours to gauge the level of information required by an individual. It then determines whether the person is deemed a 'monitor' or a 'blunter'.

Monitors

Coping style very similar to vigilant coping where individuals prefer copious amounts of information.

Morbidity

Medical complications in the postoperative period, which may result in the delayed return to 'normal' functioning.

Neuroticism

Personality trait in which the person has an anxious predisposition, i.e. may easily interpret events as anxiety-provoking.

Objective data collection

The collection of data about an experience via more rigid and formal methods thereby providing little room for speculation and debate, e.g. blood pressure measurement, body temperature, blood analysis, number of pain-killers consumed, etc.

Opioid

An opioid is any drug that activates the opioid receptors found in the brain, spinal cord and gut. There are three broad classes of opioids: (1) naturally occurring opium alkaloids, such as morphine and codeine, (2) semi-synthetics such as heroin, oxycodone and hydrocodone which are produced by modifying natural opium alkaloids, and finally (3) pure synthetics such as fentanyl and methadone which are not produced from opium. Opioids are widely used in pain management because no other effective analgesics have been found for severe pain.

Preassessment clinic

Hospital appointment before the day of admission primarily to check medical fitness for surgery/anaesthesia and provide information.

Primary appraisal

Construct central to the transactional approach to coping. Primary appraisal concerns our initial impressions of a stressful event.

Problem-focused coping

Problem-focused coping embraces strategies in which the person attempts directly to challenge the stressor by embarking on a plan of action, e.g. when faced with the prospect of day surgery a patient may wish to discover exactly what will happen to him or her, and gain information about the operation, events on the day of surgery and the length of the recovery period in order to alter, circumvent or eliminate a particular stressor.

Procedural or situational information

The sequential order of events on the day of surgery once a patient is admitted to the surgical unit, i.e. what will happen next and the order in which the events will occur. Studies in the USA often refer to this as situational information.

Propofol (Diprivan)

Propofol is a pharmacological preparation used largely as an intravenous anaesthetic agent for the induction and maintenance of general anaesthesia. Propofol is the first of a new class of intravenous anaesthetic agents called alkylphenols.

Psychodynamic approach

Approach to coping broadly based on our past experiences (beginning in childhood), which subsequently become unconsciously embedded in our everyday thoughts and actions as we grow, e.g. personality traits.

Psychoeducational intervention

Defined here as the purposeful attempt to provide tangible aspects of care aimed at enhancing an individual's psychological status, together with the planned provision of educational material.

Relaxation

Individual strategies of relaxation or a planned programme of relaxation techniques, e.g. music therapy, simple methods of distraction, hypnosis.

Repression-sensitization scale

Early theory (Byrne 1961) about extremes of coping, which later became known as vigilant and avoidant coping (Krohne 1989). Other authors have termed such an approach 'blunting and monitoring' (Miller 1987).

Secondary appraisal

Construct central to the transactional approach to coping. Secondary appraisal concerns the coping resources available to us to help master, reduce or tolerate the demands created by the stressful event.

Self-efficacy

Confidence in one's ability to behave in such a way as to produce a desirable outcome.

Sensory information

The bodily sensations that the patient is likely to experience before, during or after the surgical procedure, i.e. the likely sensations of the drugs entering the body during the initial stages of anaesthesia, degree and duration of pain, and medical equipment used in the immediate post-operative phase.

Significant level or level of significance

The phenomenon has not occurred by chance and there will be a 95–99% chance of achieving the same result if the exact study were to be repeated. It suggests that, if the recommended care gained from such significant results were to be employed within the clinical environment, similar results may be achieved.

State anxiety

Level of anxiety experienced by an individual during a current stressful encounter.

State-Trait Anxiety Inventory

Classic widely used anxiety questionnaire, which contains 20 items about state anxiety (present level during stressful encounter) and 20 items about trait anxiety (normal level as part of individual's enduring personality).

Stressor

An aspect causing or generating stress, e.g. the thought of a mask being placed over the face before general anaesthesia. Any experience deemed by the individual, real or perceived, to be the cause of increased anxiety.

Subjective data collection

The collection of data via informal methods, thereby providing the opportunity for greater individual expression about an experience, e.g. self-rated level of anxiety, doctors' and nurses' rating of patient adjustment to surgery, etc.

Therapeutic use of self

Supportive intervention characterized by the physical and emotional presence bestowed when a nurse, doctor or relative is in close proximity to a patient. However, it is not merely the physical presence but also the interaction and statements of reassurance (cognitive coping strategies) that are important.

Thiopental (formerly Thiopentone)

Thiopental is a rapid-onset, short-acting, barbiturate general anaesthetic. It induces general anaesthesia within 60 s of intravenous injection and lasts around 10–30 min. Up until fairly recently it was the most popular anaesthetic induction agent in many parts of the world. Thiopental has no analgesic effects so it is used as a single agent only for brief procedures. More commonly, it is used to induce anaesthesia before the use of other anaesthetic agents. However, in recent years it has been overtaken by propofol, particularly for day surgery.

Trait anxiety

Level of anxiety experienced by an individual when not directly involved in a stressful encounter, i.e. behaviour deemed part of the individual's enduring personality.

Transactional approach to coping

The transactional model considers the interplay between the individual and the environment. Two constructs central to this approach are 'cognitive appraisal' and 'coping'.

Trolley of procedures

List of approximately 25 intermediate surgical procedures deemed suitable for day-case surgery (Cahill 1999).

Type 'A' personality

Personality trait characterized by impatience, excessive competitive drive and bouts of hostility.

Variable

Any element within a research study, which may introduce change or differing circumstances, e.g. local and general anaesthesia. When asking a patient about anxiety and anaesthesia, the answers provided may greatly depend on the type of anaesthesia experienced.

Vigilant coping

A coping approach in which the individual has an intensified processing of threatening information. Copious levels of detailed information are frequently desired because too little will cause an increase in anxiety. Such individuals must be informed of all aspects of care so that nothing surprises them because omissions may be too anxiety provoking. Also referred to as monitoring and sensitizing coping styles.

Visual analogue scale

Numerically based scale where patients are requested, for example, to rate their anxiety, pain or satisfaction with care. This becomes an effective tool of measurement for instant recognition of individual experience, e.g. 1 no pain through to 10 worst pain.

Work of worry

A mental process, similar to mourning, that aids adjustment to a painful situation. If a patient were to undergo a surgical procedure he or she would mentally rehearse the various situations together with their possible consequences. The benefit of this would be to have accurate expectations of the possible pain and discomfort and thereby gain greater reality-based insight.

References

Aasboe, V., Raeder, J.C. and Groegaard, B. (1998) Betamethasone reduces post-operative pain and nausea after ambulatory surgery. Anesthesia and Analgesia 87: 319-323.

Agboola, O., Davies, J. and Davies, C. (1998) Laparoscopic sterilisation: The immediate and long term post-operative side effects using bupivacaine infiltration and diclofenac. Journal of One-Day Surgery 8(3): 7-9.

Agha, R., Heaton, S.R. and Roberts, D. (2004) Patient satisfaction with day-case septoplasty and septorhinoplasty. Journal of One-Day Surgery 14(1): 22-25.

Aldwinckle, R.J. and Montgomery, J.E. (2004) Unplanned admission rates and postdischarge complications in patients over the age of 70 following day case surgery. Anaesthesia 59: 57-59.

Alexander, M.F., Fawcett, J.N. and Runciman, P.J. (2001) Nursing Practice – Hospital and Home: The adult patient, 2nd edn. London: Churchill Livingstone.

Alkaissi, A., Stalnert, M. and Kalman, S. (1999) Effect and placebo effect of acupressure (P6) on nausea and vomiting after outpatient gynaecological surgery. Acta Anaesthesiologica Scandinavica 43: 270-274.

Amarnath, T.S., Coulthard, R.A. and Tate, J.J.T. (2002) Laparoscopic cholecystectomy as a 'session' surgery. Journal of Ambulatory Surgery 10: 33-36.

Anderson, E.A. (1987) Pre-operative preparation for cardiac surgery facilitates recovery, reduces psychological distress and reduces the incidence of acute post operative hypertension. Journal of Consulting and Clinical Psychology 55a: 513-520.

Anderson, L.A. and Gross, J.B. (2004) Aromatherapy with peppermint, isopropyl alcohol, or placebo is equally effective in relieving postoperative nausea. Journal of Peri-Anesthesia Nursing 19(1): 29-35.

Andrew, J.M. (1970) Recovery from surgery, with and without preparatory instruction for three coping styles. Journal of Personality and Social Psychology 15: 223-226.

Ansell, G.L. and Montgomery, J.E. (2004) Outcome of ASA3 patients undergoing day-case surgery. British Journal of Anaesthesia 92: 71-74.

Apfelbaum, J.L., Walawander, C.A., Grasela, T.H. et al. (2002) Eliminating intensive postoperative care in same-day surgery patients using short-acting anesthetics. Anesthesiology 97: 66-74.

Audit Commission for Local Authorities and the National Health Service in England and Wales (1990) A Short Cut To Better Services: Day surgery in England and Wales. London: HMSO.

Audit Commission for Local Authorities and the NHS in England and Wales (1991) Measuring Quality: The patient's view of day surgery, No. 3. London: HMSO.

Audit Commission for Local Authorities and the NHS in England and Wales (1992) All in A Day's Work: An audit of day surgery in England and Wales, No. 4. London: HMSO.

Audit Commission for Local Authorities and the NHS in England and Wales (1993) What Seems to be the Matter: Communication between hospitals and patients. London: HMSO.

Audit Commission for Local Authorities and the NHS in England and Wales (1997) Anaesthesia under Examination. London: HMSO.

Audit Commission for Local Authorities and the NHS in England and Wales (1998a) Managing Pain after Surgery: A booklet for nurses. London: HMSO.

Audit Commission for Local Authorities and the NHS in England and Wales (1998b) Day Surgery Follow-up: Progress against indicators from 'A Short Cut to Better Services'. London: HMSO.

Audit Commission for Local Authorities and the NHS in England and Wales (2001) Day Surgery: Review of national findings. No. 4. London: HMSO.

Auerbach, S.M. (1989) Stress management and coping research in the health care setting: An overview and methodological commentary. Journal of Consulting and Clinical Psychology 57: 388-395.

Augustin, P. and Hains, A.A. (1996) Effects of music on ambulatory surgery patients' pre-operative anxiety. American Operating Room Nurses' Journal 63: 750-758.

Averill, J.R. and Rosenn, M. (1972) Vigilant and non-vigilant coping strategies and psycho-physiological stress reactions during the anticipation of electric shock. Journal of Personality and Social Psychology 23: 128-141.

Avis, M. (1994) Choice cuts: An exploratory study of patients' views about participation in decision-making in a day surgery unit. International Journal of Nursing Studies 31: 289-298.

Badner, N.H., Nielson, W.R., Munk, S., Kwiatkowska, C. and Gelb, A.W. (1990) Pre-operative anxiety: Detection and contributing factors. Canadian Journal of Anaesthesia 37: 444-447.

Bahir, A., Lawaetz, O., Kjeldsen, L. and Lund, P. (2001) Convalescence and driver reaction time after tension-free inguinal hernia repair. Journal of Ambulatory Surgery 9: 19-21.

Bain, J., Kelly, H., Snadden, D. and Staines, H. (1999) Day surgery in Scotland: Patient satisfaction and outcomes. Quality in Health Care 8: 86-91.

Bandura, A. (1977) Self-efficacy: Towards a unifying theory of behavioural change. Psychological Review 84: 191-215.

Bandura, A. (1982) Self-efficacy mechanism in human agency. American Psychologist 37: 122-147.

Bar Tal, Y. and Spitzer, A. (1999) The effect on coping of monitoring, blunting, and the ability to achieve cognitive structure. Journal of Psychology 133: 395-412.

Barthelsson, C., Lutzen, K., Anderberg, B., Bringman, S. and Nordstrom, G. (2003a) Patients' experiences of laparoscopic fundoplication in day surgery. Journal of Ambulatory Surgery 10: 101-107.

Barthelsson, C., Lutzen, K., Anderberg, B. and Nordstrom, G. (2003b) Patients' experiences of laparoscopic cholecystectomy in day surgery. Journal of Clinical Nursing 12: 253-259.

Baskerville, P.A., Heddle, R.M. and Jarrett, P.E.M. (1985) Preparation for surgery: Information tapes for the patient. Practitioner 229: 677-678.

Baume, R.M., Croog, S.H. and Nalbandian, J. (1995) Pain perception, coping strategies, and stress management among periodontal patients with repeated surgeries. Perceptual and Motor Skills 80: 307-319.

Beauregard, L., Pomp, A. and Choiniere, M. (1998) Severity and impact of pain after day-surgery. Canadian Journal of Anaesthesia 45: 304-311.

Beddows, J. (1997) Alleviating pre-operative anxiety in patients: A study. Nursing Standard 11(37): 35-38.

Beers, R.A., Calimlim, J.R., Uddoh, E., Esposito, B.F. and Camporesi, E.M. (2000) A comparison of the cost-effectiveness of remifentanil versus fentanyl as an adjuvant to general anesthesia for outpatient gynecologic surgery. Anesthesia and Analgesia 91: 1420-1425.

Bernard, J.M., Faintreny, A., Leinhart, A. and Souron, R. (1996) Patient-controlled premedication by I.V. midazolam for ambulatory surgery. Acta Anaesthesiologica Scandinavica 40: 331-337.

Bernier, M.J., Sanares, D.C., Owen, S.V. and Newhouse, P.L. (2003) Pre-operative teaching received and valued in a day surgery setting. American Operating Room Nurses' Journal 77: 563-569.

Berry, D.C., Michas, I.C. and Bersellini, E. (2003) Communicating information about medication: The benefits of making it personal. Psychology and Health 18: 127-139.

Bhargava, A., Rai, P. and Shrivastava, R.K. (2003) Adult day case hallux valgus surgery – a safe and viable option. Journal of Ambulatory Surgery 10: 151–154.

Bhattacharya, S., Cameron, I.M., Mollison, J., Parkin, D.E., Abramovich, D.R. and Kitchener, H.C. (1998) Admission–discharge policies for hysteroscopic surgery: A randomised comparison of day case with in-patient admission. European Journal of Obstetrics and Gynaecology and Reproductive Biology 76: 81–84.

Biley, F.C. (1989) Nurses' perception of stress in pre-operative surgical patients. Journal of Advanced Nursing 14: 575–581.

Biley, F.C. (2000) The effects on patient well-being of music listening as a nursing intervention: A review of the literature. Journal of Clinical Nursing 9: 668–677.

Birch, B.R.P. and Miller, R.A. (1994) Walk-in, walk-out day case genito-scrotal surgery with sedation reversal. A survey of patient attitudes and morbidity. British Journal of Urology 74: 658–664.

Birch, B.R.P., Chakraborty, R. and Miller, R.A. (1993) Anxiety in patients undergoing local anaesthetic day-case cystoscopy. Journal of One-Day Surgery 3: 15–17.

Black, N. and Sanderson, C. (1993) Day surgery: Development of a questionnaire for eliciting patients' experiences. Quality in Health Care 2: 157–161.

Blatt, A. and Chen, S. (2003) Day-only laparoscopic cholecystectomy in a regional teaching hospital. Australian and New Zealand Journal of Surgery 73: 321–325.

Boada, S., Recasens, J., Papaceit, J. et al. (2002) Use of elastomeric pumps for continuous intravenous analgesia administration in ambulatory surgery pain management. Journal of Ambulatory Surgery 10: 3–7.

Boker, A., Brownnell, L. and Donen, N. (2002) The Amsterdam preoperative anxiety and information scale provides a simple and reliable measure of pre-operative anxiety. Canadian Journal of Anaesthesia 49: 792–798.

Bonanno, G.A., Davis, P.J., Singer, J.L. and Schwartz, G.E. (1991) The repressor personality and avoidant information processing: A dichotic listening study. Journal of Research in Personality 25: 386–401.

Bondy, L.R., Sims, N., Schroeder, D.R., Offord, K.P. and Narr, B.J. (1999) The effect of anaesthetic patient education on pre-operative patient anxiety. Regional Anesthesia and Pain Medicine 24: 158–164.

Boore, J.R. (1978) Prescription for Recovery. London: Royal College of Nursing.

Bostock, N. (2003) Will diagnostic and treatment centres suck the NHS dry? Primary Care Report 5(15): 5–7.

Bostrom, J., Crawford-Swent, C., Lazar, N. and Helmer, D. (1994) Learning needs of hospitalised and recently discharged patients. Patient Education and Counselling 23: 83–89.

Bostrom, J., Caldwell, J., McGuire, K. and Everson, D. (1996) Telephone follow-up after discharge from the hospital: Does it make a difference? Applied Nursing Research 9(2): 47–52.

Bottrill, P. (1994) Nursing assessment prior to day surgery. Journal of One-Day Surgery 4(2): 22–23.

Bradshaw, C., Pritchett, C., Bryce, C., Coleman, S. and Nattress, H. (1999) Information needs of general day surgery patients. International Journal of Ambulatory Surgery 7: 39–44.

Breemhaar, B. and van den Borne, H.W. (1991) Effects of education and support for surgical patients: The role of perceived control. Patient Education and Counseling 18: 199–210.

Breemhaar, B., van den Borne, H.W. and Mullen, P.D. (1996) Inadequacies of surgical patient education. Patient Education and Counseling 28(2): 31–44.

Bringman, S., Anderberg, B., Heikkinen, T. et al. (2001) Outpatient laparoscopy cholecystectomy: A prospective study with 100 consecutive patients. Journal of Ambulatory Surgery 9: 83–86.

Broadbent, E., Petrie, K.J., Alley, P.G. and Booth, R.J. (2003) Psychological stress impairs early wound repair following surgery. Psychosomatic Medicine 65: 865–869.

Brumfield, V.C., Kee, C.C. and Johnson, J.Y. (1996) Pre-operative patient teaching in ambulatory surgery settings. American Operating Room Nurses' Journal 64: 941–952.

Bruster, S., Jarman, B., Bosanquet, N., Weston, D., Erens, R. and Delbanco, T.L. (1994) National survey of hospital patients. British Medical Journal 309: 1542-1546.

Bubela, N., Galloway, S., McCay, E. et al. (1990) The patient learning needs scale: reliability and validity. Journal of Advanced Nursing 15: 1181-1187.

Burden, N., DeFazio-Quinn, D.M., O'Brien, D. and Gregory-Dawes, B.S. (2000) Ambulatory Surgical Nursing. London: W.B. Saunders.

Burns, S. (1993) Surgical nurses in out-patient clinics. Surgical Nurse 6: 6.

Butler, G., Hurley, C.A. M., Buchanan, K.L. and Smith-VanHorne, J. (1996) Pre-hospital education: Effectiveness with total hip replacement surgery patients. Patient Education and Counseling 29: 189-197.

Buttery, Y., Sissons, J. and Williams, K.N. (1993) Patients' views one week after day surgery with general anaesthesia. Journal of One-Day Surgery 3: 6-8.

Byrne, D. (1961) The repression-sensitisation scale: Rationale, reliability and validity. Journal of Personality and Clinical Studies 29: 334-349.

Caballero, C. and McWhinnie, D. (1999) From first patient contact to final discharge: The role of the laparoscopic nurse practitioner in general surgery. Journal of One-Day Surgery 9: 4-5.

Cahill, H. (1998) 'It isn't what you do, but the way that you do it': nurse practitioners in day surgery. Journal of One-Day Surgery 8(3): 11-14.

Cahill, J. (1999) Basket cases and trolleys: Day surgery proposals for the millennium. Journal of One-Day Surgery 9: 11-12.

Cahill, H. and Jackson, I. (1997) Day Surgery: Principles and nursing practice. London: Baillière Tindall.

Caldwell, L.M. (1991a) The influence of preference for information on pre-operative stress and coping in surgical out-patients. Applied Nursing Research 4: 177-183.

Caldwell, L.M. (1991b) Surgical outpatient concerns: What every peri-operative nurse should know. Association of Operating Room Nurses' Journal 53: 761-767.

Callesen, T., Bech, K., Nielsen, R. et al. (1998) Pain after groin repair. British Journal of Surgery 85: 1412-1414.

Calvin, R.L. and Lane, P.L. (1999) Peri-operative uncertainty and state anxiety of orthopaedic surgical patients. Orthopaedic Nursing 18(6): 61-66.

Cameron, A. and Masterson, A. (2000) Managing the unmanageable? Nurse Executive Directors and new role developments in nursing. Journal of Advanced Nursing 31: 1081-1088.

Canonico, S., Campitiello, F. and Santoriello, A. (2003) Feasibility and problems of day-care varicose vein surgery in elderly patients. Journal of Ambulatory Surgery 10: 163-166.

Carlisle, D. (2003) Call of the wild. Health Service Journal 113: 12-13.

Carlisle, J. (2003) Pre-operative preparation. Journal of One-Day Surgery 12(4): 55-58.

Carlisle, J. (2004) Guidelines for pre-operative testing. Journal of One-Day Surgery 14: 13-16.

Carnie, J. (2002) Patient feedback on the anaesthetist's performance during the pre-operative visit. Anesthesia and Analgesia 57: 967-701.

Carroll, B.J., Birth, M. and Phillips, E.H. (1998) Common bile duct injuries during laparoscopic cholecystectomy that result in litigation. Surgical Endoscopy 12: 310-313.

Carroll, L. (2004) Clinical skills for nurses in medical assessment units. Nursing Standard 30(18): 33-40.

Cartagena, J., Vicent, J.P., Moreno-Egea, A., Sanchez Elduayen, M.T., Aguayo, J.L. and Sanz, J. (2003) Regional anaesthesia in the outpatient treatment of bilateral inguinal hernias using totally extraperitoneal laparoscopy. Journal of Ambulatory Surgery 10: 55-59.

Carter, L. and Evans, T. (1996) Pre-operative visiting: A role for theatre nurses. British Journal of Nursing 5: 204-207.

Carver, C.S. and Scheier, M.F. (1994) Optimism and health-related cognition: What variables actually matter? Psychology and Health 9: 191-195.

Casey, D. and Ormrod, G. (2003) The effectiveness of nurse-led surgical pre-assessment clinics. Professional Nurse 18: 685-687.

Caumo, W., Schmidt, A.P., Schneider, C.N. et al. (2001) Risk factors for pre-operative anxiety in adults. Acta Anaesthesiologica Scandinavica 45: 298-307.

Caunt, H. (1992) Pre-operative nursing intervention to relieve stress. British Journal of Nursing 1: 171-174.

Challands, A., Haddock, J. and Stevens, J. (2000) Patients contact with primary care following day surgery. Journal of One-Day Surgery 10(1): 12-14.

Charalambous, C.P., Zipitis, C.S., Yarwood, S. and Hirst, P. (2003) The development of a protocol in using day surgery for minor orthopaedic trauma patients. Annals of the Royal College of Surgeons of England 85: 28-31.

Chen, X., Tang, J., White, P.F. et al. (2001) The effect of timing of dolasetron administration on its efficacy as a prophylactic antiemetic in the ambulatory setting. Anesthesia and Analgesia 93: 906-911.

Cheng, C.J.C., Smith, I. and Watson, B.J. (2003) Recovery after day surgery: A survey of anaesthetists regarding return of home fitness and street fitness. Journal of Ambulatory Surgery 10: 67-72.

Chew, T.T.H., Tan, T., Tan, S.S. and Ip-Yam, P.C. (1998) A survey of patients' knowledge of anaesthesia and peri-operative care. Singapore Medical Journal 39: 399-402.

Christopherson, B. and Pfeiffer, C. (1980) Varying the timing of information to alter pre-operative anxiety and post-operative recovery in cardiac surgery patients. Heart and Lung 9: 854-861.

Chung, F. (1995) Recovery pattern and home-readiness after ambulatory surgery. Anesthesia and Analgesia 80: 896-902.

Chung, F., Parikh, S., Theodorou, C., Dusek, B. and Cruise, C. (1994) Patient satisfaction with anesthesia after day surgery. Anesthesiology 181(3/A): A51.

Chung, F., Mezei, G. and Tong, D. (1999) Adverse events in ambulatory surgery. A comparison between elderly and younger patients. Canadian Journal of Anaesthesia 46: 309-321.

Clark, K., Voase, R., Flotcher, I.R. and Thomson, P.J. (1999) Improving patient throughput for oral day case surgery: The efficacy of a nurse-led pre-admission clinic. Journal of Ambulatory Surgery 7: 101-106.

Claxton, A.R., McGuire, G., Chung, F. and Cruise, C. (1997) Evaluation of morphine versus fentanyl for post-operative analgesia after ambulatory surgical procedures. Anesthesia and Analgesia 84: 509-514.

Clinch, C.A. (1997) Nurses achieve quality with pre-assessment clinics. Journal of Clinical Nursing 6: 147-151.

Clipperley, J.A., Butcher, L.A. and Hayes, J.E. (1995) Research utilisation: The development of a pre-operative teaching protocol. Medsurgical Nursing 4: 199-206.

Clough, T.M., Sandher, D., Bale, R.S. and Laurence, A.S. (2003) The use of a local anesthetic foot block in patients undergoing outpatient bony forefoot surgery: A prospective randomized controlled trial. Journal of Foot and Ankle Surgery 42(1): 24-29.

Clyne, C.A.C. and Jamieson, C.W. (1978) The patient's opinion of day care vein surgery. British Journal of Surgery 65: 194-196.

Cobley, M., Dunne, J.A. and Sanders, L.D. (1991) Stressful pre-operative preparation procedures: The routine removal of dentures during pre-operative preparation contributes to pre-operative distress. Anaesthesia 46: 1019-1022.

Codd, C. (1991) Are analgesics necessary for women at home following laparoscopic gynaecological day surgery? Nursing Practice 5(1): 8-12.

Cohen, S.M., Fiske, J. and Newton, J.T. (2000) The impact of dental anxiety on daily living. British Dental Journal 189: 385-390.

Coll, A.M., Ameen, J.R.M. and Mead, D. (2004a) Post-operative pain assessment tools in day surgery: Literature review. Journal of Advanced Nursing 46: 123-133.

Coll, A.M., Ameen, J.R.M. and Moseley, L.G. (2004b) Reported pain after day surgery: A critical literature review. Journal of Advanced Nursing 46: 53-65.

Coloma, M., White, P.F., Markowitz, S.D. et al. (2002) Dexamethasone in combination with dolasetron for prophylaxis in the ambulatory setting: effect on outcome after laparoscopic cholecystectomy. Anesthesiology 96: 1346-1350.

Conaghan, P.J., Figueira, E., Griffin, M.A. and Ingham Clark, C.L. (2002) Randomized clinical trial of the effectiveness of emergency day surgery against standard inpatient treatment. British Journal of Surgery 89: 423–427.

Cooil, J. and Bithell, C. (1997) Pre-operative education for patients undergoing total hip replacement: A comparison of two methods. Physiotherapy Theory and Practice 13: 163–173.

Cook, T., Fitzpatrick, R. and Smith, I. (2004) Achieving Day Surgery Targets: A practical approach towards improving efficiency in day case units in the United Kingdom. London: Advanced Medical Publications.

Correa, R., Menezes, R.B., Wong, J., Yogendran, S., Jenkins, K. and Chung, F. (2001) Compliance with postoperative instructions: A telephone survey of 750 day surgery patients. Anaesthesia 56: 481–484.

Cortis, J.D. and Lacey, A.E. (1996) Measuring the quality and quantity of information giving to in-patients. Journal of Advanced Nursing 24: 674–681.

Coslow, B.I.F. and Eddy, M.E. (1998) Effects of pre-operative ambulatory gynaecological education: Clinical outcomes and patient satisfaction. Journal of Peri-Anesthesia Nursing 13(1): 4–10.

Costa, M.J. (2001) The lived perioperative experience of ambulatory surgery patients. American Operating Room Nurses' Journal 74: 874–881.

Coulter, A., Entwistle, V. and Gilbert, D. (1998) Informing Patients. London: King's Fund.

Cox, H. and O'Connell, B. (2003) Recovery from gynaecological day surgery: Are we underestimating the process. Journal of Ambulatory Surgery 10: 114–121.

Cozzarelli, C. (1993) Personality and self-efficacy as predictors of coping with abortion. Journal of Personality and Social Psychology 65: 1224–1236.

Cruise, C.J., Chung, F., Yogendran, S. and Little, D. (1997) Music increases satisfaction in elderly outpatients undergoing cataract surgery. Canadian Journal of Anaesthesia 44(1): 43–48.

Crumlish, C.M. (1998) Coping strategies of cardiac surgery patients in the peri-operative period. Dimensions of Critical Care Nursing 17: 272–278.

Cundy, J.M. and Read, P.J.H. (1981) The acceptability of day stay for termination of pregnancy. British Journal of Clinical Practice 35: 215–218.

Cupples, S.A. (1991) Effects of timing and reinforcement of pre-operative education on knowledge and recovery of patients having coronary artery bypass graft surgery. Heart and Lung 20: 654–660.

Daltroy, L.H., Morlino, C.I., Eaton, H.M., Poss, R. and Liang, M.H. (1998) Pre-operative education for total hip and knee replacement patients. Arthritis Care and Research 11: 469–478.

Daoud, Z.A. and Hasan, M.A. (1999) Day surgery: The effect of anxiety on induction of anaesthesia and insertion of the laryngeal mask airway. Journal of One-Day Surgery 9(2): 12–13.

Darkow, T., Gora-Harper, M.L., Goulson, D.T. and Record, K.E. (2001) Impact of antiemetic selection on postoperative nausea and vomiting and patient satisfaction. Pharmacotherapy 21: 540–548.

De Beer, D.A.H. and Ravalia, A. (2001) Post-operative pain and nausea following day case gynaecological laparoscopy. Journal of One-Day Surgery 11(3): 52–53.

De Bruin, J.T., Schaefer, M.K., Krohne, H-W. and Dreyer, A. (2001) Pre-operative anxiety, coping, and intra-operative adjustment: Are there mediating effects of stress-induced analgesia? Psychology and Health 16: 253–271.

De Groot, K.I., Boeke, S., Bonke, B. and Passchier, J. (1997a) A revaluation of the adaptiveness of avoidant and vigilant coping with surgery. Psychology and Health 12: 711–717. chap 4

De Groot, K.I., Boeke, S., van den Berge, H., Duivenvoorden, H.J., Bonke, B. and Passchier, J. (1997b) The influence of psychological variables on post-operative anxiety and physical complaints in patients undergoing lumbar surgery. Pain 69(1-2): 19–25. chap 1

De Jesus, G., Abbotts, S., Collins, B. and Burvill, A. (1996) Same day surgery: Results of a patient satisfaction survey. Journal of Quality in Clinical Practice 16: 165-173.

De Lathouwer, C. and Poullier, J.P. (1998) Ambulatory surgery in 1994-1995: The state of the art in 29 Organisation for Economic Co-operation and Development (OECD) countries. Journal of Ambulatory Surgery 6(1): 43-55.

De Witte, J.L., Alegret, C., Sessler, D.I. and Cammu, G. (2002) Preoperative alprazolam reduces anxiety in ambulatory surgery patients: A comparison with oral midazolam. Anesthesia and Analgesia 95: 1601-1606.

Dent, J.A. (2003) Twelve tips for developing a clinical teaching programme in a day surgery unit. Medical Teacher 25: 364-367.

Department of Health (1991) The Patient's Charter. London: HMSO.

Department of Health (2000) The NHS Plan - Creating a 21st century NHS. London: HMSO (Cm 4818-1).

Department of Health (2001) Shifting the Balance of Power Within the NHS. London: HMSO.

Department of Health (2003) Chief Executive's Report. London: HMSO.

Department of Health (2004a) General information about Treatment Centres. www.dh.gov.uk/treatmentcentres: DoH.

Department of Health (2004b) The NHS Improvement Plan: Putting people at the heart of public services. London: DoH.

Devine, E.C. (1992) Effects of psycho-educational care for adult surgical patients: A meta-analysis of 191 studies. Patient Education and Counselling 19: 129-142.

Dewar, A., Craig, K., Muir, J. and Cole, C. (2003) Testing the effectiveness of a nursing intervention in relieving pain following day surgery. Journal of Ambulatory Surgery 10: 81-88.

Dexter, F. and Epstein, R.H. (2001) Reducing family members' anxiety while waiting on the day of surgery: Systematic review of studies and implications of HIPAA health information privacy rules. Journal of Clinical Anesthesia 13: 478-481.

Deyo, R.A., Cherkin, D.C., Weinstein, J., Howe, J., Ciol, M. and Mulley, A.G. (2000) Involving patients in clinical decisions: Impact of an interactive video program on use of back surgery. Medical Care 38: 959-969.

Dixon-Woods, M. (2001) Writing wrongs? An analysis of published discourses about the use of patient information leaflets. Social Science and Medicine 52: 1417-1432.

Doering, S., Kalzlberger, F., Rumpold, G. et al. (2000) Video-tape preparation of patients before hip replacement surgery reduces stress. Psychosomatic Medicine 62: 365-373.

Domar, A.D., Noe, J.M. and Benson, H. (1987) The pre-operative use of the relaxation response with ambulatory surgery patients. Journal of Human Stress 13: 101-107.

Done, M.L. and Lee, A. (1998) The use of a video to convey pre-anaesthetic information to patients undergoing ambulatory surgery. Anesthesia and Analgesia 87: 531-536.

Donoghue, J., Pelletier, D., Duffield, C. and Gomez-Fort, R. (1995) Laparoscopic day surgery: The process of recovery for women. Journal of Ambulatory Surgery 3: 171-177.

Donoghue, J., Pelletier, D., Duffield, C. and Torres, M. (1997) Australian men's experiences of cystoscopic day surgery. Journal of Ambulatory Surgery 5: 15-19.

Donoghue, J., Pelletier, D., Duffield, C. and Torres, M. (1998) Australian men's experiences of cystoscopic day surgery (Part 2). Journal of Ambulatory Surgery 6: 189-196.

Duggan, M., Dowd, N., O'Mara, D., Harmon, D., Tormey, W. and Cunningham, A.J. (2002) Benzodiazepine premedication may attenuate the stress response in daycase anesthesia: A pilot study. Canadian Journal of Anaesthesia 49: 932-935.

Duits, A.A., Boeke, S., Taams, M.A., Passchier, J. and Erdman, R.A.M. (1997) Prediction of quality of life after coronary artery bypass graft surgery: A review and evaluation of multiple, recent studies. Psychosomatic Medicine 59: 257-268.

Duits, A.A., Duivenvoorden, H.J., Boeke, S. et al. (1999) A structural modelling analysis of anxiety and depression in patients undergoing coronary artery bypass graft surgery: A model generating approach. Journal of Psychosomatic Research 46: 187-200.

Dunn, D. (1998) Pre-operative assessment criteria and patient teaching for ambulatory surgery patients. Journal of Peri-Anesthesia Nursing 13: 274-291.

Dusseldorp, E., Van Elderen, T., Maes, S., Meulman, J. and Kraaij, V. (1999) A meta-analysis of psycho-educational programmes for coronary heart disease patients. Health Psychology 18: 506–519.

Eachus, P. (1991) Multi-dimensional health locus of control in nurses. Journal of Advanced Nursing 16: 165–171.

Edmondson, M. (1996) Patient information. In: Penn, S., Davenport, H.T., Carrington, S., and Edmondson, M. (eds), Principles of Day Surgery. London: Blackwell Science, pp. 62–74.

Edwards, N.D., Barclay, K., Catling, S.J., Martin, D.G. and Morgan, R.H. (1991) Day case laparoscopy: A survey of post-operative pain and an assessment of the value of diclofenac. Satisfaction, Anaesthesia, Pain 46: 1077–1080.

Egbert, L.D., Battit, G.E., Welch, C.E. and Bartlett, M.K. (1964) Reduction of post-operative pain by encouragement and instruction of patients. New England Journal of Medicine 270: 825–827.

Eller, L.S. (1999) Guided imagery interventions for symptom management. Annual Review of Nursing Research 17(3): 57–84.

Ellis, J. (2002) Telephone assessment: Lines of inquiry. Health Service Journal 112: 32.

Elsass, P., Duedahl, H., Friis, B., Moller, I.W. and Bredgaard Sorensen, M. (1987a) The psychological effect of having a contact-person from the anaesthetic staff. Acta Anaesthesiologica Scandinavica 31: 584–586.

Elsass, P., Eikard, B., Junge, J., Lykke, J., Staun, P. and Feldt-Rasmussen, M. (1987b) Psychological effect of detailed pre-anaesthetic information. Acta Anaesthesiologica Scandinavica 31: 579–583.

Erdem, E., Sungurtekin, H., Sungurtekin, U., Tetik, C. and Ozden, A. (2003) Comparison of local and spinal anesthesia techniques in inguinal hernia repair. Journal of Ambulatory Surgery 10: 128–132.

Evans, D. (2002) The effectiveness of music as an intervention for hospital patients: A systematic review. Journal of Advanced Nursing 37(1): 8–18.

Eysenck, H.J. and Eysenck, S.B.G. (1975) Manual of the Eysenck Personality Questionnaire. London: Hodder & Stoughton.

Fagermoen, M.S. and Hamilton, G. (2003) Preparing patients for urological surgery. International Journal of Nursing Studies 40: 281–290.

Fareed, A. (1996) The experience of reassurance: Patients' perspectives. Journal of Advanced Nursing 23: 272–279.

Farnill, D. and Inglis, S. (1993) Patients' desire for information about anaesthesia: Australian attitudes. Anaesthesia 48: 162–164.

Faymonville, M.E., Mambourg, P.H., Joris, J. et al. (1997) Psychological approaches during conscious sedation. Hypnosis versus stress reducing strategies: A prospective randomized study. Pain 73: 361–367.

Fellowes, H., Abbott, D., Barton, K., Burgess, L., Clare, A. and Lucas, B. (1999) Orthopaedic Pre-admission Assessment Clinics. London: Royal College of Nursing.

Fenton-Lee, D., Cooke, T. and Riach, E. (1994) Patient acceptance of day surgery. Annals of the Royal College of Surgeons of England 76: 331–334.

Fetzer, S.J., Hand, M.C., Bouchard, P.A., Smith, H. and Jenkins, M.B. (2004) Evaluation of the Rhodes index of nausea and vomiting for ambulatory surgery patients. Journal of Advanced Nursing 47(1): 74–80.

Firth, F. (1991) Pain after day surgery. Nursing Times 87(40): 72–76.

Fitzpatrick, R. and Hopkins, A. (1983) Problems in the conceptual framework of patient satisfaction research: An empirical exploration. Sociology of Health and Illness 5: 297–311.

Fitzpatrick, J.M., Selby, T.T. and While, A.E. (1998) Patients' experiences of varicose vein and arthroscopy day surgery. British Journal of Nursing 7: 1107–1115.

Fleming, V.E.M. (1992) Client education: a futuristic outlook. Journal of Advanced Nursing 17: 158–163.

Fleming, W.R., Michell, I. and Douglas, M. (2000) Audit of outpatient laparoscopic cholecystectomy. Australian and New Zealand Journal of Surgery 70: 423–427.

Flood, A., Lorence, D.P., Ding, J., McPherson, K. and Black, N.A. (1993) The role of expectations in patient's reports of post-operative outcomes and improvement following therapy. Medical Care 31(Part 3): 1043-1056.

Folkman, S. (1984) Personal control and stress and coping process: A theoretical analysis. Journal of Personality and Social Psychology 46: 839-852.

Folkman, S. and Lazarus, R.S. (1980) An analysis of coping in a middle-aged community sample. Journal of Health and Social Behaviour 21: 219-239.

Folkman, S., Lazarus, R.S., Dunkel-Schetter, C., DeLongis, A. and Gruen, R.J. (1986) Dynamics of a stressful encounter: Cognitive appraisal, coping and encounter outcomes. Journal of Personality and Social Psychology 50: 992-1003.

Foulger, V. (1997) Patients' views of day-case cardiac catheterisation. Professional Nurse 12: 478-480.

Fox, E., O'Boyle, C., Barry, H. and McCreary, C. (1989) Repressive coping style and anxiety in stressful dental surgery. British Journal of Medical Psychology 62: 371-380.

Fraser, R.A., Hotz, S.B., Hurtig, J.B., Hodges, S.N. and Moher, D. (1989) The prevalence and impact of pain after day-care tubal ligation surgery. Pain 39: 189-201.

Friedman, S.B., Badere, B. and Fitzpatrick, S. (1992) The effects of television viewing on preoperative anxiety. Journal of Post-Anesthesia Nursing 7: 243-250.

Frisch, S.R., Groom, L.E., Seguin, E., Edgar, L.J. and Pepler, C.J. (1990) Ambulatory surgery: A study of patients' and helpers' experiences. American Operating Room Nurses' Journal 52: 1000-1009.

Fuller, S. (2003) Diagnosis and Treatment Centres – Lessons for the Pioneers. London: DoH.

Fung, D. and Cohen, M. (2001) What do out-patients value most in their anesthesia care? Canadian Journal of Anaesthesia 48(1): 12-19.

Gaberson, K.B. (1995) The effects of humorous and musical distraction on pre-operative anxiety. Association of Operating Room Nurses' Journal 62: 784-791.

Gagliano, M.E. (1988) A literature review on the efficacy of video in patient education. Journal of Medical Education 63: 785-792.

Gammon, J. and Mulholland, C.W. (1996) Effects of preparatory information prior to elective total hip replacement on psychological coping outcomes. Journal of Advanced Nursing 24: 303-308.

Ganapathy, S., Amendola, A., Lichfield, R., Fowler, P.J. and Ling, E. (2000) Elastomeric pumps for ambulatory patient controlled regional analgesia. Canadian Journal of Anaesthesia 47: 897-902.

Ganguli, P. (2003) Will fast-track units benefit nurses? Nursing Times 99(37): 10-11.

Garcia-Urena, M.A., Garcia, M.V., Ruiz, V.V., Carnero, F.J., Huerta, D.P. and Jimenez, M.S.C. (2000) Anesthesia and surgical repair of aponeurotic hernias in ambulatory surgery. Journal of Ambulatory Surgery 8: 175-178.

Garden, A.L., Merry, A.F., Holland, R.L. and Petrie, K.J. (1996) Anaesthesia information–what patients want to know. Anaesthesia and Intensive Care 24: 594-598.

Georgalas, C., Paun, S., Zainal, A., Patel, N.N. and Mochloulls, G. (2002) Assessing day-case septorhinoplasty: Prospective audit study using patient-based indices. Journal of Laryngology and Otology 116: 707-710.

Ghosh, S. and Sallam, S. (1994) Patient satisfaction and post-operative demands on hospital and community services after day surgery. British Journal of Surgery 81: 1635-1638.

Gilmartin, J. (2004) Day surgery: Patients' perceptions of a nurse-led pre-admission clinic. Journal of Clinical Nursing 13: 243-250.

Gnanalingham, K.K. and Budhoo, M. (1998) Day case hernia repair under local versus general anaesthetic: Patient preferences. Journal of Ambulatory Surgery 6: 227-229.

Goldmann, L., Ogg, T.W. and Levey, A.B. (1988) Hypnosis and day case anaesthesia. Anaesthesia 43: 466-469.

Goodman, H. (1997) Patients' perceptions of their education needs in the first six weeks following discharge after cardiac surgery. Journal of Advanced Nursing 25: 1241-1251.

Gould, D. and Wilson-Barnett, J. (1995) A comparison of recovery following hysterectomy and major cardiac surgery. Journal of Advanced Nursing 10: 315–323.

Greenwood, M. (1993) Patients' views of oral day surgery. British Dental Journal 175: 130–132.

Grieve, R.J. (2002) Day surgery pre-operative anxiety reduction and coping strategies. British Journal of Nursing 11: 670–678.

Grogaard, B., Kimsas, E. and Raeder, J. (2001) Wound infection in day surgery. Journal of Ambulatory Surgery 9: 109–112.

Guadagnoli, E. and Ward, P. (1998) Patient satisfaction in decision making. Social Science and Medicine 47: 329–339.

Gui, G.P.H., Cheruvu, C.V.N., Subak-Sharpe, I., Shiew, M., Bidlake, L. and Fiennes, A.G.T.W. (1999) Communication between hospital and general practitioners after day surgery: A patient safety issue. Annals of the Royal College of Surgeons of England 81(suppl): 8–9.

Guilbert, E. and Roter, D. (1997) Assessment of satisfaction with induced abortion procedure. Journal of Psychology 131: 157–166.

Gupta, A., Larsen, L., Sjoberg, I. and Lennmarken, C. (1994) Out-patients survey: A survey of anaesthesia care in a university hospital. Scandinavian Journal of Caring Sciences 8(2): 107–112.

Gupta, A., Axelsson, K., Thorn, S.E. et al. (2003) Low-dose bupivacaine plus fentanyl for spinal anesthesia during ambulatory inguinal herniorrhaphy: A comparison between 6 mg and 7.5 mg of bupivacaine. Acta Anaesthesiologica Scandinavica 47: 13–19.

Guy, R.J., Ng, C.E. and Eu, K.W. (2003) Stapled anoplasty for haemorrhoids: A comparison of ambulatory vs. in-patient procedures. Colorectal Disease 5: 29–32.

Habib, A.S. and Gan, T.J. (2001) Combination therapy for post-operative nausea and vomiting – a more effective prophylaxis. Journal of Ambulatory Surgery 9: 59–71.

Haddock, J., Challands, A., Stevens, J., Wong, C. and Walters, S. (1999) Patient controlled oral analgesia at home (PCOAH) for the management of post-operative pain following day surgery. Journal of One-Day Surgery 8(4): 3–8.

Hahm, T.S., Cho, H.S., Lee, K.H., Chung, I.S., Kim, J.A. and Kim, M.H. (2001) Clonidine premedication prevents preoperative hypokalemia. Journal of Clinical Anesthesia 14: 6–9.

Haldane, G., Stott, S. and McMenemin, I. (1998) Pouch of Douglas block for laparoscopic sterilisation. Anaesthesia 53: 589–603.

Halfens, R.J.G. (1995) Effect of hospital stay on health locus of control beliefs. Western Journal of Nursing Research 17: 156–167.

Hansen, C.H., Hansen, R, D. and Shantz, D.W. (1992) Repression at encoding: discrete appraisals of emotional stimuli. Journal of Personality and Social Psychology 63: 1026–1035.

Harju, E. (1991) Patient satisfaction among day surgery patients in a central hospital. Quality Assurance in Health Care 3(2): 85–88.

Hartfield, M.T., Cason, C.L. and Cason, G.J. (1982) Effects of information about a threatening procedure on patients' expectations and emotional distress. Nursing Research 31: 202–206.

Hartford, K., Wong, C. and Zakaria, D. (2002) Randomized controlled trial of a telephone intervention by nurses to provide information and support to patients and their partners after elective coronary artery bypass graft surgery: effects of anxiety. Heart and Lung 31: 199–206.

Hartsfield, J. and Clopton, J.R. (1985) Reducing pre-surgical anxiety: A possible visitors effect. Social Science and Medicine 20: 529–533.

Hathaway, D. (1986) Effect of pre-operative instruction on post-operative outcomes: A meta-analysis. Nursing Research 35: 269–275.

Hawkes, N. (2004) Medicine and The Media. Day Surgery 2004 15th Annual Scientific Meeting and Exhibition. University of East Anglia, Norwich.

Hawkshaw, D. (1994) A day surgery patient telephone follow-up survey. British Journal of Nursing 3: 348–350.

Hayward, J. (1975) Information – A prescription against pain. Series 2, No. 5. London: Royal College of Nursing.

Hazelgrove, J.F. and Robins, D.W. (2002) Caring for the carer: An audit of the day surgery services for carers within the Wessex Region of England. Journal of Ambulatory Surgery 8: 13–18.

Health Service Commissioner for England for Scotland and for Wales (1997) Annual Report for 1996–1997. London: HMSO.

Health Service Commissioner for England for Scotland and for Wales (2001) Annual Report for 2000–2001. London: HMSO.

Healy, J. and McWhinne, D. (2003) Pre-assessment at source. Journal of One-Day Surgery 13(1): 14–15.

Hedayati, B. and Fear, S. (1999) Hospital admission after day-case gynaecological laparoscopy. British Journal of Anaesthesia 83: 776–779.

Heikkila, J., Paunonen, M., Laippala, P. and Virtanen, V. (1998) Nurses' ability to perceive patients' fears related to coronary arteriography. Journal of Advanced Nursing 28: 1225–1235.

Hein, A., Norlander, C., Blom, L. and Jakobsson, J. (2001) Is pain prophylaxis in minor gynaecological surgery of clinical value? A double-blind placebo controlled study of paracetamol 1 g versus Lornoxicam 8 mg given orally. Journal of Ambulatory Surgery 9: 91–94.

Heiser, R.M., Chiles, K., Fudge, M. and Gray, S.E. (1997) The use of music during the immediate postoperative recovery period. American Operating Room Nurses' Journal 65: 781–875.

Heseltine, K. and Edlington, F. (1998) A day surgery post-operative telephone call line. Nursing Standard 13(9): 39–43.

Higgins, P.P., Chung, F. and Mezei, G. (2002) Post-operative sore throat after ambulatory surgery. British Journal of Anaesthesia 88: 582–584.

Hilditch, W.G., Asbury, A.J. and Crawford, J.M. (2003a) Pre-operative screening: Criteria for referring to anaesthetists. Anaesthesia 58: 117–124.

Hilditch, W.G., Asbury, A.J., Jack, E. and McGrane, S. (2003b) Validation of a pre-anaesthetic screening questionnaire. Anaesthesia 58: 874–877.

Hill, B.J. (1982) Sensory information, behavioural instructions and coping with sensory alteration surgery. Nursing Research 31: 17–21.

Hock, M., Krohne, H.W. and Kaiser, J. (1996) Coping dispositions and the processing of ambiguous stimuli. Journal of Personality and Social Psychology 70: 1052–1066.

Hodge, D. (1994) Introduction to day surgery. Surgical Nurse 7(2): 12–16.

Hodge, D. (1999) Day Surgery: A nursing approach. London: Churchill Livingstone.

Holden-Lund, C. (1988) Effects of relaxation with guided imagery on surgical stress and wound healing. Research in Nursing and Health 11: 235–244.

Horne, D.J., Vatmanidis, p. and Careri, A. (1994) Preparing patients for invasive medical and surgical procedures 1: Adding behavioural and cognitive interventions. Behavioural Medicine 20(1): 5–13.

Horvath, K.J. (2003) Postoperative recovery at home after ambulatory gynecologic laparoscopic surgery. Journal of Peri-Anesthesia Nursing 18: 324–334.

Hosie, H.E. and Nimmo, W.S. (1991) Temazepam absorption in patients before surgery. British Journal of Anaesthesia 66: 20–24.

Huang, A., Stinchcombe, C., Davies, M., Phillips, D. and McWhinne, D.L. (2000) Prospective five-year audit for day-case laparoscopic cholecystectomy. Journal of One-Day Surgery 9(4): 15–17.

Hulme, J., Waterman, H. and Hillier, V.F. (1999) The effects of foot massage on patient's perception of care following laparoscopic sterilisation as day case patients. Journal of Advanced Nursing 30: 460–468.

Hunt, M. (1987) The process of translating research findings into nursing practice. Journal of Advanced Nursing 12: 101–110.

Hunt, L., Luck, A.J., Rudkin, G. and Hewett, P.J. (1999) Day-case haemorrhoidectomy. British Journal of Surgery 86: 255–258.

Hutson, M.M. and Blaha, J.D. (1991) Patients' recall of preoperative instruction for informed consent for an operation. Journal of Bone and Joint Surgery 73A: 160–162.

Hyde, R., Bryden, F. and Asbury, A.J. (1998) How would patients prefer to spend the waiting time before their operations? Anaesthesia 53: 192–200.

Icenhour, M.L. (1988) Quality interpersonal care: A study of ambulatory surgery patients' perspectives. American Operating Room Nurses' Journal 47: 1414–1419.

Ilfeld, B.M., Morey, T.E. and Enneking, F.K. (2002) Continuous infraclavicular brachial plexus block for postoperative pain control at home: A randomized, double-blinded, placebo-controlled study. Anesthesiology 96: 1297–1304.

Inglis, A. and Daniel, M. (1995) A survey of information supplied to day-case patients. Health Bulletin 53(2): 91–93.

Ismail, W. (1997) Ambulatory hernia service: Preliminary experience in a district general hospital. Journal of One-Day Surgery 7(2): 10–14.

Issioui, T., Klein, K.W., White, P.F. et al. (2002) Cost-efficacy of rofecoxib versus acetaminophen for preventing pain after ambulatory surgery. Anesthesiology 97: 931–937.

Jackson, S. and Sweeney, B.P. (2004) The efficacy of pre-emptive tramadol in orthopaedic day-surgery. Journal of Ambulatory Surgery 11: 7–9

Jakobsen, D.H., Callesen, T., Schouenborg, L., Nielsen, D. and Kehlet, H. (2003) Convalescence after laparoscopic sterilisation. Journal of Ambulatory Surgery 10: 95–99.

Jalowiec, A., Murphy, S.P. and Powers, M.J. (1984) Psychometric assessment of the Jalowiec Coping Scale. Nursing Research 33: 157–161.

James, D. (2000) Patient perceptions of day surgery. British Journal of Perioperative Nursing 10: 466–467.

Janis, I.L. (1958) Psychological Stress. Psychoanalytic and behavioural studies of surgical patients. New York: Wiley.

Jarrett, P.E.M. (1995) Day case surgery. Surgery 13(1): 5–7.

Jarrett, P.E.M. (1997) Day case surgery: Past and future growth. Surgery 15(4): 94–96.

Jelicic, M. and Bonke, B. (1991) Pre-operative anxiety and motives for surgery. Psychological Reports 68: 849–850.

Jennings, B.M. and Sherman, R.A. (1987) Anxiety, locus of control, and satisfaction in patients undergoing ambulatory surgery. Military Medicine 152: 206–208.

Jin, F., Norris, A., Chung, F. and Ganeshram, T. (1998) Should adult patients drink fluids before discharge from ambulatory surgery? Anesthesia and Analgesia 87: 306–311.

Johnston, M. (1980) Anxiety in surgical patients. Psychological Medicine 10: 145–152.

Johnston, M. (1982) Recognition of patients' worries by nurses and by other patients. British Journal of Clinical Psychology 21: 255–261.

Johnston, M. (1987) Emotional and cognitive aspects of anxiety in surgical patients. Communication and Cognition 20: 245–260.

Johnston, M. and Vogele, C. (1993) Benefits of psychological preparation for surgery: A meta analysis. Annals of Behavioural Medicine 15: 245–256.

Johnston, M., Gilbert, P., Partridge, C. and Collins, J. (1992) Changing perceived control in patients with physical disabilities: An intervention study with patients receiving rehabilitation. British Journal of Clinical Psychology 31: 89–94.

Joshi, G.P. (2003) New concepts in recovery after ambulatory surgery. Journal of Ambulatory Surgery 10: 167–170.

Junger, A., Klasen, J., Benson, M. et al. (2001) Factors determining length of stay of surgical day-case patients. European Journal of Anaesthesiology 18: 314–321.

Junttila, K., Salantera, S. and Hupli, M. (2003) Validation of perioperative nursing data set in Finland: Focus on perioperative nursing diagnoses. Journal of Advanced Perioperative Care 1(3): 95–105.

Kaempf, G. and Amodei, M.E. (1989) The effect of music on anxiety: A research study. American Operating Room Nurses' Journal 50: 112, 114–118.

Kain, Z.N., Kosarussavadi, B., Hernandez-Conte, A., Hofstadter, M.B. and Mayes, L.C. (1997) Desire for peri-operative information in adult patients: A cross sectional study. Journal of Clinical Anesthesia 9: 467–472.

Kain, Z.N., Sevarino, F., Alexander, G.M., Pincus, S. and Mayes, L.C. (2000) Pre-operative anxiety and post-operative pain in women undergoing hysterectomy: A repeated-measures design. Journal of Psychosomatic Research 49: 417–422.

Kangas-Saarela, T., Ohukainen, J. and Koivuranta, M. (1999) Patients' experiences of day surgery – an approach to quality control. Journal of Ambulatory Surgery 7: 31–34.

Karanci, A.N. and Dirik, G. (2003) Predictors of pre- and postoperative anxiety in emergency surgery patients. Journal of Psychosomatic Research 55: 363–369.

Kaufmann, C.L. (1983) Informed consent and patient decision making: Two decades of research. Social Science and Medicine 17: 1657–1664.

Keenan, J., Henderson, M.H. and Riches, G. (1998) Orthopaedic pre-operative assessment: A two-year experience in 5,000 patients. Annals of the Royal College of Surgeons of England 80: 174–176.

Kelly, M.C. (1994) Patients' perception of day case surgery. Ulster Medical Journal 63(1): 27–31.

Kelly, H., Snadden, D. and Bain, J. (1998) Tremors from the front line day case surgery: Impact on primary care providers. Health Bulletin 56: 675–679.

Kempe, A.R. and Gelazis, R. (1985) Patient anxiety levels. Association of Operating Room Nurses' Journal 41: 390–396.

Kennedy, J.A. (1995) An audit of patients' problems after discharge from a day surgery unit. British Journal of Medical Economics 9: 51–53.

Kennedy, B.W., Thorp, J.M., Fitch, W. and Millar, K. (1992) The theatre environment and the awake patient. Journal of Obstetrics and Gynecology 12: 407–411.

Kent, G. (1996) Shared understandings for informed consent: The relevance of psychological research on the provision of information. Social Science and Medicine 43: 1517–1523.

Kerrigan, D.D., Thevasagayam, R.S., Woods, T.O. et al. (1993) Who's afraid of informed consent? British Medical Journal 306: 298–300.

Keulemans, Y., Eshuis, J., De Haes, H., De Wit, L.T. and Gouma, D.J. (1998) Laparoscopic cholecystectomy: Day-care versus clinical observation. Annals of Surgery 228: 734–740.

Kiecolt-Glaser, J.K., Marucha, P.T., Malarkey, W.B., Mercado, A.M. and Glaser, R. (1995) Slowing wound healing by psychological stress. Lancet 346: 1194–1196.

Kiecolt-Glaser, J.K., Page, G.G., Marucha, P.T., MacCallum, R.C. and Glaser, R. (1998) Psychological influences on surgical recovery. American Psychologist 53: 1209–1218.

King, B. (1989) Patient satisfaction surgery: Day surgery unit. Australian Clinical Review 9(3–4): 127–129.

King, I. and Tarsitano, B. (1982) The effect of structured and unstructured pre-operative teaching: A replication. Nursing Research 31: 324–329.

King, K.B., Rowe, M.A., Kimble, L.P. and Zerwic, J.J. (1998) Optimism, coping, and long term recovery from coronary artery surgery in women. Research in Nursing and Health 21(1): 15–26.

Klafta, J.M. and Roizen, M.F. (1996) Current understanding of patients' attitudes toward and preparation for anaesthesia: A review. Anesthesia and Analgesia 83: 1314–1321.

Klein, C.T.F. and Helweg-Larsen, M. (2002) Perceived control and the optimistic bias: A meta-analytic review. Psychology and Health 17: 437–446.

Klein, S.M. and Buckenmaier, C.C. (2002) Ambulatory surgery with long acting regional anesthesia. Minerva Anesthesiologica 68: 833–841, 841–847.

Kleinbeck, S.V.M. (2000) Dimensions of peri-operative nursing for a national specialty nomenclature. Journal of Advanced Nursing 31: 529–535.

Kleinbeck, S.V.M. and Hoffart, N. (1994) Outpatient recovery after laparoscopic cholecystectomy. Association of Operating Room Nurses' Journal 60: 394–402.

Knudsen, V.J. (1996) An audit of day surgery carers. Journal of One-Day Surgery 6(2): 5–6.

Koch, M.E., Kain, Z.N., Ayoub, C. and Rosenbaum, S.H. (1998) The sedative and analgesic sparing effect of music. Anesthesiology 89: 300–306.

Kohlmann, C-W., Weidner, G. and Messina, C.R. (1996) Avoidant coping style and verbal-cardiovascular response dissociation. Psychology and Health 11: 371-384.

Koivula, M., Panunonen-Ilmonen, M., Tarkka, M.T., Tarkka, M. and Laippala, P. (2002a) Social support and its relation to fear and anxiety in patients awaiting coronary artery bypass grafting. Journal of Clinical Nursing 11: 622-633.

Koivula, M., Tarkka, M.T., Tarkka, M., Laippala, P. and Paunonen-Ilmonen, M. (2002b) Fear and in-hospital social support for coronary artery bypass grafting patients on the day before surgery. International Journal of Nursing Studies 39: 415-427.

Kong, K.L., Donovan, I.A., Child, D.L. and Nasmyth-Miller, D. (1997) Demand on primary health care after day surgery. Annals of the Royal College of Surgeons of England 79: 291-295.

Kopp, M., Bonatti, H., Haller, C. et al. (2003) Life satisfaction and active coping style are important predictors of recovery from surgery. Journal of Psychosomatic Research 55: 371-377.

Kremer, C., Duffy, S. and Moroney, M. (2000) Patient satisfaction with outpatient hysteroscopy versus day case hysteroscopy: Randomised controlled trial. British Medical Journal 320: 279-282.

Krenzischek, D.A., L., W. and Poole, E.L. (2001) Evaluation of ASPAN's preoperative patient teaching videos on general, regional, and minimum alveolar concentration/conscious sedation anesthesia. Journal of Peri-Anesthesia Nursing 16: 174-180.

Krohne, H.W. (1978) Individual differences in coping with stress and anxiety. In: Spielberger, C.D. and Sarason, I.G. (eds), Stress and Anxiety, Vol. 5. London: Wiley.

Krohne, H.W. (1989) The concept of coping modes: Relating cognitive person variables to actual coping behaviour. Advances in Behaviour Research and Therapy 11: 235-248.

Krohne, H.W., Hock, M. and Kohlmann, C-W. (1992) Coping dispositions, uncertainty and emotional arousal. In: Strongman, K.T. (ed.), International Review of Studies on Emotion, Vol. 2. Chichester: Wiley, pp. 73-95.

Krohne, H.W., Slangen, K. and Kleemann, P.P. (1996) Coping variables as predictors of peri-operative emotional states and adjustment. Psychology and Health 11: 315-330.

Krohne, H.W., de Bruin, J.T., El-Giamal, M. and Schmukle, S.C. (2000) The assessment of surgery-related coping: The coping with surgical stress scale (COSS). Psychology and Health 15: 135-149.

Krouse, H.J. (2001) Video modelling to educate patients. Advanced Journal of Nursing 33: 748-757.

Krupat, E., Fancey, M. and Cleary, P.D. (2000) Information and its impact on satisfaction among surgical patients. Social Science and Medicine 51: 1817-1825.

Kugler, J., Tenderich, G., Stahlhut, P. et al. (1994) Emotional adjustment and perceived locus of control in heart transplant patients. Journal of Psychosomatic Research 38: 403-408.

Kulik, J.A., Mahler, H.I.M. and Moore, P.J. (1996) Social comparison and affiliation under threat: effects on recovery from major surgery. Journal of Personality and Social Psychology 71: 967-979.

Kurlowicz, L.H. (1998) Perceived self-efficacy, functional ability, and depressive symptoms in older elective surgery patients. Nursing Research 47: 219-226.

Kuusniemi, K.S., Pihlajamäki, K.K., Irjala, J.K., Jaakkola, P.W., Pitkänen, M.T. and Korkeila, J.E. (1999) Restricted spinal anaesthesia for ambulatory surgery: A pilot study. European Journal of Anaesthesiology 16: 2-6.

Lamarche, D., Taddeo, R. and Pepler, C. (1998) The preparation of patients for cardiac surgery. Clinical Nursing Research 7: 390-405.

Larner, T.R., Agarwal, D. and Costello, A.J. (2003) Day-case holmium laser enucleation of the prostate for gland volumes of < 60 mL: Early experience. British Journal of Urology International 91: 61-64.

Lau, H., Wong, C., Goh, L.C., Patil, N.G. and Lee, F. (2002) Prospective randomized trial of pre-emptive analgesics following ambulatory inguinal hernia repair: Intravenous ketorolac versus diclofenac suppository. Australia and New Zealand Journal of Surgery 72: 704-727.

Law, M.L. (1997) A telephone survey of day-surgery eye patients. Journal of Advanced Nursing 25: 355-363.

Law, W.L., Tung, H.M., Chu, K.W. and Lee, F.C. (2003) Ambulatory stapled haemorrhoidectomy: A safe and feasible surgical technique. Hong Kong Medical Journal 9: 103-107.

Lawrence, K., McWhinnie, D., Jenkinson, C. and Coulter, A. (1997) Quality of life in patients undergoing inguinal hernia repair. Annals of the Royal College of Surgeons for England 79(1): 40-45.

Lazarus, R.S. (1966) Psychological Stress and the Coping Process. New York: McGraw-Hill.

Lazarus, R.S. and Folkman, S. (1987) Transactional theory and research on emotions and coping. European Journal of Personality 1: 141-169.

Leach, M., Zernike, W. and Tanner, S. (2000) How anxious are surgical patients? Australian Confederation of Operating Room Nurses 13(1): 28-35.

Lee, A., Chui, P.T. and Gin, T. (2003) Educating patients about anesthesia: A systematic review of randomized controlled trials of media-based interventions. Anesthesia and Analgesia 96: 1424-1431.

Lee, D., Henderson, A. and Shum, D. (2004) The effect of music on preprocedure anxiety in Hong Kong Chinese day patients. Journal of Clinical Nursing 13: 297-303.

Leigh, B. (1995) Day case surgery - the paradoxical revolution. British Journal of Health Care Management 1: 409-410.

Leino-Kilpi, H. and Vuorenheimo, J. (1993) Peri-operative nursing care quality. Association of Operating Room Nurses' Journal 57: 1061-1071.

Leino-Kilpi, H., Iire, L., Suominen, T., Vuorenheimo, J. and Valimaki, M. (1993) Client and information: A literature review. Journal of Clinical Nursing 2: 331-340.

Leinonen, T., Leino-Kilpi, H. and Jouko, K. (1996) The quality of intra-operative nursing care: The patient's perspective. Journal of Advanced Nursing 24: 843-852.

Leinonen, T., Leino-Kilpi, H., Stahlberg, M-R. and Lertola, K. (2001) The quality of peri-operative care: development of a tool for the perceptions of patients. Journal of Advanced Nursing 35: 294-306.

Leith, S.E., Hawkshaw, D. and Jackson, I.J.B. (1994) A national survey of the importance and drug treatment of pain and emesis following day surgery. Journal of One-Day Surgery 4(2): 24-25.

Lemos, P., Regalado, A., Marques, D. et al. (2003) The economic benefits of ambulatory surgery relative to inpatient surgery for laparoscopic tubal ligation. Journal of Ambulatory Surgery 10: 61-65.

Lepage, C., Drolet, P., Girard, M., Grenier, Y. and DeGagne, R. (2001) Music decreases sedative requirements during spinal anesthesia. Anesthesia and Analgesia 93: 912-916.

Lepczyk, M., Raleigh, E., H. and Rowley, C. (1990) Timing of pre-operative patient teaching. Journal of Advanced Nursing 15: 300-306.

Levesque, L., Grenier, R., Kerouac, S. and Reidy, M. (1984) Evaluation of a pre-surgical group program given at two different times. Research in Nursing and Health 7: 227-236.

Levin, R.F., Malloy, G.B. and Hyman, R.B. (1987) Nursing management of post-operative pain: Use of relaxation techniques with female cholecystectomy patients. Journal of Advanced Nursing 12: 463-472.

Lewin, J.M.E. and Razis, P.A. (1995) Prescribing practice of take-home analgesia for day case surgery. British Journal of Nursing 4: 1047-1051.

Lewis, C. and Bryson, J. (1998) Does day case surgery generate extra workload for primary and community health service staff? Annals of the Royal College of Surgeons of England 80: 200-202.

Ley, P. and Florio, T. (1996) The use of readability formulas in health care. Psychology, Health and Medicine 1: 7-28.

Limb, R.I., Rudkin, G.E., Luck, A.J., Hunt, L. and Hewett, P.J. (2000) The pain of haemorrhoidectomy: A prospective study. Journal of Ambulatory Surgery 8: 129-134.

Lindeman, C.A. and Van Aernam, B. (1971) The effects of structured and unstructured pre-operative teaching. Nursing Research 20: 319-332.

Linden, I. and Engberg, I.B. (1995) Patients' opinions and experiences of ambulatory surgery: A self-care perspective. Journal of Ambulatory Surgery 3: 131-139.

Linden, I. and Engberg, I.B. (1996) Patients' opinions of information given and post-operative problems experienced in conjunction with ambulatory surgery. Journal of Ambulatory Surgery 4: 85-91.

Linden, W., Stossel, C. and Maurice, J. (1996) Psychological interventions for patients with coronary artery disease: A meta-analysis. Archives of Internal Medicine 156: 745-752.

Lindwall, L. and von Post, I. (2003) Patients' and nurses' experiences of perioperative dialogues. Journal of Advanced Nursing 43: 246-253.

Lisko, S.A. (1995) Development and use of videotaped instruction for pre-operative education of the ambulatory gynaecological patient. Journal of Post-Anaesthesia Nursing 10: 324-328.

Lithner, M. and Zilling, T. (1998) Does pre-operative information increase the well-being of the patient after surgery? Nursing Science and Research in the Nordic Countries 18: 31-39.

Lithner, M. and Zilling, T. (2000) Pre and postoperative information needs. Patient Education and Counseling 40(1): 29-37.

Litt, M.D., Nye, C. and Shafer, D. (1995) Preparation for oral surgery: Evaluating elements of coping. Journal of Behavioural Medicine 18: 435-459.

Litt, M.D., Kalinowski, L. and Shafer, D. (1999) A dentist fears typology of oral surgery patients: matching patients to anxiety interventions. Health Psychology 18: 614-624.

Liu, E.H. and Tan, S. (2000) Patients' perception of sound levels in the surgical suite. Journal of Clinical Anesthesia 12: 298-302.

Liu, R., Barry, J.E.S. and Weinman, J. (1994) Effects of background stress and anxiety on post-operative recovery. Anaesthesia 49: 382-386.

Lonsdale, M. and Hutchison, G.L. (1991) Patients' desire for information about anaesthesia. Anaesthesia 46: 410-412.

Losiak, W. (2001) Can patterns of coping explain more? A study of coping and emotions in surgical stress. Anxiety, Stress and Coping 14: 213-235.

Ludwick-Rosenthal, R. and Neufeld, R.W.J. (1993) Preparation for undergoing an invasive medical procedure: Interacting effects of information and coping style. Journal of Consulting and Clinical Psychology 61: 156-164.

Lydon, A., McGinley, J., Cooke, T., Duggan, P.F. and Shorten, G.D. (1998) Effect of anxiety on the rate of gastric emptying of liquids. British Journal of Anaesthesia 81: 522-525.

MacAndie, C. and Bingham, B.J.G. (1998) Day case nasal surgery: Patient satisfaction and the impact on general practitioner workload. Journal of One-Day Surgery 7(3): 7-11.

Macario, A., Weinger, M., Carney, S. and Kim, A. (1999) Which clinical anesthesia outcomes are important to avoid? The perspective of patients. Anesthesia and Analgesia 89: 652-658.

McCallum, J., Nakamura, T., Bye, R. and Jackson, D. (2000) Day surgery for older people (70+): selection versus outcome effects. Journal of Ambulatory Surgery 8(3): 143-149.

McCarthy, S.C., Lyons, A.C., Weinman, J., Talbot, R. and Purnell, D. (2003) Do expectations influence recovery from oral surgery? An illness representation approach. Psychology and Health 18: 109-126.

McCleane, G.J. and Cooper, R. (1990) The nature of pre-operative anxiety. Anaesthesia 45: 153-155.

McCleane, G.J. and Watters, C.H. (1990) Pre-operative anxiety and serum potassium. Anaesthesia 45: 583-585.

Macdonald, M. and Bodzak, W. (1999) The performance of a self-managing day surgery nurse team. Journal of Advanced Nursing 29: 859-868.

McGaw, C.D. and Hanna, W.J. (1998) Knowledge and fears of anaesthesia and surgery: The Jamaican perspective. West Indian Medical Journal 47(2): 64-67.

McHugh, G.A. and Thoms, G.M. (2002) The management of pain following day-case surgery. Anaesthesia 57: 270-275.

Mackenzie, J.W. (1989) Daycase anaesthesia and anxiety: A study of anxiety profiles amongst patients attending a day bed unit. Anaesthesia 44: 437-440.

Mackintosh, C. and Bowles, S. (1998) Audit of post-operatively pain following day case surgery. British Journal of Nursing 7: 641–645.

Mahler, H.I.M. and Kulik, J.A. (1990) Preferences for health care involvement, perceived control and surgical recovery: A prospective study. Social Science and Medicine 31: 743–751.

Mahler, H.I.M. and Kulik, J.A. (1998) Effects of preparatory videotapes on self-efficacy beliefs and recovery from coronary bypass surgery. Annals of Behavioral Medicine 20(1): 39–46.

Mahler, H.I.M. and Kulik, J.A. (2000) Optimism, pessimism and recovery from coronary bypass surgery: Prediction of affect, pain and functional status. Psychology, Health and Medicine 5: 347–358.

Mahler, H.I.M. and Kulik, J.A. (2002) Effects of a videotape information intervention for spouses on spouse distress and patient recovery from surgery. Health Psychology 21: 427–437.

Mahler, H.I.M., Kulik, J.A. and Hill, M.R. (1993) A preliminary report on the effects of videotape preparations for coronary artery bypass surgery on anxiety and self-efficacy: A simulation and evaluation with college students. Basic and Applied Social Psychology 14: 437–453.

Male, C.G. (1981) Anxiety in day surgery patients. British Journal of Anaesthesia 53: 663pp.

Malin, N. and Teasdale, K. (1991) Caring versus empowerment: Considerations for nursing practice. Journal of Advanced Nursing 16: 657–662.

Malkin, K.F. (2000) Patients' perceptions of a pre-admission clinic. Journal of Nursing Management 8: 107–113.

Mallett, J. and Bailey, C. (1996) The Royal Marsden NHS Trust Manual of Clinical Nursing Procedures. London: Blackwell Science.

Malster, M. and Parry, A. (2000) Day Surgery. In: Manley, K. and Bellman, L. (eds), Surgical Nursing – Advancing Practice. London: Churchill Livingstone.

Malster, R.M.J., Schofield, S., Solly, J.E., Harris, P.I. and Sutton, A.M. (1998) From beginning to end: An audit of the patient's experience of day surgery. Journal of One Day Surgery 7(4): 18–21.

Man, A.K., Yap, J.C., Kwan, S.Y., Suen, K.L., Yip, H.S. and Chen, P.P. (2003) The effect of intra-operative video on patient anxiety. Anaesthesia 58: 64–68.

Manias, E. (2003) Pain and anxiety management in the post-operative gastro-surgical setting. Journal of Advanced Nursing 41: 585–594.

Manyande, A. and Salmon, P. (1992) Recovery from minor abdominal surgery: A preliminary attempt to separate anxiety and coping. British Journal of Clinical Psychology 31: 227–237.

Manyande, A., Chayen, S., Priyakumar, P. et al. (1992) Anxiety and endocrine responses to surgery: Paradoxical effects of pre-operative relaxation training. Psychosomatic Medicine 54: 275–287.

Manyande, A., Berg, S., Gettins, D. et al. (1995) Pre-operative rehearsal of active coping imagery influences subjective and hormonal responses to abdominal surgery. Psychosomatic Medicine 57: 177–182.

Maranets, I. and Kain, Z.N. (1999) Pre-operative anxiety and intra-operative anesthetic requirements. Anesthesia and Analgesia 89: 1346–1351.

Markanday, L. (1997) Day Surgery for Nurses. London: Whurr.

Markland, D. and Hardy, L. (1993) Anxiety, relaxation and anaesthesia for day case surgery. British Journal of Clinical Psychology 32: 493–504.

Markovic, M., Bandyopadhyay, M., Vu, T. and Manderson, L. (2002) Gynaecological day surgery and quality of care. Australian Health Review 25(3): 52–59.

Marquardt, H.M. and Razis, P.A. (1996) Pre-packed take-home analgesia for day case surgery. British Journal of Nursing 5: 1114–1118.

Marshall, S. and Chung, F. (1997) Assessment of 'home readiness': Discharge criteria and post-discharge complications. Ambulatory Anaesthesia 10: 445–450.

Martelli, M.F., Auerbach, S.M., Alexander, J. and Mercuri, L.G. (1987) Stress management in the health care setting: Matching interventions with patient coping styles. Journal of Consulting and Clinical Psychology 55: 201–207.

Martens-Lobenhoffer, J., Eisenhardt, S., Troger, U., Rose, W. and Meyer, F.P. (2001) The effect of anxiety and personality on the pharmacokinetics of oral midazolam. Anesthesia and Analgesia 92: 621-624.

Martikainen, M., Kangas-Saarela, T., Lopponen, A. and Salomaki, T. (2000) One-week recovery profiles after spinal, propofol, isoflurane and desflurane anaesthesia in ambulatory knee arthroscopy. Journal of Ambulatory Surgery 8: 139-142.

Martin, D. (1996) Pre-operative visits to reduce patient anxiety: A study. Nursing Standard 10(23): 33-38.

Mathews, A. and Ridgeway, V. (1981) Personality and surgical recovery: A review. British Journal of Clinical Psychology 20: 243-260.

Mathews, A. and Ridgeway, V. (1984) Psychological preparation for surgery. In: Steptoe, A., and Mathews, A. (eds), Health Care and Human Behaviour. London: Harcourt Brace Jovanovich, pp. 231-259.

Mavrias, R., Peck, C. and Coleman, G. (1990) The timing of pre-operative preparatory information. Psychology and Health 5: 39-45.

Mealy, K., Ngeh, N., Gillen, P., Fitzpatrick, G., Keane, F.B.V. and Tanner, A. (1996) Propranolol reduces the anxiety associated with day case surgery. European Journal of Surgery 162: 11-14.

Mechanic, D. (1980) The experience and reporting of common physical complaints. Journal of Health and Social Behaviour 21: 146-155.

Meeker, M.H. and Rothrock, J.C. (1999) Alexander's Care of the Patient in Surgery, 11th edn. London: Mosby.

Mehanna, H.M., Hattie, K., McLintock, T.T.C. and MacKenzie, K. (2001) Adult day-case tonsillectomy-a prospective study. Journal of One-Day Surgery 11(2): 10 -12.

Menon, N.K. (1998) Patient satisfaction with direct access vasectomy service. British Journal of Family Planning 24: 105-106.

Menon, S.T. (2002) Toward a model of psychological health empowerment: Implications for health care in multicultural communities. Nurse Education Today 22(1): 28-39.

Meredith, P. (1993) Patient satisfaction with communication in general surgery: Problems of measurement and improvement. Social Science and Medicine 37: 591-602.

Michaels, J.A., Reece-Smith, H. and Faber, R.G. (1992) Case-control study of patient satisfaction with day-case and in-patient inguinal hernia repair. Journal of the Royal College of Surgeons of Edinburgh 37(2): 99-100.

Milgram, S. (1974) Obedience to Authority. London: Tavistock.

Miller, G.E. and Cohen, S. (2001) Psychological interventions and the immune system: A meta-analytic review and critique. Health Psychology 20(1): 47-63.

Miller, S.M. (1980) When is a little information a dangerous thing? Coping with stressful events by monitoring versus blunting. In: Levine, S., and Ursin, H. (eds), Coping and Health. London: Plenum Press, pp. 145-169.

Miller, S.M. (1987) Monitoring and blunting: Validation of a questionnaire to assess styles of information seeking under threat. Journal of Personality and Social Psychology 52: 345-353.

Miller, S.M. and Mangan, C.E. (1983) Interacting effects of information and coping style in adapting to Gynaecologic stress: Should the doctor tell all? Journal of Personality and Social Psychology 45: 223-236.

Miller, S.M., Combs, C. and Stoddard, E. (1989) Information, coping and control in patients undergoing surgery and stressful medical procedures. In: Steptoe, A. and Appels, A. (eds), Personal Control and Health. Chichester: Wiley, pp. 107-130.

Miller, S.M., Rodoletz, M., Schroeder, C.M., Mangan, C.E. and Sedlacek, T.V. (1996) Applications of the monitoring process model to coping with severe long-term medical threats. Health Psychology 15: 216-225.

Miller, S.M., Mischel, W., Schroeder, C.M. et al. (1998) Intrusive and avoidant ideation among females pursuing infertility treatment. Psychology and Health 13: 847-858.

Mills, R.T. and Krantz, D.S. (1979) Information, choice and reactions to stress: A field experiment in a blood bank with laboratory analogue. Journal of Personality and Social Psychology 37: 608-620.

Miluk-Kolasa, B., Obminski, Z., Stupnicki, R. and Golec, L. (1994) Effects of music treatment on salivary cortisol in patients exposed to pre-surgical stress. Experimental and Clinical Endocrinology 102: 118-120.

Miluk-Kolasa, B., Matejek, M. and Stupnicki, R. (1996) The effects of music listening on changes in selected physiological parameters in adult pre-surgical patients. Journal of Music Therapy 33(3): 208-218.

Miluk-Kolasa, B., Klodecka, R.J. and Stupnicki, R. (2002) The effect of music listening on perioperative anxiety levels in adult surgical patients. Polish Psychological Bulletin 33(2): 55-60.

Minatti, W.R., Perriello, J., Dicaprio, M., Pierini, L. and Mendiburo, A. (2002) Postoperative outcomes in ambulatory surgery: Are they the same, worse or better? Journal of Ambulatory Surgery 10: 17-19.

Miro, J. and Raich, R.M. (1999a) Effects of a brief and economical intervention in preparing patients for surgery: Does coping style matter? Pain 83: 471-475.

Miro, J. and Raich, R.M. (1999b) Preoperative preparation for surgery: An analysis of the effects of relaxation and information provision. Clinical Psychology and Psychotherapy 6: 202-209.

Mishel, M.H. (1981) The measurement of uncertainty in illness. Nursing Research 30: 258-263.

Mitchell, M.J. (1994) Pre-operative and post-operative psychological nursing care. Surgical Nurse 7(3): 22-25.

Mitchell, M.J. (1997) Patients' perceptions of pre-operative preparation for day surgery. Journal of Advanced Nursing 26: 356-363.

Mitchell, M.J. (1999a) Patient's perceptions of day surgery: A literature review. Journal of Ambulatory Surgery 7: 65-73.

Mitchell, M.J. (1999b) Summary of studies into adult patient's perceptions of day surgery. Journal of Ambulatory Surgery 7: 75-100.

Mitchell, M.J. (2000) Psychological preparation for patients undergoing day surgery. International Journal of Nursing Studies 8(1): 19-29.

Mitchell, M.J. (2001) Constructing information booklets for day-case patients. Journal of Ambulatory Surgery 9: 37-45.

Mitchell, M.J. (2003a) Impact of discharge from day surgery on patients and carers. British Journal of Nursing 12: 402-408.

Mitchell, M.J. (2003b) Patient anxiety and modern elective surgery: A literature review. Journal of Clinical Nursing 12: 806-815.

Mitchell, M.J. (2004) Methodological challenges in the psychological study of recovery from modern surgery. Nurse Researcher 12(1): 64-75.

Mitchell, M.J. (2005) Nurse Education in Practice Journal. In press.

Mitchell, R.B., Kenyon, G.S. and Monks, P.S. (1999) A cost analysis of day-stay surgery in otolaryngology. Annals of the Royal College of Surgeons of England 82(suppl): 85-92.

Mitra, S., Bodzak, W. and Turner, A. (2003) The impact of day care surgery on general practitioner services: An update study. Journal of One-Day Surgery 13(1): 12-13.

Moerman, N., Van Dam, F.S.A.M. and Oosting, J. (1992) Recollections of general anaesthesia: A survey of anaesthesiological practice. Acta Anaesthesiologica Scandinavica 36: 767-771.

Moerman, N., Van Dam, F.S.A.M., Muller, M.J. and Oosting, H. (1996) The Amsterdam pre-operative anxiety and information scale. Anesthesia and Analgesia 82: 445-451.

Mogg, K., Mathews, A., Bird, C. and MacGregor-Morris, R. (1990) Effects of stress and anxiety on the processing of threat stimuli. Journal of Personality and Social Psychology 59: 1230-1237.

Mok, E. and Wong, K.Y. (2003) Effects of music on patient anxiety. American Operating Room Nurses' Journal 77: 396-410.

Montori, A. (1998) Minimally invasive surgery. Endoscopy 30: 244-252.

Moon, L.B. and Backer, J. (2000) Relationships among self-efficacy, outcome expectancy, and postoperative behaviors in total joint replacement patients. Orthopaedic Nursing 1(2): 77-85.

Moon, J.S. and Cho, K.S. (2001) The effects of handholding on anxiety in cataract surgery patients under local anaesthesia. Journal of Advanced Nursing 35: 407-415.

Moore, A. (2003) No problem. Nursing Standard 17(42): 16-17.

Moore, J., Ziebland, S. and Kennedy, S. (2002) 'People sometimes react funny if they're not told enough': Women's views about the risks of diagnostic laparoscopy. Health Expectations 5: 302-309.

Morales, R., Esteve, N., Casas, I. and Blanco, C. (2002) Why are ambulatory surgical patients admitted to hospital? Ambulatory Surgery 9: 197-205.

Morris, J. (1995) Monitoring post-operative effects in day-surgery. Nursing Times 91(10): 32-34.

Mott, A.M. (1999) Psychologic preparation to decrease anxiety associated with cardiac catheterisation. Journal of Vascular Nursing 17(2): 41-49.

Motyka, M., Motyka, H. and Wsolek, R. (1997) Elements of psychological support in nursing care. Journal of Advanced Nursing 26: 909-912.

Mukumba, S., Wright, M. and Punchihewa, V.G. (1996) Notes on a unlimited telephone helpline. Journal of One-Day Surgery 6(3): 14.

Mullen, B. and Suls, J. (1982) The effectiveness of attention and rejection as coping styles: A meta-analysis of temporal differences. Journal of Psychosomatic Research 26: 43-49.

Mumford, M.E. (1997) A descriptive study of the readability of patient information leaflets designed by nurses. Journal of Advanced Nursing 26: 985-991.

Mumford, E., Schlesinger, H.J. and Glass, G.V. (1982) The effects of psychological intervention on recovery from surgery and heart attacks: An analysis of the literature. American Journal of Public Health 72: 141-151.

Munafo, M.R. and Stevenson, J. (2003) Selective processing of threat-related cues in day surgery patients and prediction of post-operative pain. British Journal of Health Psychology 8: 439-449.

Murdoch, J.A.C. and Kenny, G.N.C. (1999) Patient-maintained propofol sedation as premedication in day-case surgery: Assessment of a target-controlled system. British Journal of Anaesthesia 82: 429-431.

Myles, P.S., Williams, D.L., Hendrata, M., Anderson, H. and Weeks, A.M. (2000) Patient satisfaction after anaesthesia and surgery: Results of a prospective survey of 10,811 patients. British Journal of Anaesthesia 84: 6-10.

Myles, P.S., Iacono, G.A., Hunt, J.O. et al. (2002) Risk of respiratory complications and wound infection in patients undergoing ambulatory surgery: smokers versus nonsmokers. Anesthesiology 97: 842-847.

Neale, J.M. and Liebert, R.M. (1986) Science and Behaviour: An introduction to methods of research, 3rd edn. London: Prentice-Hall.

Nettina, S.N. (1996) Lippincott Manual of Nursing Practice, 6th edn. Philadelphia: Lippincott.

NHS Management Executive (1993) Report by the Day Surgery Task Force. London: HMSO (updated in 1994).

NHS Management Executive (1996) Professional Roles in Anaesthetics: A scoping study. London: HMSO.

NHS Management Executive (2000) Professional Roles in Anaesthesia. London: Department of Health.

NHS Management Executive Value for Money Unit (1991) Day Surgery: Making it happen. London: HMSO.

NHS Modernisation Agency (2002) Operating Theatre and Pre-operative Assessment for Programme National Team. London: HMSO.

NHS Modernisation Agency (2003) Treatment Centres (www.modern.nhs.uk/treatmentcentres). London: HMSO.

NHS Modernisation Agency (2004) 10 High Impact Changes for Service Improvement and Delivery. London: HMSO.

Nichols, K.A. (1985) Psychological care by nurses, paramedical and medical staff: Essential developments for general hospitals. British Journal of Medical Psychology 58: 231–240.

Nielsen, K.C., Greengrass, R.A., Pietrobon, R., Klein, S.M. and Steele, S.M. (2003) Continuous interscalene brachial plexus blockade provides good analgesia at home after major shoulder surgery-report of four cases. Canadian Journal of Anaesthesia 50(1): 57–61.

Nilsson, U., Rawal, N., Unestahl, L.E., Zetterberg, C. and Unosson, M. (2001) Improved recovery after music and therapeutic suggestions during general anaesthesia: A double-blind randomised controlled trial. Acta Anaesthesiologica Scandinavica 45: 812–817.

Nishimori, M., Moerman, N., Fukuhara, S. et al. (2002) Translation and validation of the Amsterdam pre-operative anxiety and information scale (APAIS) for use in Japan. Quality of Life Research 11: 361–364.

Nkyekyer, K. (1996) Day-case laparoscopy in a Ghanaian teaching hospital: the patients' perspective. Tropical Doctor 26(4): 147–150.

Noon, B.E. and Davero, C.C. (1987) Patient satisfaction in a hospital-based day surgery setting. American Operating Room Nurses' Journal 46: 306–312.

Nyamathi, A. and Kashiwabara, A. (1988) Pre-operative anxiety. Association of Operating Room Nurses' Journal 47(1): 164–169.

O'Connor, S.J., Gibberd, R.W. and West, P. (1991) Patient satisfaction with day surgery. Australian Clinical Review 11(4): 143–149.

O'Hara, M.W., Ghoneim, M.M., Hinrichs, J.V., Mehta, M.P. and Wright, E.J. (1989) Psychological consequences of surgery. Psychosomatic Medicine 51: 356–370.

O'Neill, O. (2002) The efficacy of music therapy on patient recovery in the post-anaesthetic care unit. Journal of Advanced Perioperative Care 1(1): 19–26.

Oberle, K., Allen, M. and Lynkowski, P. (1994) Follow up of same day surgery patients: A study of patient concerns. Association of Operating Room Nurses' Journal 59: 1016–1018, 1021–1025.

Oetker-Black, S.L., Teeters, D.L., Cukr, P.L. and Rininger, S.A. (1997) Self-efficacy enhanced preoperative instruction. American Operating Room Nurses' Journal 66: 854–861.

Ong, E.L., Chiu, J.W., Chong, J.L. and Kwan, K.M. (2000) Volatile induction and maintenance (VIMA) versus total intravenous anaesthesia (TIVA) for minor gynaecological procedures. Journal of Ambulatory Surgery 8: 37–40.

Oordt, M.S. (2001) Managing severe gas mask anxiety with a cognitive-behavioural approach: An illustrative case study and treatment protocol. Military Psychology 13: 165–176.

Ormrod, G. and Casey, D. (2004) The educational preparation of nursing staff undertaking pre-assessment of surgical patients – a discussion of the issues. Nurse Education Today 24: 269–276.

Otte, D.I. (1996) Patients' perspectives and experiences of day surgery. Journal of Advanced Nursing 23: 1228–1237.

Padilla, G.V., Grant, M.M., Rains, B.L. et al. (1981) Distress reduction and the effects of preparatory teaching films and patient control. Research in Nursing and Health 4: 375–387.

Papanikolaou, M.N., Voulgari, A., Lykouras, L. et al. (1994) Psychological factors influencing the surgical patients' consent to regional anaesthesia. Acta Anaesthesiologica Scandinavica 38: 607–611.

Parahoo, K. (1997) Nursing Research: Principles, process and issues. London: Macmillan.

Parent, N. and Fortin, F. (2000) A randomized, controlled trial of vicarious experience through peer support for male first-time cardiac surgery patients: impact on anxiety, self-efficacy expectation, and self-reported activity. Heart and Lung: Journal of Acute and Critical Care 29: 389–400.

Parlow, J.L., Meikle, A.T., van Vlymen, J. and Avery, N. (1999) Post-operative nausea and vomiting after ambulatory laparoscopy is not reduced by promethazine prophylaxis. Canadian Journal of Anaesthesia 46: 719–724.

Parsons, E.C., Kee, C.C. and Gray, P. (1993) Peri-operative nursing caring behaviours. Association of Operating Room Nurses' Journal 57: 1106-1114.

Peerbhoy, D., Hall, G.M., Parker, C., Shenkin, A. and Salmon, P. (1998) Patients' reactions to attempts to increase passive or active coping with surgery. Social Science and Medicine 47: 595-601.

Pellino, T., Tluczek, A., Collins, M. et al. (1998) Increasing self-efficacy through empowerment: preoperative education for orthopaedic patients. Orthopaedic Nursing 17(4): 48-59.

Perez, E.M., Barriga, R., Rodriguez, M.A., Larranaga, E., Figueroa, J.M. and Serrano, P.A. (2000) Ambulatory surgery for groin hernia: The Gilbert repair. Journal of Ambulatory Surgery 8: 135-138.

Peterson, C. and Stunkard, A.J. (1989) Personal control and health promotion. Social Science and Medicine 28: 819-828.

Petticrew, M., Black, N.A. and Moore, L. (1995) Day surgery dilatation and curettage: Patients' experiences. Journal of Ambulatory Surgery 3: 185-188.

Pfisterer, M., Ernst, E.M., Hirlekar, G. et al. (2001) Post-operative nausea and vomiting in patients undergoing day-case surgery: An international, observational study. Journal of Ambulatory Surgery 9: 13-18.

Philip, B.K. (1992) Patients' assessment of ambulatory anaesthesia and surgery. Journal of Clinical Anaesthesiology 4: 355-358.

Pickett, C. and Clum, G.A. (1982) Comparative treatment strategies and their interaction with locus of control in the reduction of post-surgical pain and anxiety. Journal of Consulting and Clinical Psychology 50: 439-441.

Pineault, R., Contandriopoulos, A-P., Valois, M., Bastian, M-L. and Lance, J-M. (1985) Randomised clinical trial of one-day surgery: Patient satisfaction, clinical outcomes and costs. Medical Care 23: 171-182.

Pollard, J.A. (2004) Responding to the market in a surgicentre. Journal of One-Day Surgery 14(3): 79-80.

Pollock, I. and Trendholm, J. (1997) All in a day's work. Which?: Independent Consumer Guide February: 14-17.

Poole, E.L. (1993) The effects of post-anesthesia care unit visits on anxiety in surgical patients. Journal of Post-Anesthesia Nursing 8: 386-394.

Price, J. and Leaver, L. (2002) ABC of psychological medicine: Beginning treatment. British Medical Journal 325: 33-35.

Priest, H.M. (1999) Psychological care in nursing education and practice: A search for definition and dimensions. Nurse Education Today 19(1): 71-78.

Purhonen, S., Turunen, M., Ruohoaho, U.M., Niskanen, M. and Hynynen, M. (2003) Supplemental oxygen does not reduce the incidence of postoperative nausea and vomiting after ambulatory gynecologic laparoscopy. Anesthesia and Analgesia 96: 91-96.

Radcliffe, S. (1993) Pre-operative information: The role of the ward nurse. British Journal of Nursing 2: 305-309.

Raftery, J. and Stevens, A. (1998) Day case surgery trends in England: The influences of target settings and of general practitioner fundholding. Journal of Health Service Research Policy 3: 149-152.

Rai, M.R. and Pandit, J.J. (2003) Day of surgery cancellations after nurse-led pre-assessment in an elective surgical centre: The first 2 years. Anaesthesia 58: 692-699.

Raikkonen, K., Mathews, K.A., Flory, J.D., Owens, J.F. and Gump, B.B. (1999) Effects of optimism, pessimism, and trait anxiety on ambulatory blood pressure and mood during everyday life. Journal of Personality and Social Psychology 76: 104-113.

Ramachandra, V. (1994) Day surgery pain. Journal of One-Day Surgery 3(4): 14-15.

Ramsay, M.A. E. (1972) A survey of pre-operative fear. Anaesthesia 27: 396-402.

Ratcliffe, F., Lawson, R. and Millar, J. (1994) Day-case laparoscopy revisited: Have post-operative morbidity and patient acceptance improved? Health Trends 26(2): 47-49.

Rawal, N., Hylander, J., Nydahl, P.A., Olofsson, I. and Gupta, A. (1997) Survey of post-operative analgesia following ambulatory surgery. Acta Anaesthesiologica Scandinavica 41: 1017-1022.

Rawal, N., Allvin, R., Axelsson, K. et al. (2002) Patient-controlled regional analgesia (PCRA) at home: Controlled comparison between bupivacaine and ropivacaine brachial plexus analgesia. Anesthesiology 96: 1290-1296.

Ray, C. and Fitzgibbon, G. (1981) Stress arousal and coping with surgery. Psychological Medicine 11: 741-746.

Read, D. (1990) Day surgery: A consumer survey. New Zealand Medical Journal 103: 369-371.

Recart, A., Issioui, T., White, P.F. et al. (2003) The efficacy of celecoxib premedication on postoperative pain and recovery times after ambulatory surgery: A dose-ranging study. Anesthesia and Analgesia 96: 1631-1635.

Redman, B.K. (1993) Patient education at 25 years: Where we have been and where we are going. Journal of Advanced Nursing 18: 725-730.

Rees, S. and Tagoe, M. (2002) The efficacy and tolerance of local anaesthesia without sedation for foot surgery. Foot 12: 188-192.

Reid, J.H. (1997) Meeting the informational needs of patients in a day surgery setting: An exploratory level study. British Journal of Theatre Nursing 7(4): 19-24.

Richert, A.J. (1981) Sex differences in relation of locus of control and reported anxiety. Psychological Reports 49: 971-974.

Ridgeway, V. and Mathews, A. (1982) Psychological preparation for surgery: A comparison of methods. British Journal of Clinical Psychology 21: 271-280.

Ridner, S.H. (2004) Psychological distress: Concept analysis. Journal of Advanced Nursing 45: 536-545.

Robaux, S., Bouaziz, H., Cornet, C., Boivin, J.M., Lefevre, N. and Laxenaire, M.C. (2002) Acute post-operative pain management at home after ambulatory surgery: A French pilot survey of general practitioners. Anesthesia and Analgesia 95: 1258-1262.

Robins, K., McManus, E. and Jackson, I. (2000) Audit-Safety of analgesic prescribing in day case surgery. Journal of One-Day Surgery 9(3): 18-19.

Rogers, M. and Reich, P. (1986) Psychological intervention with surgical patients. Advanced Psychosomatic Medicine 15: 23-50.

Rosdahl, C.B. and Kowalski, M.T. (2003) Textbook of Basic Nursing, 8th edn. London: Lippincott Williams & Wilkins.

Rose, K., Waterman, H., Toon, L., McLeod, D. and Tullow, A. (1999) Organising day surgery for cataract: Selecting the outcome measures. Ophthalmic Nursing: International Journal of Ophthalmic Nursing 2(4): 14-20.

Rosenbaum, M. and Piamenta, R. (1998) Preference for local or general anesthesia, coping dispositions, learned resourcefulness and coping with surgery. Psychology and Health 13: 823-845.

Roth, S. and Cohen, L.J. (1986) Approach, avoidance, and coping with stress. American Psychologist 41: 813-819.

Rothrock, J.C. (1989) Peri-operative nursing research. Part I: Pre-operative psycho-educational interventions. Association of Operating Room Nurses' Journal 49: 597-619.

Rotter, J. (1966) Generalised expectancies for internal vs. external control of reinforcement. Psychological Monographs 80(1): 1-26.

Royal College of Surgeons of England (1992) Guidelines for Day Case Surgery. London: HMSO.

Royal College of Surgeons of England and East Anglia Regional Health Authority (1995) New Angles on Day Surgery. NHS Executive: East Anglian Regional Clinical Audit Office.

Royal College of Surgeons of England and Royal College of Nursing (1999) Assistants in Surgical Practice: A discussion document. London: Royal College of Surgeons.

Royal College of Surgeons of England and Royal College of Psychiatrists (1997) Report on the Working Party on the Psychological Care of Surgical Patients (CR55). London: RCS and RCP.

Ruckley, C.V., Garraway, W.M., Cuthbertson, C., Fenwick, N. and Prescott, R.J. (1980) The community nurse and day surgery. Nursing Times 76: 255–256.

Rudkin, G.E., Bacon, A.K., Burrow, B. et al. (1996) Review of efficiencies and patient satisfaction in Australian and New Zealand day surgery units: A pilot study. Anaesthesia and Intensive Care 24: 74–78.

Rudolfsson, G., Hallberg, L.R.M., Ringsberg, K.C. and von Post, I. (2003a) The nurse has time for me: The perioperative dialogue from the perspective of patients. Journal of Advanced Perioperative Care 1(3): 77–84.

Rudolfsson, G., Ringsberg, K.C. and von Post, I. (2003b) A source of strength – nurses' perspectives of the perioperative dialogue. Journal of Nursing Management 11: 250–257.

Russell, I.T., Devlin, H.B., Fell, M., Glass, N.J. and Newell, D.J. (1977) Day-case surgery for hernias and haemorrhoids. Lancet i: 844–847.

Ruuth-Setala, A., Leino-Kilpi, H. and Suominen, T. (2000) How do I manage at home? Where do Finnish short-stay patients turn for help, support and company after discharge, and why? Journal of One-Day Surgery 10(1): 15–18.

Ryan, D.W. (1975) A questionnaire survey of pre-operative fears. British Journal of Clinical Practice 29: 3–6.

Salmon, P. (1992a) Psychological factors in surgical stress: Implications for management. Clinical Psychology Review 12: 681–704.

Salmon, P. (1992b) Surgery as a psychological stressor: Paradoxical effects of pre-operative emotional state on endocrine response. Stress Medicine 8: 193–198.

Salmon, P. (1993) The reduction of anxiety in surgical patients: An important nursing task of medicalisation of preparatory worry. International Journal of Nursing Studies 30: 323–330.

Salmon, P. and Hall, G.M. (1997) A theory of post-operative fatigue. Journal of the Royal Society of Medicine 90: 661–664.

Salmon, P., Evans, R. and Humphrey, D.E. (1986) Anxiety and endocrine changes in surgical patients. British Journal of Clinical Psychology 25: 135–141.

Salmon, P., Shah, R., Berg, S. and Williams, C. (1994) Evaluating customer satisfaction with colonoscopy. Endoscopy 26: 342–346.

Salvage, J. (1990) The theory and practice of the 'New nursing'. Nursing Times 86(1): 42–45.

Sanderson, I.M. (1998) The clinical negligence scheme for trusts: A review of its present function. Clinical Risk 4(2): 35–43.

Sandin, R.H., Enlund, G., Samuelsson, P. and Lennarken, C. (2000) Awareness during anaesthesia: A prospective case study. Lancet 355: 707–711.

Scheier, M.F. and Carver, C.S. (1992) Effects of optimism on psychological and physical well-being: Theoretical overview and empirical update. Cognitive Therapy and Research 16: 201–228.

Schoessler, M. (1989) Perceptions of pre-operative education in patients admitted the morning of surgery. Patient Education and Counseling 14: 127–136.

Schroder, K.E.E. and Schwarzer, R. (1998) Coping as a mediator from recovery from cardiac surgery. Psychology and Health 13(1): 83–97.

Schultz, A.A., Andrews, A.L., Goran, S.F., Mathew, T. and Sturdevant, N. (2003) Comparison of acupressure bands and droperidol for reducing post-operative nausea and vomiting in gynecologic surgery patients. Applied Nursing Research 16: 256–265.

Schwartz-Barcott, D., Fortin, J.D. and Kim, H.S. (1994) Client/Nurse interaction: Testing for its impact on pre-operative instruction. International Journal of Nursing Studies 31: 23–35.

Schwarz, N., Banditt, P., Gerlach, K.L. and Meyer, F.P. (2002) Absorption kinetics of paracetamol are not influenced by high anxiety levels in preoperative patients. International Journal of Clinical Pharmacology and Therapeutics 40: 419–421.

Schweizer, K., Beck-Seyffer, A. and Schneider, R. (1999) Cognitive bias of optimism and its influence on well-being. Psychological Reports 84: 627–636.

Schwender, D., Kunze-Kronawitter, H., Dietrich, P., Klasing, S., Forst, H. and Madler, C. (1998) Conscious awareness during general anaesthesia: Patients' perceptions, emotions, cognition and reactions. British Journal of Anaesthesia 80: 133-139.

Scioli, A., Chamberlin, C.M., Samor, C.M., Lapointe, A.B., Campbell, T.L. and Macleod, A.R. (1997) A prospective study of hope, optimism and health. Psychological Reports 81(Part 1): 723-733.

Scriven, A. and Tucker, C. (1997) The quality and management of written information presented to women undergoing hysterectomy. Journal of Clinical Nursing 6(2): 107-113.

Seeman, M. and Seeman, T.E. (1983) Health behaviour and personal autonomy: A longitudinal study of the sense of control in illness. Journal of Health and Social Behaviour 24: 144-160.

Segerstrom, S.C., Taylor, S.E., Kemeny, M.E. and Fahey, J.L. (1998) Optimism is associated with mood, coping and immune change in response to stress. Journal of Personality and Social Psychology 74: 1646-1655.

Shafer, A., Fish, M.P., Gregg, K.M., Seavello, J. and Kosek, P. (1996) Preoperative anxiety and fear: A comparison of assessments by patients and anesthesia and surgery residents. Anesthesia and Analgesia 83: 1285-1291.

Shaw, C., McColl, E. and Bond, S. (2003) The relationship of perceived control to outcomes in older women undergoing surgery for fractured neck of femur. Journal of Clinical Nursing 12(1): 117-123.

Sherman, A., Higgs, G.E. and Williams, R.L. (1997) Gender differences in the locus of control construct. Psychology and Health 12: 239-248.

Shertzer, K.E. and Keck, J.F. (2001) Music and the PACU environment. Journal of Peri-Anesthesia Nursing 16: 90-102.

Shevde, K. and Panagopoulos, G. (1991) A survey of 800 patients' knowledge, attitudes, and concerns regarding anesthesia. Anesthesia and Analgesia 73: 190-198.

Shipley, R.H., Butt, J.H., Horwitz, B. and Farbry, J.E. (1978) Preparation for a stressful medical procedure: Effect of amount of stimulus pre-exposure and coping style. Journal of Consulting and Clinical Psychology 46: 499-507.

Shipley, R.H., Butt, J.H. and Horwitz, B. (1979) Preparation to re-experience a stressful medical examination: Effect of repetitious videotape exposure and coping style. Journal of Consulting and Clinical Psychology 47: 485-492.

Shuldham, C. (1999a) A review of the impact of pre-operative education on recovery from surgery. International Journal of Nursing Studies 36: 171-177.

Shuldham, C. (1999b) Pre-operative education-a review of the research design. International Journal of Nursing Studies 36: 179-187.

Shuldham, C.M., Cunningham, G., Hiscock, M. and Luscombe, P. (1995) Assessment of anxiety in hospital patients. Journal of Advanced Nursing 22(1): 87-93.

Siew, L.B., Ling, S.M., Aziz, S.B. and Chin, Y.S. (2000) A descriptive and comparative study of preoperative teaching on patient's satisfaction, self-efficacy and anxiety levels in elective surgical patients. Professional Nurse (Singapore) 27(2): 37-39.

Sigurdardottir, A.K. (1996) Satisfaction among ambulatory surgery patients in two hospitals in Iceland. Journal of Nursing Management 4(2): 69-74.

Sime, A.M. (1976) Relationship of pre-operative fear, type of coping, and information received about surgery to recovery from surgery. Journal of Personality and Social Psychology 34: 716-724.

Singleton, R.J., Rudkin, G.E., Osborne, G.A., S., W.D. and Williams, J.A.R. (1996) Laparoscopic cholecystectomy as a day surgery procedure. Anaesthesia and Intensive Care 24: 231-236.

Smith, A.F. and Pittaway, A.J. (2002) Premedication for anxiety in adult day surgery (Cochrane Review). In: The Cochrane Library - Issue 3. Oxford: Update Software.

Smith, A.R. (2000) Post-operative complications following minimal access surgery. Best Practice and Research in Clinical Obstetrics and Gynecology 14: 123-132.

Smith, J. (1998) Patient satisfaction survey: Inguinal hernia repair performed in a primary setting. Journal of One-Day Surgery 8(1): 10-16.

Smith, R. and Draper, P. (1994) Who is in control? An investigation of nurse and patient beliefs relating to control of their health care. Journal of Advanced Nursing 19: 884-892.

Snyder, M. and Chlan, L. (1999) Music therapy. Annual Review of Nursing Research 17(1): 3-25.

Spector, P.E. and Sistrunk, F. (1979) Reassurance: A mechanism by which the presence of others reduces anxiety. Journal of Social Psychology 109: 119-126.

Spielberger, C.D., Gorsuch, R.L., Lushene, R., Vagg, P.R. and Jacobs, G.A. (1983) Manual for the State-Trait Anxiety Inventory for Adults. Palo Alto, CA: Consulting Psychologists Press.

Spitellie, P.H., Holmes, M.A. and Dommino, K.B. (2002) Awareness during anesthesia. Anesthesiology Clinics of North America 20: 317-332.

Spitzer, A. (1998) Moving into the information era: Does the current nursing paradigm still hold? Journal of Advanced Nursing 28: 786-793.

Stanley, B.M., Walters, D.J. and Maddern, G.J. (1998) Informed consent: How much information is enough? Australian and New Zealand Journal of Surgery 68: 788-791.

Steelman, V.M. (1990) Intra-operative music therapy. American operating Room Nurses' Journal 52: 1026-1034.

Stengrevics, S., Sirois, C., Schwartz, C.E., Friedman, R. and Domar, A.D. (1996) The prediction of cardiac surgery outcome based upon pre-operative psychological factors. Psychology and Health 11: 471-477.

Stephenson, M.E. (1990) Discharge criteria in day surgery. Journal of Advanced Nursing 15: 601-613.

Stephenson, P. (2002) In a day's work. Health Service Journal 112: 9-10.

Stevens, K. (1990) Patients' perceptions of music during surgery. Journal of Advanced Nursing 15: 1045-1051.

Stevens, J., van de Mortel, T. and Leighton, D. (2001) Generating theory from the client's experience of same day laparoscopic sterilisation. Australian Journal of Holistic Nursing 8(1): 23-30.

Stockdale, A. and Bellman, M. (1998) An audit of post-operative pain and nausea in day case surgery. European Journal of Anaesthesiology 15: 271-274.

Storm, H., Myre, K., Rostrup, M., Stokland, O., Lien, M.D. and Raeder, J.C. (2002) Skin conductance correlates with peri-operative stress. Acta Anaesthesiologica Scandinavica 46: 887-895.

Strickland, B.R. (1978) Internal-external expectancies and health related behaviours. Journal of Consulting and Clinical Psychology 46: 1192-1211.

Strull, W.M., Lo, B. and Charles, G. (1984) Do patients want to participate in medical decision making? Journal of the American Medical Association 252: 2990-2994.

Suls, J. and Fletcher, B. (1985) The relative efficacy of avoidant and nonavoidant coping strategies: A meta analysis. Health Psychology 4: 249-288.

Suls, J. and Wan, C.K. (1989) Effects of sensory and procedural information on coping with stressful medical procedures and pain: A meta analysis. Journal of Consulting and Clinical Psychology 57: 372-379.

Suls, J., David, J.P. and Harvey, J.H. (1996) Personality and coping: three generations of research. Journal of Personality and Clinical Studies 64: 711-735.

Swindale, J.E. (1989) The nurse's role in giving pre-operative information to reduce anxiety in patients admitted to hospital for elective minor surgery. Journal of Advanced Nursing 14: 899-905.

Tang, J., Chen, X., White, P.F. et al. (2003) Antiemetic prophylaxis for office-based surgery: Are the 5-HT3 receptor antagonists beneficial? Anesthesiology 98: 293-298.

Taylor, S.E. and Lobel, M. (1989) Social comparison activity under threat: Downward evaluation and upward contacts. Psychological Review 96: 569-575.

Teasdale, K. (1989) The concept of reassurance in nursing. Journal of Advanced Nursing 14: 444-450.

Teasdale, K. (1993) Information and anxiety: A critical reappraisal. Journal of Advanced Nursing 18: 1125-1132.

Teasdale, K. (1995a) The nurse's role in anxiety management. Professional Nurse 10: 509–512.

Teasdale, K. (1995b) Theoretical and practical considerations on the use of reassurance in the nursing management of anxious patients. Journal of Advanced Nursing 22(1): 79–86.

Thagaard, K.S., Steine, S. and Raeder, J. (2003) Ondansetron disintegrating tablets of 8 mg twice a day for 3 days did not reduce the incidence of nausea or vomiting after laparoscopic surgery. European Journal of Anaesthesiology 20: 153–157.

Thapar, P., Korttila, K.T. and Apfelbaum, J.L. (1994) Assessing recovery after day-case surgery. Current Anaesthesia and Critical Care 5: 155–159.

Thatcher, J. (1996) Follow-up after day surgery: How well do patients cope? Nursing Times 92(37): 30–32.

Thomas, J.J. (1995) Reducing anxiety during phase I cardiac rehabilitation. Journal of Psychosomatic Research 39: 295–304.

Thomas, H. and Hare, M.J. (1987) Day case laparoscopic sterilisation–time for a rethink. British Journal of Obstetrics and Gynaecology 94: 445–448.

Thomas, S., Singh, J., Bishnoi, P.K. and Kumar, A. (2001) Feasibility of day-care open cholecystectomy: Evaluation in an in-patient model. Australia and New Zealand Journal of Surgery 71(2): 93–97.

Thompson, K., Melby, V., Parahoo, K., Ridley, T. and Humphreys, W.G. (2003) Information provided to patients undergoing gastroscopy procedures. Journal of Clinical Nursing 12: 899–911.

Thoms, G.M., McHugh, G.A. and Lack, J.A. (2002) What information do anaesthetists provide for patients? British Journal of Anaesthesia 89: 917–919.

Thomson, P.J., Fletcher, I.R., Briggs, S., Barthram, D. and Cato, G. (2003) Patient morbidity following oral day surgery–use of a post-operative telephone questionnaire. Journal of Ambulatory Surgery 10: 122–127.

Tierney, A.J., Worth, A. and Watson, N. (1999) Informational needs pre- and post-discharge: A qualitative study of the perceptions and experiences of patients and carers. Report to the NHS Executive Research and Development Programme – Primary and secondary interface. University of Edinburgh.

Tix, A.P. and Frazier, P.A. (1998) The use of religious coping during stressful life events: Main effects, moderation and mediation. Journal of Consulting and Clinical Psychology 66: 411–422.

Tong, D. and Chung, F. (1999) Post-operative pain control in ambulatory surgery. Surgical Clinics of North America 79: 401–430.

Tongue, B. and Stanley, I. (1991) A video-based information system for patients. Health Trends 23(1): 11–12.

Towey, R.M., Stanford, B.J., Ballard, R.M. and Gilbert, J.R. (1979) Morbidity of day-case gynaecological surgery. British Journal of Anaesthesia 51: 453–455.

Towse, A. and Danzon, P. (1999) Medical negligence and the NHS: an economic analysis. Health Economics 8(2): 93–101.

Trimm, D. (1997) Spousal coping during the surgical wait. Journal of Peri-Anesthesia Nursing 12: 141–151.

Tromp, F., van Dulmen, S. and van Weert, J. (2004) Interdisciplinary pre-operative patient education in cardiac surgery. Journal of Advanced Nursing 47: 212–222.

Ture, H., Eti, Z., Adil, M., Kara, O.F. and Gogus, Y. (2003) The incidence of side effects and their relation with anesthetic techniques after ambulatory surgery. Journal of Ambulatory Surgery 10: 155–159.

Tusek, D., Church, J.M. and Fazio, V.W. (1997) Guided imagery as a coping strategy for perioperative patients. American Operating Room Nurses' Journal 66: 644–649.

Van Balen, F. and Verdurmen, J. (1999) Medical anxiety and the choice for treatment: The development of an instrument to measure fear of treatment. Psychology and Health 14: 927–935.

van den Berg, A.A. (2003) Towards needleless induction of anaesthesia. Anaesthesia 58: 806–807.

van der Zee, K.I., Huet, R.C., Gallandat, Cazemier, C. and Evers, K. (2002) The influence of the premedication consult and preparatory information about anesthesia on anxiety among patients undergoing cardiac surgery. Anxiety, Stress and Coping 15: 123-133.

van Weert, J., van Dulmen, S., Baer, P. and Venus, E. (2003) Interdisciplinary preoperative patient education in cardiac surgery. Patient Education and Counselling 49: 105-114.

Van Wijk, M.G.F. and Smalhout, B. (1990) A postoperative analysis of the patient's view of anaesthesia in a Netherlands' teaching hospital. Anaesthesia 45: 679-682.

Vilos, G.A. (2002) Laparoscopic bowel injuries: Forty litigated gynaecological cases in Canada. Journal of Obstetrics and Gynaecology Canada 24: 224-230.

Vogele, C. and Steptoe, A. (1986) Physiological and subjective stress responses in surgical patients. Journal of Psychosomatic Research 30: 205-215.

Vogelsang, J. (1990) Continued contact with a familiar nurse affects women's perceptions of the ambulatory surgical experience: A qualitative-quantitative design. Journal of Post-Anaesthetic Nursing 5: 315-320.

Volicer, B.J. (1973) Perceived stress levels of events associated with the experience of hospitalisation: Development and testing of a measurement tool. Nursing Research 22: 491-497.

Volicer, B.J. and Bohannon, W.M. (1975) A hospital stress rating scale. Nursing Research 24: 352-359.

Voulgari, A., Papanikolaou, M.N., Lykouras, L., Alevizos, B., Alexiou, E. and Christodoulou, G.N. (1994) Prevention of post-operative anxiety and depression. Bibliotheca Psychiatric 165: 49-55.

Waisel, D.B. and Truog, R.D. (1995) The benefits of the explanation of risks of anaesthesia in the day surgery patient. Journal of Clinical Anesthesia 7: 200-204.

Walker, J.A. (2002) Emotional and psychological pre-operative preparation in adults. British Journal of Nursing 11: 567-575.

Walker, J.A., McIntyre, R.D., Schleinitz, P.F. et al. (2003) Nurse-administered propofol sedation without anesthesia specialists in 9152 endoscopic cases in an ambulatory surgery center. American Journal of Gastroenterology 98: 1744-1750.

Wallace, L.M. (1984) Psychological preparation as a method of reducing the stress of surgery. Journal of Human Stress 10(2): 62-77.

Wallace, L.M. (1986a) Communication variables in the design of pre-surgical preparatory information. British Journal of Clinical Psychology 25: 111-118.

Wallace, L.M. (1986b) Pre-operative state anxiety as a mediator of psychological adjustment to and recovery from surgery. British Journal of Medical Psychology 59: 253-261.

Wallace, L.M. (1986c) Day-case laparoscopy: Patient preferences, adjustment and management. Journal of Psychosomatic Obstetrics and Gynecology 5: 207-216.

Wallston, K.A., Malcarne, V.L., Flores, L. et al. (1999) Does god determine your health? The god locus of health control scale. Cognitive Therapy and Research 23: 131-142.

Walsgrove, H. (2004) Piloting a nurse-led gynaecology pre-operative assessment clinic. Nursing Times 100(3): 38-41.

Walsh, D. and Shaw, D.G. (2000) The design of written information for cardiac patients: A review of the literature. Journal of Clinical Nursing 9: 658-667.

Wang, S-M., Peloquin, C. and Kain, Z.N. (2001) The use of auricular acupuncture to reduce pre-operative anxiety. Anesthesia and Analgesia 93: 1178-1180.

Wang, S-M., Kulkarni, L., Dolev, J. and Kain, Z.N. (2002) Music and preoperative anxiety: A randomized, controlled study. Anesthesia and Analgesia 94: 1489-1494.

Watson, B. and Allen, J.G. (2003) Spinal anaesthesia in day surgery – an audit of the first 400 cases. Journal of One-Day Surgery 12(4): 59-62.

Watt-Watson, J., Chung, F., Chan, V.W.S. and McGillion, M. (2004) Pain management following discharge after ambulatory same-day surgery. Journal of Nursing Management 12: 153-161.

Webb, C. and Hope, K. (1995) What kind of nurses do patients want? Journal of Clinical Nursing 4: 101-108.

Webber, G.C. (1990) Patient Education: A Review of the Issues. Medical Care 28(Part 2): 1089-1103.

Wedderburn, A.W., Morris, G.E. and Dodds, S.R. (1996) A survey of post-operative care after day case surgery. Annals of the Royal College of Surgeons of England 78(2): 70-71.

Wells, J.K., Howard, G.S., Nowlin, W.F. and Vargas, M.J. (1986) Pre-surgical anxiety and post-surgical pain and adjustment: Effects of a stress inoculation procedure. Journal of Consulting and Clinical Psychology 54: 831-835.

Weltz, C.R., Klein, S.M., Arbo, J.E. and Greengrass, R.A. (2003) Paravertebral block anesthesia for inguinal hernia repair. World Journal of Surgery 27: 425-429.

Wicklin, N. and Forster, J. (1994) The effects of a personal versus a factual approach video-tape on the level of pre-operative anxiety of same day surgery patients. Patient Education and Counselling 23(2): 107-114.

Wikinski, S., Lombardo, M., Medina, J.H. and Rubio, M.C. (1994) Lack of anxiolytic effect of diazepam in pre-anaesthetic medication. British Journal of Anaesthesia 72: 694-696.

Wilkinson, D., Bristow, A. and Higgins, D. (1992) Morbidity following day surgery. Journal of One-Day Surgery 2(1): 5-6.

Williams, R.D. and Clark, A.J. (2000) A qualitative study of women's hysterectomy experience. Journal of Women's Health and Gender Based Medicine 9(2): S15-S25.

Williams, A., Ching, M. and Loader, J. (2003) Assessing patient satisfaction with day surgery at a metropolitan public hospital. Australian Journal of Advanced Nursing 21(1): 35-41.

Willis, C.E., Watson, J.D., Harper, C.V. and Humphreys, W.G. (1997) Does day surgery embarrass the primary health care team?: An audit of complications and consultations. Journal of Ambulatory Surgery 5(2): 71-75.

Willsher, P.C., Urbach, G., Cole, D., Schumacher, S. and Litwin, D.E.M. (1998) Outpatient laparoscopic surgery. Australia and New Zealand Journal of Surgery 68: 769-773.

Wilson, J.F. (1981) Behavioural preparation for surgery: Benefit or harm? Journal of Behavioural Medicine 4(1): 79-102.

Wilson-Barnett, J. (1976) Patient's emotional reactions to hospitalisation: An exploratory study. Journal of Advanced Nursing 1: 351-358.

Wilson-Barnett, J. (1984) Interventions to alleviate patients' stress: A review. Journal of Psychosomatic Research 28(1): 63-72.

Winter, M., J., Paskin, S. and Baker, T. (1994) Music reduces stress and anxiety of patients in the surgical holding area. Journal of Post-Anesthesia Nursing 9: 340-343.

Winwood, M.A. and Jago, R.H. (1993) Anxiety levels following anaesthesia for day case surgery. Anaesthesia 48: 581-584.

Wittenberg, M.I., Lark, T.L., Butler, C.L. et al. (1998) Effects of oral diazepam on intravenous access in same day surgery patients. Journal of Clinical Anesthesia 10(1): 13-16.

Wolfer, J.A. and Davies, C.E. (1970) Assessment of surgical patients' pre-operative emotional condition and post-operative welfare. Nursing Research 19: 402-414.

Woodhouse, M., King, T.A. and Challiner, A. (1998) Impact of day surgery on community services. Journal of One-Day Surgery 8(1): 3-4.

Yellen, E. and Davis, G.C. (2001) Patient satisfaction in ambulatory surgery. American Operating Room Nurses' Journal 74: 483-486.

Young, L. and Humphrey, M. (1985) Cognitive methods of preparing women for Hysterectomy: Does a booklet help? British Journal of Clinical Psychology 24: 303-304.

Young, R., de Guzman, C.P., Mantis, M.S. and McClure, K. (1994) Effect of pre-admission brochures on surgical patients' behavioural outcomes. Association of Operating Room Nurses' Journal 60: 232-241.

Yount, S. and Schoessler, M. (1991) A description of patient and nurse perceptions of pre-operative teaching. Journal of Post-Anaesthesia Nursing 6: 17-25.

Ziemer, M.M. (1983) Effects of information on post-surgical coping. Nursing Research 32: 282-287.

Zigmond, A.S. and Snaith, R.P. (1983) The hospital anxiety and depression scale. Acta Psychiatrica Scandinavica 67: 361-370.

Zvara, D.A., Manning, M., Stewart, T., McKinley, A.C. and Cran, W. (1994) Pre-operative anesthetic concerns: Perceptions versus reality in men and women. Anesthesiology 81(3A): A1260.

Zvara, D.A., Mathes, D.D., Brooker, R.F. and McKinley, A.C. (1996) Video as a patient teaching tool: Does it add to the pre-operative anesthetic visit? Anesthesia and Analgesia 82: 1065–1068.

Index

LIVERPOOL
JOHN MOORES UNIVERSITY
AVRIL ROBARTS LRC
TEL. 0151 231 4022